HEALTH CARE
FOR THE
OTHER
AMERICANS

HEALTH CARE
FOR THE
OTHER
AMERICANS

Vern L. Bullough, R.N., Ph.D.
Dean
Natural and Social Sciences
State University College at Buffalo

Bonnie Bullough, R.N., Ph.D.
Dean
School of Nursing
State University of New York at Buffalo

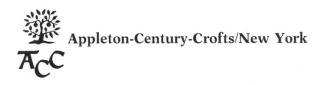 Appleton-Century-Crofts/New York

82 83 84 85 86 / 10 9 8 7 6 5 4 3 2 1

Prentice-Hall International, Inc., London
Prentice-Hall of Australia, Pty. Ltd. Sydney
Prentice-Hall of India Private Limited, New Delhi
Prentice-Hall of Japan, Inc., Tokyo
Prentice-Hall of Southeast Asia (Pte.) Ltd., Singapore
Whitehall Books Ltd., Wellington, New Zealand

Library of Congress Cataloging in Publication Data

Bullough, Bonnie.
  Health care for the other Americans.

  Updated ed. of: Poverty, ethnic identity,
and health care. 1972.
  Bibliography: p.
  Includes index.
  1. Minorities—Medical care—United States.
2. Poor—Medical care—United States.
I. Bullough, Vern L.   II. Title. [DNLM:
1. Delivery of health care. Minority groups.
WA 300 B938h]
RA448.4.B84   1981   362.1   81-17026
ISBN 0-8385-3664-6   AACR2
ISBN 0-8385-3663-8 (pbk.)

Design: Jean M. Sabato
Production Editor: Carol Pierce
PRINTED IN THE UNITED STATES OF AMERICA

CONTENTS

Preface   vii

1 Overview of the Problem: Poverty, Ethnic Identity and Health Care   1

2 Immigrant Minority Groups   15

3 Black Americans   34

4 The Spanish-Speaking Minority Groups   65

5 Native Americans   92

6 New Immigrants and Old Traditions   116

7 Poverty and Hunger Transcend Racial Lines..   133

8 Mental Health and Mental Illness   157

9 Discrimination and Segregation   178

10 Improving Health Care Delivery   199

Bibliography   230

Index   267

v

PREFACE

Health Care for the Other Americans is an update of *Poverty, Ethnic Identity and Health Care* published almost a decade ago. That work documented the disadvantages faced by the poor in achieving good health as stemming from two problems: poverty and ethnicity. We argued that poverty was by far the most important barrier— both to good health and to good health care. Membership in an ethnic minority group, however, clearly was identified as a factor which could add to the impact of poverty. This basic conceptualization has been retained in this volume, although the book has been renamed to reflect the fact that this is an extensive revision of the earlier work.

During the time span between the first book an this one some significant improvements in the health care of the poor have occurred. Consequently, this edition finished on a hopeful note, although the remaining problems faced by the society in achieving equity in the access to good health care are clearly identified. Most of the work of rewriting was done in 1980. Just as the book went to press the administration in Washington, D.C. changed. While it is too early to assess the long-range impact of the philosophy of the Reagan administration on the health of the disadvantaged Americans including the poor, the elderly, and members of ethnic minority groups, it is clear the impact will be a negative one. How negative is still unclear. Whether the reversal will be long lasting and devastating or temporary is also unclear. We hope that what we face is a temporary reversal in a long-range movement towards a more healthy society.

We wish to acknowledge the help of our long time senior editor and friend, Charles Bollinger, for his continuing support. The help of editors Leslie Boyer and Carol Pierce was also appreciated. Expert typing of the manuscript was done by Judy Stolzman and Mary Boldt.

HEALTH CARE
FOR THE
OTHER
AMERICANS

1

Overview of the Problem: Poverty, Ethnic Identity, and Health Care

One measure of a society's level of civilization could be the way it treats its temporarily or permanently disadvantaged members: infants, aged, sick, and minority group members. If this is a true measure, the United States still has a long way to go in achieving the "good life." For example, a baby born in the United States has 14 chances in 1,000 of not surviving its first year, while a baby born in Sweden has 8 chances in 1,000 of not surviving.[1] Despite the fact that we spend more money on health care than any other country[2]— in absolute terms and a greater proportion (9 percent) of our gross national product—our infant mortality rates remain higher than those of most other industrialized countries.

This is not to deny that the United States has made significant strides in decreasing infant mortality rates. In 1900, our infant mortality rate was 100: that is, we lost 100 infants out of every 1,000 live births. By 1935, that rate had been cut to 55.7.[3] This sharp decline was related to discoveries made in the late nineteenth century that bacteria and other microorganisms caused communicable disease. This knowledge facilitated the development of isolation techniques, hospital nursing that made hospitalization less hazardous, improved sanitation in cities, and the development of immunization techniques against the major childhood diseases.[4] The passage of the Social Security Act in 1935 helped distribute public health services more broadly by furnishing federal grants-in-aid to states to develop local public health programs. By 1950, the infant mortality rate had fallen to 29.2 per 1,000 live births and the United States ranked sixth in the world.[5]

Although the infant mortality rate has continued to decline, the strides made by the United States have been less dramatic than those of other industrialized countries. Our infant mortality rate in 1950 marked a sort of plateau, as one by one the advanced nations of the world have passed us. By 1963, we had fallen to fourteenth place, with a rate of 25.2 deaths per 1,000 live births. In 1980, our infant mortality rate was 12.5 which was a significant improvement.[6] Yet when the United States is compared with other nations, it's rate is not the lowest. Table 1 shows the world-wide infant mortality rates in 1977. As can be noted, the relative ranking of the United States was seventeenth when compared with the ranking of other countries with the same or less wealth.

The question that must be asked is: Why do we not have the lowest infant mortality rate? Since we have by far the largest gross national product, the mortality figures cannot be attributed to our lack of economic development. Nor is our higher infant mortality rate due to lack of medical knowledge, since our medical expertise and research capabilities are second to none. Rather, it seems obvious that our drop in comparative position is due to the unequal distribution of materials, resources, and health care, as well as to our system of priorities, which places emphasis upon highly specialized tertiary care, including the more dramatic types of health services such as heart transplants, rather than on the actual application of knowledge already at hand. Thus, the mortality rate for white infants in 1977 was 12.3 per 1,000 live births, while the rate for nonwhite infants was 21.7[7] When income alone is used as a variable, the figures are comparable, and it is the high death rates for disadvantaged babies that pulls down the overall American statistics.[8]

An examination of Table 1 will indicate that those countries that have passed the United States have several things in common. They tend to be countries with fairly homogenous populations, no steep differences in income levels, and some system of national health insurance that delivers adequate health care to everyone, not just those who can buy it on the open market. In the United States, in spite of the fact that illness is likely to be more common and lead to disability and death among the poor, medical care for low-income people is inferior in both quality and quantity to that received by the more well-to-do members of society.

These differences in the life expectancy for infants by race and

TABLE 1
COMPARATIVE INFANT
MORTALITY RATES 1977

Country	Infant Mortality Rate*
Iceland*	8.0
Sweden	8.0
Denmark	8.9
Japan	8.9
Finland	9.1
Norway	9.2
Netherlands	9.5
Switzerland†	9.8
France	11.4
Belgium	11.9
Singapore	12.4
Canada	12.4
Australia	12.5
East Germany	13.1
Hong Kong	13.5
England and Wales	13.7
United States	14.0

The infant mortality rate is expressed here in terms of infant death per every 1,000 births (death during the first year of life).
†The statistics for the countries Iceland and Switzerland are based on 1976 figures; all other countries are based on data representing the year 1977.*
1. *United Nations: Demographic Yearbook 1978. New York, United Nations, 1979, Chart 15, pp. 286–289.*
2. *U. S. Bureau of the Census: World Population 1977: Recent Demographic Estimate for the Countries and Regions of the World. Washington, D.C., 1978.*

income are illustrative of the problems addressed in this book. In addressing these problems, three major factors are examined: (1) the poverty experienced by a significant portion of our population, (2) the barriers to good health that are related to an ethnic minority status, and (3) the less than adequate health care delivery system. Although these three factors are treated as separate concepts, in the real world this separation is not always possible.

Two case studies, based on observations spanning three decades

of nursing experience, may be offered to illustrate the interrelation-
ship of poverty and ethnicity as they impact on health care. These
two experiences also suggest a contrast in the discriminatory patterns of the 1950s and the late 1970s. Some ground was gained in
the reform movements of the 1960s and 1970s, but there are still
problems facing our society if we are to achieve the "good life" for
our citizenry. The first anecdote is recounted from notes kept while
one of the authors (BB) served as a public health nurse on Chicago's
South Side:

> In 1953, rats mutilated and killed an infant in an area next
> to the district in which I was working. In my own district, they
> chewed the hand of a small black newborn infant named Wil-
> liam Henry.[9] William's mother and four siblings lived in a dug-
> out basement under a dilapidated row house. Mrs. Henry had
> been awakened in the middle of the night by the cries of her
> baby and found two huge grey rats on top of him. When she
> snatched him up, his hand was a bleeding mass of mangled
> flesh. She took her baby to Cook County Hospital for emergency
> care.
>
> Cook County, however, was more than an hour away by bus
> and, in order to get there, she borrowed money from her neigh-
> bors to take a taxi. Because she was afraid to leave her other
> four children alone at home, she took all of them with her and
> they spent the night in the emergency room, waiting for the
> baby to be treated and admitted. Most of William's hand could
> be saved, although he lost the distal portion of three fingers.
> When William was discharged from the hospital, the Health De-
> partment was notified. I was sent to visit the family. I found
> them living in a basement that had probably never been meant
> to be used as a residence.

Most of the houses in this particular area had been built 60 to 70
years earlier, long before electrical outlets were a standard feature
in a home, and when food storage posed serious problems. The base-
ments in these houses had been designed to store food and coal, and
the original owners probably never thought of these dugouts as possible residences. It obviously was not a suitable place for five children to live.

> I felt the rats would attack the infant again unless some-
> thing was done. I called the office of the city housing inspector,
> met with officials in the urban renewal office, and had long
> discussions with my own supervisor. In spite of all my efforts,
> some of which became quite frantic, no public official could be

talked into doing anything about the rats, and there seemed to be no other housing available at the level the Henry family could afford.

Rather, it should be said, there was low-income housing available in Chicago at that time, but it was not available to blacks—even those who were quite well to do. The Chicago ghetto had burst the officially imposed boundaries in the years following the 1947 U.S. Supreme Court decision that made restrictive covenants unenforceable. Even with the help of the ever-present block busters, the informal pressure against integration in housing or a rapid expansion of the ghetto had kept the "black belt" much too small for the number of people seeking housing. This meant that housing for blacks rented at about twice the price per room of that available for whites. Inevitably, landlords broke up apartments into smaller and smaller units, rented out storage areas, and expected several families to share a bathroom and kitchen.

Mrs. Henry lived in this ghetto and, like many of her neighbors, she was on welfare. Her welfare checks were smaller than those of families of comparable size because she had tried to keep the arrival of her new baby a secret. She was convinced that her social workers would cut off her aid entirely if it became known that she had conceived again without finding a stable male breadwinner for the family.

The house above the Henrys' basement was scheduled to be torn down as part of a large urban renewal project. The official at the Office of Urban Renewal whom I contacted explained that his department might eventually use its influence to place the Henrys in public housing, since finding other kinds of replacement housing on the open market for such a large family, at a price they could afford, was next to impossible. However, the official refused to speed up the process or even let Mrs. Henry know that she had a chance to obtain public housing, because he felt it would be "bad for neighborhood morale." He explained to me that the only way to get "those old mamas off their cans" was to frighten them with the bulldozer. He stated there were not enough public housing units to accommodate all the people who were displaced by urban renewal projects, so that his job of finding replacement housing was much easier if he could convince the people in the buildings scheduled to be cleared that they would have to find an apartment for themselves or face the prospect of being in the house when the wrecking crew arrived. Most of the tenants in the buildings already razed had relocated themselves by moving into other slum housing or by doubling up with relatives.

The doubling up had added to the slum problem by creating overcrowding, which is a major factor in the rapid deterioration of the central-city ghetto housing. Not only does such crowding rapidly wear out a building, but when large numbers of families use a single facility, such as a kitchen, it is difficult to fix responsibility for keeping the area clean or repaired.

As far as rats were concerned, the slum clearance project was a major factor in creating the problem in the first place. The large luxury buildings being built on the cleared land were virtually rat-proof. The displaced rats, like the displaced people, made their way to nearby slum areas. Because of increased concentration, the appetites of the rats soon outstripped the available uncollected garbage supplies and they turned to attacking infants in their cribs.

> Several families in the area had built heavy screen cages over their children's beds and, sometimes at night, they would hear rats gnawing on the screens. Mrs. Henry, however, lacked money to buy screens and apparently also had little talent as a carpenter. After the baby came home from the hospital, she tried to keep herself awake at night to guard him, but soon the state of chronic exhaustion made this difficult. In a desperate attempt to do something constructive to help her, I begged two half-grown cats from another family I knew and took them to her. Before a week was past, the rats had eaten the cats.

The Henry family was black and poor. This particular combination of circumstances rendered them relatively powerless to deal with their problems. Affluent black families could afford somewhat better housing, while poor white families could secure much better housing for the same amount of money. Because the Henrys were poor, they had no family physician, and because they were black, no South Side emergency room would then treat William.[10] They faced poverty, discrimination, and an inadequate health care delivery system. It was an impossible combination.

In 1979, this same author was hired to serve as an expert witness in a malpractice suit carried by a law firm that accepted cases from people with disadvantaged backgrounds. The patient was a middle-aged black laborer who was treated for a leg injury in a negligent manner.

The case started one evening a year earlier when the patient, whom we shall call Mr. Jones, went out to investigate a noise in the back yard. In the process, he caught his foot in a gopher hole and dislocated his leg. His wife applied ice bags and helped him elevate his leg. In spite of this, by morning the pain was intense. Mr. Jones went to a local physician who was known to accept the kind of health insurance he carried and with whom he had had some contact. After some delay with x-rays, the physician sent him to an orthopedic surgeon. For some reason, the surgeon did not see him until the next day, when emergency surgery was done on the knee.

After the operation, Mr. Jones was admitted to a hospital ward, where the nurses had difficulty palpating a pedal pulse. They also noted the affected foot was cold to the touch. They called the surgeon, who was quoted as suggesting that perhaps the patient had a congenital absence of pulse in that foot. The next day the "family" physician visited Mr. Jones, but he said the case was now in the hands of the surgeon. The nurses continued to chart the absent pulse and the other symptoms of vascular problems. They were obviously worried but felt impotent to force the two physicians to do more. Finally, after three days, they called the hospital chief of staff. As a consequence, a vascular surgeon was called and the patient was returned to surgery for an attempted repair of the popliteal artery. Postoperatively, the nurses found the pedal pulse ambiguous and the foot remained cold. They called the vascular surgeon, the orthopedic surgeon, and the family physician, all of whom did nothing more. The nursing staff continued to fuss about their inability to force any better solution to Mr. Jones' problem, but, fearful of offending the three physicians, they did not call the chief of staff again.

In a few days, the cast on Mr. Jones' leg softened and purulent drainage appeared; in another week, the stench from the leg was so bad that Mr. Jones had to be transferred to a private room. In another week, small flies were noticed exiting from the wound. A month after the original injury a midthigh amputation was done. The case was settled out of court, so no formal charges of negligence were proven. However, all three physicians seemed to have shared some aspect of negligence, and the hospital nurses, in spite of their concern and continued accurate charting of the deteriorating condition of the leg, were considered negligent. The hospital paid damages because the nurses did not call the chief of staff earlier and more often. Thus, in many respects, this case supports the landmark Darling case, which held the hospital and nursing staff responsible for the care that is given by everyone, including the doctors.[11] The fact that the principals in the case were willing to give a settlement to Mr. Jones suggests a beginning sense of responsibility on the part of the health care delivery system. Mr. Jones, however, still lost his leg.

In many respects, growth in the malpractice movement is an expression of concern by consumers for the inadequacies in the health care delivery system. It is a way of communicating with the health care industry that has ignored more polite efforts to communicate. Mr. Jones' case fits in with this general movement. However, one cannot help but speculate whether or not the first delay the day after the injury and the second delay after the orthopedic surgery would have occurred if Mr. Jones had been more affluent, more knowledgeable, or white.

Obviously, this is certainly a more subtle discriminatory pattern than that experienced in 1953 by William Henry. Mr. Jones lived in a small single-family house in a pleasant California suburban neighborhood. He was admitted to the nearest community hospital, rather than a distant county hospital. He was in a room with patients of other ethnic backgrounds, until the gangrenous process in his leg demanded that he be moved. Individual nurses from a variety of ethnic backgrounds tried to help him, although ineffectively. He was able to find a malpractice attorney who carried his case. The changes over time suggest that discrimination related to poverty and ethnicity is lessening and becoming more subtle, but there are still discriminatory patterns.

CHANGING NATURE OF HEALTH CARE

In some ways, the modern health care delivery system is less able to accommodate the disadvantaged patient than the delivery system of the nineteenth century. Since the turn of the century, the nature of medicine has changed from being more or less custodial to materially assisting in the cure of the patient. During the same period, hospitals changed from eleemosynary institutions run by religious or charitable bodies to centers of scientific medicine, and some of them have even become profit-making institutions.

Such changes have also modified the relationship of the physician to the patient. At the turn of the century, physicians had a one-to-one relationship with their patients, and it was not unusual for the local physician to vary the fees according to the economic circumstances of the patients. Moreover, the qualifications for becoming a physician were not particularly arduous or time-consuming, and the physician's income was not proportionately much different from that of the grocer or other small merchants. This meant that physicians were likely to live in all parts of the city, although the wealthier ones undoubtedly lived in the higher-income areas, since their wealth came from serving upper-income patients. Childbirth was most likely to take place under the supervision of the midwife, and, in the care of the critically ill, the nurse was as important as the physician. Slum dwellers or poor people in the city never saw a physician until they were seriously ill, and then they were likely to depend upon a charity hospital for care. In fact, hospitals were regarded as places for poor patients to go, and they were often attached to a medical school or had a number of volunteer physicians who donated their services. Well-to-do people were treated in their own homes, under the supervision of a private-duty nurse.

During the course of the twentieth century, more and more of the medical tasks became institutionalized. Childbirth, which previously had been centered in the home, moved into the hospital. Developments in anesthesia, obstetrical surgery, special equipment, and better aseptic techniques, as well as the changing nature of the American family, all contributed to the move. So did the invention of the incubator, as well as other devices for infant care that could only be found in the hospitals. Scientific breakthroughs in the nineteenth and twentieth centuries made operative wounds less prone to become infected, and hundreds of new surgical techniques allowed the surgeon to operate on the chest, brain, heart, and other parts of the body that earlier would not have been probed. In addition to the improvements in asepsis and anesthesia, the perfection of transfusion aided the development of surgery. The invention of x-ray equipment, the electro-encephalograph, radioactive-isotopes techniques, CAT (computerized automated tomography) scanning equipment, and numerous other tools for treatment and diagnosis led to greater and greater concentration of patients in the hospitals in order to make better use of the investment required to operate such equipment. Further encouraging the growth of hospitals was the development of health insurance, an innovation primarily born during the depression of the 1930s. In the United States, health insurance usually paid only for claims incurred during hospitalization, and many diagnostic and minor surgical procedures that could have been performed in the doctor's office were transferred to the hospital.

Increasingly, the government entered the medical field, not always with the intended results. The results of government intervention are recounted in some detail in the course of this book, but the end result has been to establish what Arnold S. Relman, editor of the *New England Journal of Medicine*, in 1980 called the *medical industrial complex*.[12] The term gives new meaning to a warning issued by President Dwight D. Eisenhower at the end of his terms in office (1952–1960) about the military industrial complex. The military industrial complex had been built up by the government in collaboration with private industry largely on the cost-plus basis, that is, industry was guaranteed a profit for all of its military work, and there was little need to cut cost, consider more effective alternatives, or even analyze how much of a defense industry the country needed. The government, the military, and the industry were all working together, and industry was becoming rich and lazy as a result.

The same thing has happened in the medical field, as private industry, largely on a cost-plus basis through government-guaranteed insurance policies, has begun to gain great wealth from the health field, although there is little examination of just how much the patient is benefiting. Relman used the term *medical industrial complex* to describe the most rapidly growing segment of the nation's economy: proprietary hospitals, proprietary nursing homes and clinics, and diagnostic laboratories, which in 1979 grossed an estimated 40 billion dollars. Relman estimated that about 1,000 hospitals are run for profit, about 15 percent of the nongovernmental acute-care facilities. Seventy-seven percent of the 10,000 nursing homes are profit, and one third of the diagnostic laboratories are run by profit-making companies. Newly established profit-making companies are also entering business to do mobile CAT scanning, dental care, treat alcoholism, and carry out many other rehabilitation programs that the federal government funds. Forty percent of the patients on hemodialysis are customers of profit-making units, something that was first made possible by the 1972 amendment to the Social Security Act. Some of the profits are more indirect. Physicians often own the pharmacy located in their medical building and get a percentage of the profits; many own the other allied businesses associated with health care today, which in turn are paid for by public monies, so that more and more of government money is going to fewer and fewer people. At the same time, many physicians refuse to treat patients on Medicare or Medicaid. Hospitals, while nominally accepting them as patients, demand that they contribute significant sums out of their own pocket to pay for anesthesia, special surgical procedures, or any number of other services. The result is that the private hospitals and even some of the nonprofit hospitals, where certain classes of physicians are allowed to set hospital policy, are "skimming the cream" off patient populations, catering to middle-class affluent patients with acute problems while leaving more difficult and labor-intensive cases to the government sectors.

Almost every development in medicine has added to its expense. Education for physicians has been upgraded radically during the twentieth century; at first, the length of training was increased, while proportionately the number of physicians in the population was deliberately decreased. The result was a rapid growth in physicians' income. Most of the changes in the nature of training were initiated by the American Medical Association in a conscious effort to upgrade both medical services and incomes of individual practitioners, although at the same time it potentially improved the quality of care. *Potential* is a key word because, as this book argues, the potential has not always been realized. As part of the effort to upgrade, medical schools themselves have changed. Fewer and fewer medical schools utilize the county hospitals as the main source of "guinea pig" patients, simply because so many of the patients in such hospitals are no longer "interesting" medical problems. They are routinely sick people. Instead, medical schools have moved on to the university campus, where "teaching beds" have replaced charity beds. Inevitably, interns and residents want to work at the frontiers of medical knowledge; therefore, in order to attract them, the ordinary hospital has to pay for their services or establish special medical teaching wards and get a university affiliation, all of which has added to the cost of medical care.

Developments in medicine coincided with similar changes in nursing. In the years following World War II, the nature of the hospital training school changed, as more and more nurses went to collegiate or community-college schools of nursing. In the period before World War II, the vast majority of hospitals had been run by student nurses, who received little more than their board, room, and "education" for their work. With the upgrading of nursing schools, hospitals were no longer able to recruit a supply of underpaid student laborers, and, increasingly, professional staffs replaced student nurses. This meant that hospitals had to pay for their staffs, and the cost of hospitalization rose accordingly.

These and other changes in medicine and nursing led to a growing crisis in medical care. Add to them the disabilities inherent in a discriminatory system and the crisis reaches epidemic proportions. Unfortunately, the United States has never developed any comprehensive plan to deal with this medical crisis. In fact, the whole history of medical care of the poor in this country indicates that there has never been any well-thought-out plan; rather, health programs have taken the path of least resistance. In most cases, such programs did not take into account the welfare of the poor patients as a prime consideration. Even the public health measures in the United States have most often been instituted in those areas that concern middle- and upper-class Americans and not to satisfy the health needs of the poor. The fact that American public health has concentrated either in the area of the least resistance or in areas most popular to middle- and upper-income groups is evident from the emphasis given to sanitation, immunization, and epidemiology.

Once the contagious nature of certain diseases was established by such men as Louis Pasteur and Robert Koch, it was relatively easy to convince citizens and taxpayers to support wide-scale sanitation and immunization efforts, because it was obvious that infectious diseases spread to all segments of society. Though the poor benefited greatly from such programs, it was the fact that immunizing the poor child cut down the spread of disease to the middle-class child that made such measures so politically potent. The middle-class bias in control of contagious disease is perhaps nowhere more evident than in the types of disease public health officials worked the hardest to control. Poliomyelitis is a good case in point, because it was probably more likely to leave its crippling aftereffects in the richer areas than the poor. In the crowded urban slums, the disease was quickly passed around so that children had frequent exposures while they were young and often developed mild cases that gave lasting immunity without the crippling aftereffects. Middle- and upper-class children who were more protected tended to contract the disease at a later age and were often likely to be permanently crippled—as was so dramatically demonstrated by the case of President Franklin D. Roosevelt. Following President Roosevelt's lead, the March of Dimes raised money to finance a vigorous research program, as well as to buy equipment and give treatment to poliomyelitis victims. Ultimately, the program led to the Salk vaccines and indirectly to the Sabin vaccines. On the other hand, tuberculosis research and therapy received very little public support—although it was a far more dangerous disease, killing 33,633 people in 1950 compared to poliomyelitis, which killed 1,686. Tuberculosis, however, was a disease that mainly stayed in the slums—where it killed rather than gave immunity.[13] Today, tuberculosis is still common among the less affluent minority groups, such as Indians, Mexican Americans, and blacks, but it is not very common among affluent whites.

This is not to say that the public health movement has focused on certain diseases or problems out of any malicious neglect, but simply that funds and resources are limited, problems are vast, and it is politically feasible to concentrate on some things to the exclusion of others. When poor people are recipients of programs designed specifically for the poor, the emphasis is usually either consciously or unconsciously in a noncontroversial area, such as the care of infants, pregnant mothers, or crippled children. In many cases, these programs, most of which were established in the 1930s, took over existing charitable enterprises that had already focused public attention on the problem. It was also easy for public health programs to enter into areas where public institutions already existed, such as the school health program. To set up brand new institutions to deal with health problems was much more difficult to accomplish.

The result is that medical care for the poor today is very spotty. Pregnant mothers and well babies receive the most attention, school children are the focus of some programs, and, with the advent of Medicare, senior citizens also receive some care. People with rare diseases receive outstanding care because they are of interest to medical schools or to hospital staffs that have teaching beds at their disposal. For the rest, however, even with Medicare and Medicaid, present care is inadequate. The factors present in the current crisis in health care will receive somewhat more detailed analysis in this book, but obviously the answer to the crisis involves a rethinking of our whole health care delivery system.

REFERENCES

1. United Nations. Demographic Yearbook 1978. New York: United Nations, 1979, Chart 15, pp. 286–289.
2. Hamburg, D. A. & Brown, S. S. Science Base and the Social Context of Health Maintenance: An Overview. *Science*, 1978, *200*, 847–849.
3. Shapiro, S., Schlesinger, E. R., & Nesbitt, Jr., R. E. L. Infant, Perinatal, Maternal and Childhood Mortality in the United States. Cambridge: Harvard University Press, 1968.
4. Bullough, V. & Bullough, B. The Care of the Sick: The Emergence of Modern Nursing. New York: Prodist, 1978.
5. Shapiro, Schlesinger, & Nesbitt. op. cit.
6. U. S. Department of Health and Human Services, National Center for Health Statistics, *Monthly Vital Statistics Report* 1981, 30:2.
7. U.S. Bureau of Census. Statistical Abstract of the United States: 1979. Washington, D.C.: U. S. Government Printing Office, 1979, p. 75, Table 108.
8. Stickle, G. The Health of Mothers and Babies: How Do We Stack Up? *The Family Coordinator*, 1977, *26*, 205–210. Brooks, C. H. Social, Economic and Biologic Correlates of Infant Mortality in City Neighborhoods. *Journal of Health and Social Behavior*, 1980, *21*, 2–11.
9. This is a fictitious name to protect William's privacy, although considering the opportunities available to a slum child of that time it is doubtful that he or many of his peers would have become a health professional, a sociologist, or readers of books such as this one. One of the characteristics of our present problem in health care delivery is that

the victims of the inequities of the system are also cut off from the educational opportunities that would have allowed them to read the scholarly literature about their problems.

10. It should be noted that legislation passed in recent years would make illegal the open exclusion of William from emergency care because he was black.

11. Darling vs. Charleston Community Hospital 200 NE 2d 253 (1965). The Darling Case. *Journal of the American Medical Association,* 1968, *206,* 1875.

12. See: Relman, A. L. *New England Journal of Medicine,* 1980, *23.* See also: *Science,* 1980, *210,* 612–613.

13. Simmons, O. G. Implications of Social Class for Public Health. In J. R. Folta & E. S. Deck (Ed.), A Sociological Framework for Patient Care (1st ed.). New York: Wiley, 1966.

2

Immigrant Minority Groups

Technically, a minority is any racial, religious, occupational, or other group constituting less than a numerical majority of the population. In this sense, all of us belong to various kinds of minorities. Sometimes a numerical majority can technically be defined as equivalent to a minority because they lack the kinds of power that usually go with majority status. A good example of this is the case of blacks and mixed-race people (coloreds) in the Union of South Africa. Many of the people in the women's movement in the United States have said that women have the status of a minority, even if numerically they are a majority. Essentially, when we discuss minority status, we are dealing with those groups that need protection and encouragement from the overpowering majority that controls the government, since they are often looked down upon because of racial, religious, or other reasons. The Constitution of the United States includes special protections for minorities through its due process and equal protection clauses, as well as through its guaranteed freedoms of speech, religion, and assembly.

In the early history of the United States, minority status was based mostly upon religion, but in the nineteenth century it came to be identified with place of national origin as well as religion; in the twentieth century, racial and economic factors have more often been the basis for designation as a minority. Within the past few

15

decades, sex has also been added to the list, as has such special conditions as being physically handicapped. Every high school student knows that America has been made up by different groups of immigrants, but it is not always so evident that these immigrants were themselves for a time minority group members and had many of the same problems as today's minority group members. Emigration was a traumatic experience. It took people out of their traditional environments and replanted them in strange settings, among strange people with even stranger customs. Old modes of behavior were no longer adequate to meet the new and quite different problems of life. The responses of the newly arrived prospective citizen were not easy or automatic, for emigration had changed the underlying nature of the social structure to which the person had been accustomed, and neither the complex of institutions nor the societal patterns that formerly guided the immigrant were present.

Though some immigrants became rapidly assimilated into the culture of the new country, most of them tried to find people with like ways and customs, settling down together, fearful almost that, if they did not retain at least some of the old ways, they themselves would be lost. In the long run, this in-group identification of the members of minorities has been both a strength and a weakness for our society. The competing minority groups consciously or unconsciously helped us to achieve our own particular type of pluralistic democracy, because the diversity of groups tended to prevent any one faction from achieving a monopoly of power. Even the basic constitutional guarantee of freedom of religion was due in part to the fact that Americans could not agree upon one single religion. On the other hand, ethnic status—based upon religious, national, or racial identity—has also been used as a basis for exploitation and conflict.

Usually, as the members of the minority group achieved a measure of power and economic success, they were all too willing to discriminate against the newer minority groups, denying them access to the more pleasant neighborhoods, the better jobs, an adequate education, and even health care. Inevitably, this discrimination led to conflict, because the deprived groups had imbibed too much of the American dream to be contented with their second-class status, and they too struggled for their share of the good life. In part, for the past 100 years the history of the United States has been the history of successive minority groups attempting to move up in American society and the reaction of the older established groups in opposing them.

Although in many ways the American experience is unique, this is not the only country with minority groups based on ethnic identity. In Europe, minority ethnic populations have been created many times by changing national boundaries. With each new conquest, indigenous peoples in the conquered territories have had to adjust to new national identities and have often been pressured to adopt the dominant culture of their new nation. In some disputed areas, these changes in national identity have occurred with painful regularity. Alsace-Lorraine has been French, German, French, German, and French in the past century. Poland, which was part of Russia until the end of World War I, found its boundaries moved westward after World War II, taking in areas that had been German and losing much of its eastern territory to Russia. There are German-speaking minorities in northern Italy, and Italian-speaking groups in Yugoslavia; Hungarian-speaking groups in Romania; and the list could go on. Europe has also seen mass migrations of people, such as the French-speaking Huguenots into Prussia during the seventeenth century. Sometimes minorities exist peacefully; at other times there are almost mass genocides, as happened to the Armenians in Turkey in the post–World War I period or to the people in Vietnam, Laos, and Cambodia today. Not all minority groups respond to their minority status in the same way. Louis Wirth, a pioneering investigator into minority group problems, proposed a four-fold classification of minority groups based upon their dominant aims: (1) pluralistic, (2) assimilationist, (3) secessionist, and (4) militant. A minority group with a pluralistic aim "seeks toleration for its differences on the part of the dominant group," while an assimilationist minority "craves the fullest opportunity for participation in the life of the larger society." Secessionists, on the other hand, want "to achieve political as well as cultural independence from the dominant group," while a militant minority sets its sights on "domination over others."[1]

In an earlier era, before nationalism became such a potent force, most European minority groups were pluralistic in their aims, content with retaining their own language and religion but not particularly vigorous in trying to change their situation. With time, pluralism often led to assimilation, as the minority groups accepted the culture of the nation that had conquered them. One of the most notable examples was the city of Strasbourg in France, which until its seizure by the French in 1681 had been German-speaking and Protestant but over a period of time became French-speaking and Catholic. With the rise of nationalism, which gathered tremendous strength in the nineteenth century, many minority groups became more militant and sought domination by their group over others, as the Germans and Hungarians did in the Austro-Hungarian Empire before World War I, while some groups sought self-identity, as did the Serbs, the Croats, the Romanians, and others who felt themselves subjugated. There are a few minorities, such as the Basques in Spain and France, who have maintained their identity for thousands of years.

Aiding the growth of nationalism was the expansionist policies of the European imperialistic countries, notably England, France, and Spain. Many of the conquered peoples had never thought of themselves as national groups, but their common resentment against conquering powers often led to the growth of such feelings. This has created all kinds of problems in today's world, although in some areas the problem is greater than in other areas because of the nature of European penetration. In many of the conquered lands, the imperialist powers were content with economic exploitation and they never became an important part of the culture of the conquered peoples. In some areas, however, the Europeans sent out permanent settlers, reducing the indigenous people to a minority status. This occurred with the Indians in the Americas, the Maoris of New Zealand, the Bushmen of Australia, and the native Hawaiians.

In the United States, only the Indians and the Spaniards of the Southwest became minorities by conquest of their homeland. The other American minorities, to which all the rest of us belong, were willing or unwilling immigrants. The most unwilling to come were the slaves who were brought here and exploited by the European settlers. Other groups of immigrants might also have been reluctant to come, including some of the convicts transported to Georgia or the Chinese imported to build the railroads, but most others came willingly. It could be expected that the willing immigrants would feel more open to assimilation than conquered peoples, and this in fact seems to have been the case. It should be emphasized, however, that many of the Europeans and Asians who came to this country did not intend to stay and settle. Instead, they were sojourners who planned to accumulate some wealth and return to their homelands, and, in point of fact, large numbers of them did return—although not always with the wealth they had dreamed of taking back. Although the statistics describing emigration rates from the United States are not as complete as those describing immigration in the nineteenth century, early twentieth-century figures indicate that the emigration rate from the United States was not insignificant. For example, in the eight-year period ending in 1915, there were approximately eight million immigrants, but there were four million people who left the country.[2] It has been estimated that about 30 percent of the American immigrants who entered the country between 1821 and 1924 eventually returned to their homeland.[3] It would seem that these sojourners would cling more to the old-country customs than people who were planning to stay permanently, and this had an influence upon the immigrant communities. Moreover, there were probably many millions of others who intended to return to their homeland but because of various circumstances never made it. Nevertheless, the goal of returning to the homeland undoubtedly encouraged many of them to keep alive their old culture, thus slowing down the rate of assimilation and increasing the generation gap between them and their American-born children.

Adding to the gap between immigrant groups and other Americans was the fact that the homeland of immigrants differed from one era to another. During the colonial period, most of the immigrants were from the British Isles, with the largest single identity being Scotch Irish. The Scotch Irish had been relocated in Ireland from the Scottish lowlands during the seventeenth century, but, discontented with an unfavorable land tenure system, they came to the American colonies in increasing numbers during the eighteenth century and settled along the frontier. During this same period, there were also a large number of German-speaking settlers from a variety of German states and the German cantons of Switzerland, as well as some Dutch, Swedish, and French Huguenot settlers.[4] Even in this early stage in the settlement of the colonies the tendency for the various groups to form ethnic enclaves could be noted. One of the most striking examples of this separatism took place in Pennsylvania, where the Scotch Irish and German communities grew up alongside each other.[5] The continuation of separate ethnic communities is still obvious in Pennsylvania, where some of the Older Order Amish and other Mennonites still manage to cling to many of the customs of the eighteenth century.

Refugees from the French Revolution swelled the number of immigrants at the end of the eighteenth century, but it was not until the nineteenth century that large-scale migration to this country occurred. The first wave followed in the aftermath of the Napoleonic Wars, and there were increases during each successive decade until the 1850s, when more than two million Europeans migrated to this country. Although every country in Europe contributed to this outward flow, the majority of immigrants were from the northern and western parts of Europe. The reasons for setting out for America varied. There was a rapid expansion of population in Europe during the period, putting a premium upon land, and increasing numbers of people had heard of the opportunities available in America. Political discontent played a role, as evidenced by the German migration following the failure of the Revolution of 1848, and so did religion (witness the converts to the Mormon Church), but the most important motive was an economic one, as Europeans sought land, jobs, and a better life. Great national tragedies also played a part in the displacement of populations. The potato blight hit Ireland's main food crop between 1845 and 1849, causing widespread famine and driving many of the survivors to seek new homes and opportunities in America.

The nineteenth-century newcomer was different from his eighteenth-century counterpart in the area of settlement. Most eighteen-century immigrants had headed for the undeveloped frontier where land was available, while the nineteenth-century immigrants, with a number of exceptions, settled first in the cities and sought employment in the developing industries. The newly arrived people moved into the rapidly growing cities' low-rent areas (*slum* is the term we now use), usually located in and around the business or factory district of the city, as the more well-to-do residents had moved farther out. Adjustment to the new world and to new conditions was never easy. Affluent or successful people seldom emigrated to America, so those who did leave home tended to have meager resources, and what little money they did have was used on transportation to the new land. In fact, this was one of the reasons these people so often settled in the city rather than in the countryside in the nineteenth and twentieth centuries: many of them lacked the resources to go much farther.

Strangers in the immediate world around them, the immigrants fought the loneliness of their condition and created a variety of formal and informal institutions to help them adjust. Usually, they settled in the same neighborhood as their former countrymen. In the process, they created Germantowns, New Irelands, or Little Polands. Eventually, as these settlers became successful, some of them were able to move out into more comfortable neighborhoods. The old ethnic neighborhood was then taken over by new immigrants who, like their predecessors, were attracted by the cheap rents and central location. As the changeover took place, the new arrivals filtered into the district, occupying house after house as they became vacant, until the whole character of a Germantown had changed into a Little Italy or an Irish enclave had given way to a Russian Jewish ghetto. This challange to the old settled groups by the new was often associated with hostility and conflict.

The immigrants were also exploited. Sometimes this exploitation was by individuals of the same ethnic group, whose experience or facility with English enabled them to deal with the more established

Americans. Often, however, the manipulation was done by outsiders who had little sympathy with or understanding of the new immigrant group, but could use the group's naiveté, poverty, and lack of English language skills to exploit them. Unfortunately, the very tendency of the immigrants to "ghettoize" themselves made them more exploitable. The land near the center of the city might eventually have great value, but only in terms of the land and not for the existing structures. Inevitably, the existing housing tended to become dilapidated, and essential repairs were neglected as the owners waited for their land to appreciate. The newcomers lacked the economic or political power to demand improvements. Moreover, the fact that they were segregated made it possible to neglect essential services in their areas without inconveniencing other usually richer and more politically powerful citizens, so that municipal services—such as garbage collection, street repairs, and police protection—were inferior to those supplied the residents of the newer sections of the city.[6] Schooling for the children of the new immigrants was inferior to that given to pupils whose parents lived in the more affluent sections of the city: buildings were older, staffs smaller, and the children left school at an earlier age than did children who came from families who were higher on the socioeconomic ladder.[7]

If this account sounds like a description of some of the major urban areas in the United States today, particularly in the North and Midwest, it is because immigration has continued and "flight" of the richer and more well-to-do from the central cities continues to be a problem. The immigrants of today might come from other sections of the United States (the black migration into the northern industrial cities from the rural south that took place in the 1940s and 1950s, and the Puerto Rican and Appalachian migration that followed it) or from outside American borders, as do the vast numbers of recent migrants from Mexico, Latin America, Cuba, and Southeast Asia now entering the country.

The tendency of each new group of immigrants to form enclaves based on ethnic identity also made it possible for other Americans to accuse them of "clannishness" and to argue that immigrants lived in squalor because they liked it that way. Inevitably, when members of the groups did accumulate enough capital to buy homes or rent more comfortable quarters, the racist justifications for their earlier exploitation gave them a negative image that worked to exclude them from the outer sections of the city by informal pressures, agreement, and even laws and deed restrictions. Irish immigrants in particular were targets for discriminatory action during the mid-nineteenth century, because they were the first large group of Catholics to come to this country and many of them had arrived in the most abject poverty. Though the United States had been founded by religious refugees, most of them were Protestants who had built-in fears of "popery," which the large influx of Irish (and to a lesser extent German) Catholics aroused to fever pitch. Even in the colonial period, many of the colonies had charged the captain of ships who brought Catholic immigrants an extra head tax.[8]

In spite of the prejudice against them, the Irish were eventually able to make their way into better-paying jobs in the building trades, as policemen, or as minor political officials. Their paychecks became their weapons against discrimination and they gradually moved out of the central city slum areas. However, the ingrained nature of the prejudice against them was probably not fully eradicated until John F. Kennedy, an Irishman and a Catholic, was elected President of the United States, thus following in the footsteps of Dwight David Eisenhower, who was of German background. Spiro T. Agnew also became a symbolic breakthrough for the more recent Greek immigrants.

As the Irish moved out of the central city slum areas, they were replaced by newer groups: Italians, Hungarians, Bohemians, Poles, Russians, and new waves of Germans, Swedes, and others. Again, the new immigrants—employed in the most menial and low-paying jobs—were able only to rent quarters in the most deteriorated sections of the city. Few of the immigrants from eastern and southern Europe were Protestants or even Catholics. Large numbers were either Orthodox- or Byzantine-rite Christians or Jews, so that their religious identity proved an additional source of prejudice from both Protestant and Catholic Americans.

Those people most accustomed to minority status were the Jews. The word *ghetto*, which is used by sociologists and other scholars to describe segregated residential areas, was originally used to describe the Jewish section of European cities. It is believed that the word had its origin in Venice, which in the late Middle Ages had set apart a portion of the city as the Jewish quarter.[9] This ghettoization of Jews in Europe had been partly voluntary (for religious and cultural reasons), partly protective (because of periodic outbreaks of hostility toward Jews), but mainly for legal reasons. As the Jewish communities had grown and the boundaries had remained unchanged, the European ghettos crammed more and more people into a small space. Ghettoization also prevented the Jews' assimilation into the general culture of the surrounding communities. In fact, large numbers of Jews in Poland and Russia did not speak the languages of these countries but instead spoke Yiddish.

With this background, Jewish immigrants came to the United States already prepared for ghetto life. They settled primarily in the large urban areas, with New York City serving as the home of more than half of the new Jewish immigrants.[10] Though there had been earlier waves of Jewish settlers from Spain and Portugal (via Brazil) and from Germany, after 1881 the largest groups came from Russia (including Poland) as refugees from the periodic pogroms and other persecutions. The already existing Jewish community helped the poverty-stricken refugees survive, but it also helped cut them off from contact with other ethnic groups. Orthodox Jews—and most of the immigrants were Orthodox—were not supposed to ride to the synagogue on the sabbath, and this meant that the devoted Jew could not move far from the synagogue. Successful second- and third-generation descendants of the immigrants who wanted to move out into more comfortable neighborhoods, yet remain Jewish, were forced to move the synagogue with them or change their religion to suit the realities of American life. Both of these things took place, with Conservative and Reform Judaism developing, but the nature of the European experience in the ghetto and the outside pressures of the non-Jewish community made the assimilation of Jewish minorities slower than some of the other groups.[11] They also suffered greater discrimination in jobs, housing, and public accommodation than their Christian countrymen who were often contemporary immigrants. For example, college fraternities and sororities long excluded Jews because they were non-Christian, even in nonsectarian state universities. Many colleges and universities put a quota on entrance for non-Christians.

The wave of Jewish immigrants was just part of a flood of people seeking new opportunities in the United States in the decade between 1900 and 1910. Immigration reached a peak in these years as more than eight million people arrived in this country, a figure not matched even by the flood of refugees in the 1970s and 1980s. Inevitably, the great waves of immigrants created hostility toward the open-immigration policy and there was a growing racism toward the new immigrants. As the Indians were the only indigenous Americans, it became necessary to rationalize the hostility on grounds other than simple immigrant status. To this end, science, or rather "pseudoscience," contributed a new justification. Sociology, which was only beginning to emerge as an independent discipline, made generalizations about the immigrant that have proved shocking to the sociologist of today. Nevertheless, through analyzing criminality, intemperance, poverty, and disease, these early sociologists found that the immigrant was associated with all social problems. This meant that either society was at fault or the newcomer, and it proved much too tempting to blame the problems on the immigrant. Sociologists adopted the dictum that social characteristics were dependent upon racial differences, and a succession of books were published demonstrating that the flaws in the biological constitution of the newer immigrants were responsible for every evil that beset America—from pauperism, to depression, to homosexuality. Historians, novelists, and politicians joined this movement and a body of literature grew up expounding the innate biological superiority of Northern Europeans, with corollary argument that all other peoples were of physically and/or mentally inferior stock.[12] Joining with the emerging social scientist in the racist cause were labor union leaders, who saw the new immigrant as a means for employers to undercut wages and undermine the craftsmen who then dominated organized labor.

The first group actually to be restricted were the Chinese, with passage of the Exclusion Act in 1882, which many of its supporters regarded as only temporary. The legislation was passed in response to the virulent anti-Chinese feelings of Californians, who were convinced that the Chinese "coolies" were suppressing wages. Local discriminatory legislation had been passed earlier and the Chinese residents had been subjected to numerous incidents of mob violence. Rather than a temporary act, however, the Chinese Exclusion Act proved a harbinger of things to come. In 1894, the Immigration Restriction League was formed in Boston to limit the number of admissions and to select from among the potential applicants only the superior stocks related to the "American Aryans." Various prohibited categories were adopted. In 1882, Congress had also barred idiots, criminals, and others likely to become public charges. In 1891, this had been extended to take in believers in anarchism and in polygamy (aimed at the Mormons), as well as contract laborers. Adding to the anti-immigrant pressure was the fear of radicalism by the business community, a fear flamed by the Haymarket Riot in 1886 in Chicago, which culminated in a bomb blast that killed several policemen. Five of the six anarchists accused of the bombing were immigrants. World War I gave added fuel to the growing xenophobic tendencies. In 1917, at the height of the "100 percent Americanism" groundswell, a literacy test requiring every newcomer to the United States to demonstrate his or her ability to read was enacted into law over the veto of President Woodrow Wilson. It seems clear that many of the sponsors of the legislation assumed that the literacy test would limit the influx from southern and eastern Europe, where elementary education was not very well established, without excluding those from northern and western Europe, the ancestral homes of most Americans.

Eastern and southern Europeans, however, quickly demonstrated their ability to acquire the necessary literacy, and the demand for revision of the 1917 legislation mounted for a variety of different reasons. For example, Christian groups with large missionary establishments in China urged that the legislation be changed. This was because the 1917 legislation had not eliminated the Chinese exclusion and it was felt that missionary efforts in China were handicapped. One of the alternatives to the literacy test that had been proposed was a quota system based on the percentage of immigrants from a particular country already resident in the United States. This system had the advantage of not being aimed at Orientals in particular and also of preserving the power of existing immigrant groups. In 1921, Congress adopted a scheme that limited the total of each group of newcomers to three percent of the number from their nation who were living in the United States. Asiatics still received harsh treatment under the act and this heightened rather than eased antagonisms in the Orient. In 1924, a further restriction was imposed by basing quotas upon the proportion of residents present in the population in 1890—before the large-scale Polish, Russian, Italian, Serbian, Greek, and Jewish immigration occurred. This act also completely excluded Japanese immigrants.

With the 1924 act, the period of mass migration into the United States basically ended and even the anti-Jewish pogroms of Adolf Hitler did not change the system. Millions of Jews were killed who might have lived had the United States been willing to amend its immigration policy to accept refugees, something that did not happen until 1952.

The 1952 revision also modified the immigration law to admit a few Asians, although most of the Asians who became citizens under this provision had been residents of the United States for much of their lives. The refugee provision of the act allowed Hungarians, Cubans, Vietnamese, Koreans, and others caught up in the turmoil of today's world to be admitted. In 1965, there was a further modification so that unfilled quotas based on the percentage of nationals in the population in 1890 could be used by "preference" immigrants whose national quotas had been exhausted. Preference immigrants were those who would be reunited with their families or who had skills and talents needed in the country. It was this provision that led the so-called "underdeveloped countries" to complain of a "brain drain," since so many physicians, scientists, nurses, and other such professionals were allowed to become citizens of the

United States rather than return to or remain in their homeland after completing schooling. In 1968, there was a further revision, with a yearly limit of 170,000 set for immigrants from countries outside the Western Hemisphere (20,000 maximum from any one country), and a total of 120,000 immigrants from the Western Hemisphere to be admitted on a first-come-first-served basis. This last restriction put a limitation on immigrants from Latin America, which had led to increasing numbers of people from south of the border crossing into the country illegally as undocumented aliens. Just how many undocumented aliens there are is debatable, but some sources put it in the millions.

Though there were limitations put on the number of refugees, 17,400 per year, there were a number of special circumstances under which the Attorney General could exercise a power called *parole authority*. It was under this authority that a number of Hungarians entered the country between 1956 and 1958 and under which 260,000 Cuban refugees entered the country between 1965 and 1973. The special parole authority has been used to allow thousands of Soviet and East European refugees into the United States. After the fall of the Saigon government in South Vietnam, some 250,000 Indochinese were allowed into the United States, as well as other refugees from Laos, Cambodia, and in 1980, again from Cuba. As of this writing there is an attempt to again put limitations on the number of refugees who can be admitted. Only after consulting Congress can the President admit a large number of refugees.

Most of the immigrants in the past arrived in America in an exhausted state, worn out by lack of rest, poor food, and cramped quarters on ships, and unaccustomed to new conditions. In the early part of the nineteenth century, sea travel itself was exhausting. The journey from Liverpool to New York averaged about 40 days, although favorable winds might shorten the time somewhat. On the other hand, unfavorable ones might lengthen it to two to three months. Wrecks were frequent and disastrous. In one year in the 1830s, 17 vessels foundered on the run from Liverpool to Quebec alone. Fire was an ever-present danger, and so was disease. Great numbers of immigrants came steerage class and vessels before the Civil War were pitifully small, some three hundred tons crammed with anywhere from four hundred to a thousand passengers. Though there were cabins for the well-to-do, most travelers lived below decks in the hold, about seventy-five feet long, twenty-five feet wide, and six feet high. Each family received a daily ration of water, to which larger and larger doses of vinegar was added to conceal the odor. In steerage, the passengers furnished their own provisions, and if they ran out they either went hungry or had to buy from the ship's captain at prices they could not afford. It was not until mid-century that the United States government would specify the supplies that had to be taken onboard for each passenger.[13]

The only ventilation below the deck was through the hatches, which were battened down in rough weather. When the air was not stifling hot, it was bitter cold, since it was not possible to light a fire. Rats were at home in the dirt and disorder. The results were cholera, dysentery, yellow fever, smallpox, measles, and a sort of generic "ship fever" that might be anything. The normal mortality on crossing the Atlantic was about 10 percent, although some years it was closer to 20 percent.

Some changes for the better came in mid-century. The introduction of steam in the 1840s and the appearance of the Cunard Line and its imitators took over the upper-class passenger business and left the immigrant trade to the sailing ships, which were consequently forced to improve accommodations. After 1870, the new emphasis on merchant fleets led France, Germany, England, and Italy to build larger ships and to give subsidies to the operators of lines bearing their flags. Under these circumstances, the price of steerage passage on a steamship fell to as little as twelve dollars and included food. By 1900, the traveler could count on a crossing of little more than a week in vessels of ten to twenty thousand tons. It was still not an easy trip, since the ships were overcrowded, there was lack of privacy, and the food was poor, but much larger proportions survived the voyage. Still, it is no wonder that so many were so exhausted that they stayed at the port of embarcation without going on into the interior. Those who did move on used the railroads and often remained at the junction points on the route—for example, Buffalo, Cleveland, Pittsburgh, Chicago, St. Louis, and Milwaukee—even though they had originally intended to go elsewhere.

Increasingly, in fact, the immigrants came to settle in the cities, and rural small town America saw proportionately fewer of the new masses of people that came in the last part of the nineteenth and first part of the twentieth centuries. This occurred in spite of the fact that great numbers of immigrants had originally left with the intention of farming and tilling the soil. In fact, unless they had money and resources, or organized expeditions (as the Mormons did), few of them managed to escape from the cities. Most of them, even though of peasant origin and knowing only how to farm, became trapped in the city, able only to sell their strength, since they had little of the skills needed for other jobs. It was the immigrants who built the canals, the railroads, and the early highways that, in the days before big earth-moving equipment was available, required masses of men. The factories and mines also offered employment opportunities, and some immigrants became machine operators. Many also opened businesses to serve their fellow immigrants as storekeepers, butchers, bakers, and so forth.

Trapped in the city, however, life was still hard and death rates were high. New York City and the other major Atlantic ports, where the immigrant concentration was greatest, crowded newcomers into tenements. In the interior of the country, smaller units were more the norm, but it was not unusual to stuff six families into units built for one. This overcrowding helped to spread disease; tuberculosis rates were particularly high among the foreign-born population. The immigrants were also pushed into the least desirable places to live. In Chicago, they were pushed beside the slaughterhouses; in Boston, they were hemmed in by the docks and markets of the North End; and in other towns, they located near the railroad switching yard. One of the great problems in tenements was that of sanitation. Many of the early buildings had been built without privies at all. From the middle of the nineteenth century onward, when most tenements were built with privies or water closets (which washed away the sewage), these were located outside in the back yards and alleys. For those people who lived on the sixth floor, this arrangement was very inconvenient. Later on, as the modern flush toilet was developed, the newer tenements were built with inside toilets, usually two on each floor. However, these were open to all comers but charged to the care of none and left to the neglect of all. In the winter the pipes overflowed, and weeks might go by before matters were set right. Some of the tenements thereafter retained the odor of human excrement through the rest of their history.

Filth was inescapable. Open drains were common and, even in a city as large as Chicago, it was not until well into the twentieth century that some of the sewers were covered, so that until that time fly-borne diseases were quite prevalent. Since an adequate water supply was difficult to obtain, it was often necessary to carry tubs and jugs from taps in the alley. Water was connected to toilets first, and in many cases water for drinking and bathing still had to be carried from a public faucet outside. Illness was rampant, drunkenness was common, and behavioral disorders and neuroses—all classed as "insanity" in that day—were ever-present. America, however, was slow to deal with the problems. The New York State Senate in 1858 appointed a committee to look into the need for municipal health measures. It attributed the high rate of mortality in New York City at that time to the:

. . . overcrowded condition of tenement houses, the want of practical knowledge of the proper mode of constructing such houses,
deficiency of light, imperfect ventilation, impurities in domestic
economy, unwholesome food and beverages, insufficient sewage
(i.e., sewers), want of cleanliness in the streets and at the
wharves and piers, to a general disregard of sanitary precautions, and finally, to the imperfect execution of existing ordi-
nances and the total absence of a regularly organized sanitary
police.[14]

Finally, in 1866, the Metropolitan Board of Health was established, and soon after this New York City was given its own department. Much of the early activity of the Board was motivated by the
concept that disease was caused by dirt, and investigators concentrated on reporting defective plumbing or ventilation and tried to
control contagious disease through environmental sanitation.

Immigrants, and slum dwellers in particular, were hard hit by
the various epidemics in the United States in the nineteenth century. Cholera epidemics hit in 1832, 1848 to 1849, 1866, and 1873.
Yellow fever was more or less endemic during much of the nineteenth century, as was smallpox. Diphtheria and scarlet fever were
major causes of death among children, and, during the 40-year period from 1840 to 1880, scarlet fever was particularly virulent.

Actual control of the contagious diseases was dependent upon
the development of the germ theory by Louis Pasteur and others
during the last part of the nineteenth century. The new science of
bacteriology reached the United States in the 1880s and gradually
more effective preventive measures were taken against epidemics.
The epidemics, as well as illness in general, were more likely to hit
the immigrant than the more affluent Americans, primarily because
of the nature of the living conditions. However, medical care of the
poor was also inferior to that given to the more well-to-do people. As
indicated earlier, hospitals were primarily charitable institutions;
they were not particularly clean, and, through most of the nineteenth century, they lacked any kind of trained nursing care. They
were usually the institutions of last resort, and many people felt
that going to the hospital meant that they were dying. Well-to-do
people were cared for by servants or by physicians themselves at
home, where there was less chance of the spread of infection.[15]

Communities did little in an organized way to care for the
health needs of the poor. Instead, they relied upon various charitable institutions. Probably the most important medical institution
for the poor was the dispensary that had appeared in England in the
late eighteenth century and been imported to Philadelphia in 1786.

Growth of the dispensary movement was slow before the Civil War, but rapid thereafter. By 1874, there were 29 dispensaries in New York City, treating some 213,000 patients. By 1900, some 876,000 patients were being treated in the New York City dispensaries. Most dispensaries had a resident physician who performed minor surgery, pulled teeth, and treated minor medical complaints. Mostly, what the physician did was issue prescriptions, and it was the routine and exclusive dependence on drug therapy that distinguished the medicine of the poor from that of the middle class. As dispensaries grew in size, the staff increased, but almost all operated on a shoestring budget of no more than four to five thousand dollars a year. Only in New York did the dispensaries receive any city or state money. Supplementing the resident physician were often a resident druggist apothecary and a number of younger physicians just starting out in practice who were assigned to visit patients too ill to visit the dispensary. Established medical practitioners in the community often acted as consultants and volunteers.[16]

The cultural and social gap between patient and medical attendant was wide and deep. Most physicians were young and at least from middle-class backgrounds, while their patients were usually poor and immigrants. To the physician, the patient often seemed undesirable, filthy, drunken, and alien. A dispensary physician in 1850 proclaimed that the Irish were particularly violent and disease prone, adding,

> I am fearful [this] will continue to be the case, since no form of legislation can reach them, or force them to change their habits for those more conducive to cleanliness and health.[17]

The dispensary movement began to decline in the twentieth century as the hospitals grew, aided in large part by the emergence of hospital nursing. Many of the tasks done by the dispensaries were also taken over by the public health nurse. Physicians who had used the dispensaries as a sort of internship for medical practice now moved into hospital-centered internships and residencies. If anything, however, the cultural gap between the patients and physicians widened. In the early 1900s, the distinguished Boston physician Richard Cabot, examining his own reactions to foreign-born patients at the Massachusetts General Hospital, noted that the

> ... chances are ten to one that I shall look out of my eyes and see, not Abraham Cohen, but a Jew. ... I do not see this man at all. I merge him in the hazy background of the average Jew.

But . . . if I am a little less blind than usual to-day . . . I may notice something in the way his hand lies on his knee, something that is queer, unexpected. That hand . . . it's a muscular hand, it's a prehensible hand; and whoever saw a Salem Street Jew with a muscular hand before? . . . I saw him. Yet he was not more real than the thousands of others whom I had seen and forgotten,—forgotten because I never saw them, but only their ghostly outline, their generic type, the racial background out of which they emerged.[18]

Prejudice was probably less in dealing with infants and young children or with pregnant women than with adults. In 1859, the New York Infirmary for Women and Children appointed a "sanitary visitor" to give simple practical instruction to "poor mothers on the management of infants, and the preservation of the health of families," but this effort was soon submerged in the Civil War. During the Panic (or depression) of 1873, the New York Diet Kitchen set up food stations to feed the poor, and as conditions improved the food station became a milk station for babies. Nathan Strauss, a private philanthropist, began to establish a system of milk stations in 1893, which by 1902 were distributing 250,000 bottles monthly. The milk stations were visualized by some of the reformers as the basis for a maternal and child-care center. Leading efforts for this were a husband-and-wife team, Wilbur and Elsie Cole Phillips, who had laid the groundwork for their experiment in Milwaukee and carried it to fruition in Cincinnati. Ultimately, the projects both in Milwaukee and Cincinnati were terminated because Phillips and many of those working with him were Socialists and their efforts were opposed by the medical and political establishment. The more successful efforts took place in New York City, where nurses became a main element in the local health district.[19]

Nurses were also active in another movement that worked to better conditions among the new immigrant, the settlement house movement, which also served as a modern community clinic. A settlement house differed from other social agencies in that it was concerned about the neighborhood as a whole. It differed from the dispensaries and the health centers in that the physician was not the controlling influence. Originally, the settlement house sought to develop relationships among the community groups of different cultural, religious, and social characteristics, and to help people act together to improve their living conditions and environments. Lillian Wald summed up the aims as "fusing these people who come to us from the Old World Civilization into . . . a real brotherhood among men."[20] Wald and her partner Mary Brewster were nurses, and their settlement, the Henry Street Settlement, shares the distinction with Hull House in Chicago as being the most famous settlement houses of their time.[21]

Both settlements emphasized health care and education and did much to develop the professions of social work and public health. Wald as well as others recognized that ill health and physical disability were the "most constant attendants of poverty," and it was estimated that a serious disabling condition existed in about three-fourths of the families needing charity. Though the settlement house movement, and particularly Hull House and the Henry Street Settlement, are now looked upon with universal favor and even reverence, in their own day they were considered to be quite radical. They helped to develop autonomous neighborhood organizations, and the leaders of the movement, including many nurses, saw the poverty of the immigrants as something that could be corrected. Both Lillian Wald and Jane Addams were politically oriented and urged and fought for protective labor legislation, child welfare laws, compensation for workers when injured, and various other forms of government intervention to deal with the problems of the poor, all of which were regarded as alien and radical ideas by the more affluent segment of society. Most of what these early reformers advocated have since become part of the American way of life, but the problems of poverty, minority status, and alienation still exist, only in slightly different forms.

Half a century has passed since the end of the large-scale European migration to this country, and new minority groups have emerged, many of them from cultures even more alien to traditional American ideology. Some of the problems and prejudices faced by these new groups are similar to those encountered by the European immigrants, although there are some essential differences between those problems and the problems faced by blacks, Mexican Americans, Puerto Ricans, Koreans, Cubans, and others who are the new immigrants and new minority groups. Knowing that we have gone through some of these problems before, however, helps put both the similarities and the differences in context.

REFERENCES

1. Wirth, L. The Problem of Minority Groups. In R. Linton (Ed.), The Science of Man in the World Crisis. New York: Columbia University Press, 1945, pp. 345–372.
2. Warne, F. J. The Tide of Immigration. New York: D. Appleton, 1916, p. 205.

3. Carr-Saunders, A. M. World Population. Oxford: Clarendon Press, 1936, p. 49.
4. Jones, M. A. American Immigration. Chicago: University of Chicago Press, 1960, pp. 22–27.
5. Ibid., p. 49.
6. Wald, L. The House on Henry Street. New York: Henry Holt, 1915, pp. 1–25, Burgess, E. W. Urban Areas. In T. V. Smith & L. White (Eds.), Chicago: An Experiment in Social Science Research. Chicago: University of Chicago Press, 1929, pp. 113–138.
7. Greer, C. Public Schools: The Myth of the Melting Pot. Saturday Review, 1969, 84–86, 102–103.
8. Jones, op. cit., p. 43.
9. Wirth, L. The Ghetto. Chicago: University of Chicago Press, 1928, p. 2
10. Ibid., pp. 150–151.
11. Gordon, M. Assimilation in American Life: The Role of Race, Religion and National Origin. New York: Oxford University Press, 1964, p. 123 passim.
12. Gossett, T. F. Race: The History of an Idea in America. Dallas: Southern Methodist University Press, 1963, pp. 287–309.
13. Handlin, O. The Uprooted. Boston: Atlantic-Little, Brown, 1952, pp. 37–62.
14. Rosen, G. A History of Public Health. New York: MD Publications, 1958, p. 244.
15. Bullough, V. & Bullough, B. Care of the Sick: Emergence of Modern Nursing (3rd ed.). New York: Prodist, Neale Watson, 1978 pp. 75–153.
16. See: Rosenberg, C. E. Social Class and Medical Care in 19th-Century America: The Rise and Fall of the Dispensary. *Journal of the History of Medicine*, 1974, *29*, 32–54. This was reprinted in J. W. Leavitt & R. L. Numbers (Eds.), Sickness and Health in America. Madison: University of Wisconsin Press, 1978, pp. 157–171.
17. Quoted by Rosenberg, in Leavitt and Numbers, p. 164.
18. Cabot, R. C. Social Service and the Art of Healing. New York: Dodd, Mead, 1931, pp. 4–7.
19. Rosen, G. The First Neighborhood Health Center Movement—Its Rise and Fall. *American Journal of Public Health*, 1971, *61*, 1620–1635.
20. Duffus, R. L. Lillian Wald: Neighbor and Crusader. New York: Macmillan, 1939, p. 147.
21. Wald, op. cit., Addams, J. Twenty Years at Hull House. New York: Macmillan, 1912.

3

Black Americans

Since its beginnings in the eighteenth century, the modern business and industrial complex has depended upon a supply of cheap labor to carry out the more burdensome and lower-paying tasks. Traditionally, workers to perform these jobs have been recruited from the farm and the village. When rural areas were not able to meet the demands for workers, countries such as England turned to parts of their Empire, particularly to Ireland, but in recent years West Indians, Pakistani, and Indians have come to England in great numbers. Since World War II, other countries, such as Germany and Switzerland, have recruited large numbers of Italians, Greeks, Yugoslavs, and people from other nations where industrialization has not been so advanced. Most of these workers sign to work for a stipulated length of time and leave their families behind. In a sense, they are today's counterpart to the sojourners and other temporary immigrants to the United States in the past.

In the United States, the lower ranking industrial workers traditionally have come either from the small towns and the farms or from among the recent immigrants. The movement from the rural areas to the industrial cities reached flood-tide proportions in the twentieth century, in part because of periodic restrictions on immigration, but also because the mechanization of the farm eliminated many of the farm workers and made the lot of the small farmer more and more difficult. Not all sections of the United States have undergone industrialization at the same pace; during most of the century, the great industrialization took place along the coastal areas and around the Great Lakes. This meant that, until very recently, migration within the United States took place not only from the farm to the city but from the South, one of the poorer and least industrialized sections of the country, to the North and the West, and from the farm belt in the interior of the country to centers of industry along the coast and the Great Lakes. In the past decade, the South and the West have also begun to industrialize at a more rapid pace, and some of the immigrants moving to these areas are from the older industrial areas of the Northeast and the Great lakes. This movement has caused a crisis of falling population in some of the older industrial cities, such as Cleveland, Detroit, Buffalo, Chicago, and New York City.

In general, those residents of the rural areas most likely to move to the city were either the young, the dissatisfied, or those who lacked property and investment. Inevitably, many of them went through periods of readjustment as severe as those faced by immigrants from other countries. The so-called "Oakies" and "Arkies" who migrated to California during the 1920s and 1930s were met with hostility and exploitation. To the Californians, their culture seemed at the time to be almost an alien one.[1] Facing even greater prejudice in their migration northward during the 1940s and 1950s were the blacks, who were not only less educated than the "Oakies" of the 1930s but also had the difficulty of skin color and the burden of past slavery and subjugation to overcome. Replacing the "Oakies" of the 1930s as the most poverty-stricken section of white America were the residents of Appalachia, many of whom have moved to the city seeking employment as the coal fields and farms of Appalachia began to fail. Even if the prominence of coal is re-established, new mining techniques employ far less workers than in the past, and there is still a shortage of jobs in Appalachia.

Another source of cheap labor, both in the city and in the country, has been the Spanish-speaking migrants from Puerto Rico, who are American citizens, and those from Mexico and Central America, who cross the borders both legally and illegally to find work. There are also large numbers of indigenous Spanish-speaking peoples in the Southwest whose homes had been annexed to the United States in the nineteenth century but who still lack real facility in English. This is due to the fact that Spanish speakers were so plentiful in some of the barrios that residents were not forced to learn English, and there was no commitment by educational authorities to provide adequate schooling. Still another indigenous group with real minority status is the native Americans, the Indians, many of whom live in poverty on reservations or in the slums of the city. Other visible minorities, such as the Oriental Americans, also face problems, although there are many variations. Both the Japanese and the older Chinese Americans are better off than blacks, Spanish-speaking Americans, or Indians, and compare favorably to the descendants of immigrants from Europe. Recent Chinese immigrants, as well as those from Thailand, Korea, Cambodia, and the Philippines, have undergone much the same experience as earlier groups of immigrants. Some members of these "new" groups who came in as special refugees were extremely well-to-do, but most refugees came with little more than the clothing they wore and what they could carry. The Oriental newcomers have been joined by refugees and immigrants from the Arab countries of the Middle East, by Samoans from the South Pacific, by Jews from Russia, and by vast numbers of Armenians, Iranians, Indians, and peoples from various countries in Central and South America. The best way to look at the problems of the various groups is to examine some of them separately, and the remainder of this chapter will be devoted to discussing blacks.

BLACKS

Blacks had come to America early, perhaps with Columbus, although there is some scholarly dispute as to whether Pedro Alonzo Nino, the navigator of the Niña was an African or not. It is known for certain that several members of the French and Spanish exploring parties were black; for example, Jean Baptiste Point du Sable, the founder of Chicago, was black.[2] The overwhelming majority of black Africans who came to this country, however, were different from other immigrants in that they came unwillingly on slave ships. Slavery was big business in American colonial history, and many an American fortune, particularly those in New England, was built upon the transportation of slaves from the West Indies, where they had been brought by the British. During the seventeenth century, Dutch, French, Portuguese, and English companies were active in the African slave trade, but by the eighteenth century the English had achieved dominance.

Slaves were captured or bought from Arab tradesmen in West Africa, primarily from the Gold Coast (modern Ghana) or the Congo (modern Zaire). They were then chained together and packed into ships for the passage across the Atlantic. Almost every difficulty that the willing European immigrant encountered was compounded for the black prisoner, who faced greater overcrowding, less adequate food, and a general feeling of hopelessness. Probably no more than half of the slaves who were loaded onto ships in Africa actually reached their destination, at least in any condition to work, and work was almost essential to their continued survival. Large numbers died of disease, committed suicide, or were permanently disabled by the ravages of disease or from the injuries they received. Until fairly late in the slave trade, profits were so great that the traders tried simply to stuff more people onto their ships to compensate for anticipated loss of life rather than humanize conditions.

It was the development of the sugar crop in the Caribbean islands that had first made the American slave trade so profitable, the West Indies being the destination of the early slave ships. Here, slaves were "seasoned" or taught their new work roles under the whips of overseers. It was from the West Indies that the slaves were transported to the American colonies, a trade that rapidly increased after 1792 with the invention of the cotton gin. Cotton became an important money crop in the South at the very time that sugar was becoming less important in the West Indies.

To America's credit, there were always powerful critics of the slave trade, and they managed to abolish the practice in the United States as of January 1, 1808. Great Britain abolished it first in 1806 but in stronger terms in 1811. Since the British controlled the seas as well as the west coast of Africa, their effort to abolish the trade proved more effective and by the middle of the nineteenth century, it had been nearly eliminated. The elimination of the slave trade removed one abuse, but it did not necessarily improve the lot of the slave, who now had to work harder. Moreover, some of the areas of the United States took to encouraging the breeding of slaves, selling the surplus to other areas. The abolition of the slave trade also did not end the practice of hiring contract laborers, whom the British recruited in India, China, and elsewhere and transported to various ports. Contract laborers from China, for example, built the western portion of the transcontinental railroad across the United States. Though nominally under contract, in fact many of the indentured laborers were recruited by unscrupulous means, and all too often their contracts for return to their homeland were not honored.

It was the British, nonetheless, who led the effort to eliminate actual slavery. In 1833, slavery was officially abolished in British possessions, although the act was only to take place after slaves had been trained to take jobs in society. In the British West Indies, for example, it was not until 1838 that all slaves were free. Slowly, other European states followed the British example, with France emancipating its slaves in 1848, Portugal in 1858, and Holland in 1863, although in most cases freedom was given only gradually. Mexico abolished slavery in 1829, and Brazil in 1871, but the full effect was not felt in Brazil until 1888. Black slavery continued to exist in the Spanish possessions of Cuba and Puerto Rico and in the Philippines until these colonies were taken over or given their independence by the United States in the aftermath of the Spanish American War.

As every school child has learned, the struggle for emancipation in the United States was long and bitter, as well as extremely divisive. In large part, this was due to the fact that slavery was not particularly profitable in New England, the Middle Atlantic States, or the developing West, and thus came to be a phenomenon largely concentrated in the cotton-growing South. The fact that emancipation occurred only in conjunction with the Civil War made the Southerners much more antagonistic to blacks and complicated the life of the newly freed slave much more than might have been the case if the owners had been given compensation for their "property" as they had in the British colonies. All these events left their mark on the life of the American black, the overwhelming majority of whom had roots in the American South.

IMPACT OF SLAVERY

Franklin Frazier, a pioneer black sociologist, held that the trauma of the terrifying trip across the Atlantic, the brutal breaking-in experience in the West Indies or under the American plantation overseers, plus the humiliating experience of slavery itself, virtually destroyed the African cultural heritage. Further adding to the destruction was the fact that slaves were forced to use English to communicate with each other because their tribal origins and languages varied so much. Dispersement of tribal groups was a more or less formal policy because it was believed it would cut down on the dangers of insurrection.[3] Slavery also weakened the African family, if only because slaves were often forbidden to marry. Even where unions could and did take place, they could be violated by the owners of the slave, who could and did seize a woman for his own sexual pleasure or break up a potential family by selling off some of its members. Inevitably, the collective personality shaped by these experiences had little resemblance to the proud and independent African tribe that had been the slave's ancestor.[4]

Without denying the trauma and humiliation suffered by the black slave immigrants, other scholars, such as the anthropologist Melville Herskovits, have effectively argued that American blacks still managed to retain some of their past tradition. Herskovits studied African culture traits, compared them with culture traits of blacks in the New World, and found similarities in language, religion, music, and numerous other aspects of culture. Though the slaves learned English, they used African patterns in speech and intonation and somehow managed to keep alive folk tales and magical practices that they had brought with them from Africa. Though such carryovers were more evident in the West Indies and in Latin America than in the large urban ghettoes of the American North, they still existed.[5]

As studies on Africa and blacks have progressed, the insights of Herskovits have been verified. Despite the fact that slaves were brutally removed from their past, thrust unwillingly into a radically different life pattern, and denied opportunities to form associations, they continued to view their experiences from the point of view of their past, and their culture was vibrant enough and ingrained enough to allow them to do so. In fact, the rich cultural heritage of American blacks, however brutalized they might have been, has enriched all of American culture.[6]

Medical and nursing care for the ill slave was somewhat ambiguous. Most masters insisted that, as property, the slave immediately inform the person in charge when they were sick so the malady might be treated before it worsened. Many blacks, however, were reluctant to submit to the often harsh prescription and remedies of eighteenth-and nineteenth-century white medical practice and preferred self-treatment or turned to black herb and root doctors or to influential conjurers. Generally, the white owner was concerned about sick slaves if only because they represented a financial investment that required protection. Many masters undoubtedly had humanitarian motives, and even those that did not realized that certain illnesses could easily spread to their own families if not properly treated and contained. The difficulty was that the plantation overseer was in the impossible position of needing to produce as much labor as possible from the slaves, using punishment when necessary, and at the same time having to care for slaves' illnesses and protect them from exposure, exhaustion, and accident. The plantation overseer was taskmaster, judge, physician, and nurse simultaneously, but his first duty was to turn out the work. Often, actual nursing care was done by the slave-owner's wife or daughter, although post–Civil War southerners have tended to over-romanticize the woman's role and sacrifices as nurse. The overseer's wife often also assisted.

A former slave, Baily Cunningham, recalled late in his life that, when he was a slave, his mistress "had three kinds of medicine that would cure everything": vinegar nail, a drink made from leaving one pound of nails overnight in a jug of vinegar, and which was used to cure aches and pains in the stomach or back; rosin pills, prepared from raw pine rosin; and tar, used for tooth or ear aches. Cunningham added that his mistress never called a physician.[7]

One of the things that slave masters were always on the watch for was malingering. Todd L. Savitt has written that most owners believed that, if a slave complained of illness, he or she was only acting like a true black in feeling "poorly" to escape work.[8] One way of getting at this "problem" was to make the medicine worse than the complaint. Charles Grandy recalled in 1937 how some eighty years earlier he had pretended to be ill when the overseer found him sleeping in the cornfield:

> When you gits sick, dey give you some kin' o' medicine called ipicac. . . . Dey make me take dat an' I got sick den sho' 'nough. Got so sick I hadda go to bed. Stayed dere three or four days too. So I got clear o' dat whippin'.[9]

One of the results of the master's perception of malingering was that a black had to be very sick to receive effective treatment. There are numerous incidents of slaves dying because the master did not believe they were ill. Several incidents have been collected from the immediate pre–Civil War period. In one case, a strong young field-hand complained to his master for a week about his poor condition, but the master refused to listen until the slave died of typhoid fever. William, a Richmond tobacco-factory hand, had jumped twelve feet from a platform to escape punishment and later died of a severe concussion. The physician who treated him believed he "was practicing deception," and even visited William at night unannounced "thinking I might probably find the mask thrown off, and my patient walking about, or enjoying himself with friends."[10]

Inevitably, many slaves turned to self-treatment. Owners seemed willing to permit this, providing the sickness did not get out of hand. Most of the black home remedies were derived from local plants, perhaps plants similar to those found in Africa, but some were also based upon conjuring, a carryover from the African witch doctor. Conjure doctors were men and women who used African tribal magic, violence, persuasion, and considerable psychology as well as medical proficiency to gain a reputation. They were viewed as healers of illnesses that white doctors could not cure and as perpetrators of sickness through "spells."

Nursing was often the duty of female slaves. One nurse, Jensey Snow, became a living legend in her home town of Petersburgh, Virginia. She was given her freedom (manumitted in 1825) for

> . . . several acts of extraordinary merit performed . . . during the last year, in nursing, & at the imminent risk of her own health & safety, exercising the most unexampled patience and attention in watching over the sick beds of several individuals of this town.

She thereupon opened a town hospital.

One of the roles in which slave women served both the black and white populations with regularity was as midwives. Most babies were delivered by midwives, and most of the midwives were black, since the experience in the slave quarters gave the necessary expertise for general practice. Mildred Graves, who was still living in Fredericksburg, Virginia, in 1939, remembered bringing many youngsters into the world during her years as a slave midwife:

> You know in dem days dey didn't have so many doctors. So treatin' de sick was always my job. Whenever any of de white folks 'roun' Hanover was goin' to have babies dey always got word to Mr. Tinsley [her master] dat dey wanted to hire me for dat time. Sho' he lef me go. . . . 'twas money fo him, you know. He would give me only a few cents, but dat was kinda good of him to do dat. Plenty niggers was hired out an' didn't get nothin'. Sometimes I had three an 'four sick at de same time, Marser used to tell me I was a valuable slave. Dey use to come for me both day an' night—you know it's a funny thing how babies has a way of comin' heah when it's dark.[12]

THE END OF SLAVERY

Emancipation did not end the problems of being black in this country. Although slavery was abolished in the aftermath of the Civil War, few of the blacks were educated, and many of them had picked up what might be called "survival traits" in slavery that made adjustment in a nonslave society difficult. Moreover, the bulk of the the white South was accustomed to blacks being slaves, and, in spite of the constitutional amendments, most whites were determined to assert their dominance over the blacks who in many parts of the South outnumbered the whites. When blacks, with the encouragement of the federal government and the presence of Union troops, assumed positions of authority, the South countered by establishing secret movements designed to keep the blacks in "their place," by terror if necessary. The Knights of the White Camelia and the Ku Klux Klan were the most powerful of the secret orders. Members, armed with guns, swords, and other weapons, patrolled some parts of the South day and night. Scattered Union troops proved wholly ineffectual in coping with the problem, and few blacks were able to face up to the threats. Many either left the South or resigned themselves to trying to seek advancement through other ways. Those blacks who did go North found that they were greeted with hostility and suspicion because most of the northerners, while antislavery, were also antiblack.

Though the dedicated abolitionists made attempts to ensure black rights in the South, they were comparatively few in number. Even though the southerners had lost the war, they were determined to rule themselves, and they believed in their minds and hearts that blacks were not qualified to rule. As the restraints imposed upon the southerners by the federal government and the presence of occupying troops were relaxed or removed, and the stringent postwar legislation repealed, the Reconstruction of the South gradually fell into the hands of the southerners, and while there were occasionally bloody racial clashes, the white southerner soon emerged dominant. In the aftermath of the disputed presidential election of 1876 between Rutherford B. Hayes and Samuel J. Tilden, an agreement was made by the Republicans to withdraw all federal troops in return for southern electoral support of Hayes. By this time, the North had grown weary of the crusade for black rights, and, while there were still some old antislavery leaders, most of the leaders of the younger generation had little zeal for the blacks and cared more about the industrial and business interests in the North and South. With the return of the old leaders in the South, most of whom identified with the Democratic Party, ways were soon found to disenfranchise blacks or to nullify their political strength, in spite of the Fifteenth Amendment to the Constitution. As soon as the political power of the blacks and their allies declined, the South turned to erecting the barrier of segregation to replace the old barrier of slavery. This so-called "Jim Crow" legislation separated blacks and whites on trains, in depots, on wharves, in barber shops, at drinking fountains, restaurants, theaters, schools, and in almost every aspect of life. This was not done without opposition, but the southern officials either executed or expelled those blacks who opposed the imposition of segregation. In the first two years of the twentieth century, there were some 214 lynchings of blacks in the South. With the law, the courts, and the execution of justice in the hands of whites, blacks, even though technically no longer slaves, had to struggle to survive and could only make feeble gropings in the direction of progress.[13] One of the basic difficulties was always the lack of black professionals in the health professions.

TRENDS WITHIN THE BLACK COMMUNITY

Because of the inherent difficulties in obtaining equality of educational opportunities for blacks, the Booker T. Washington solution seemed attractive to many. Washington, who had become head of the Tuskegee Institute in 1881, believed that whites, southern whites in particular, had to be convinced that the education of blacks was in the true interest of the South before basic Southern support would be forthcoming. In a rather fatherly fashion, he counseled blacks to respect the law, cooperate with the white authorities in maintaining peace, and to train themselves to become farmers, mechanics, and domestic servants, until they had improved themselves sufficiently to be ready for better things. Washington emphasized and taught habits of thrift, patience, perserverance, the cultivation of good manners, and in the process won the support of many whites, northerners as well as southerners, who saw his plan as a formula for peaceful race relations in the South. Though Washington believed in the ultimate attainment of equality and integration, many of his white supporters, skeptical of the capacity of blacks to become completely assimilated, viewed his scheme as leading the blacks to their proper place in American life, a position that they felt should be inferior to that of the whites. Others of his white supporters were so happy with his gradualism that they never bothered about his ultimate goals.

One of the leading opponents of the Washington philosophy was W. E. B. DuBois, a Harvard-educated, northern-born black, who went to the South to teach and do research on Southern blacks. DuBois believed that it was impossible for blacks, no matter what their level in society, to defend themselves without the vote. He also held that Washington's advice to blacks to stay in rural areas did not face up to the reality of the ongoing industrialization and urbanization in America. In 1905, a group of black men under the leadership of DuBois, determined to secure full citizenship, met in conference at Niagara Falls, Canada. There they wrote a platform demanding freedom of speech and criticism, suffrage, abolition of all distinctions based on race, recognition of basic principles of human brotherhood, and respect for the workingman. The group called itself the Niagara Movement. Following a race riot in Springfield, Illinois, in August 1908, the founders of the movement joined with various older surviving abolition movements, as well as other groups interested in bettering the lot of blacks, to sponsor a conference on Lincoln's birthday in 1909. Out of this came the National Association for the Advancement of Colored People (NAACP), most of whose first officers were white. The term *colored* was then the term most often used by educated blacks to describe themselves, just as *Negro* became the more popular term in later years, while *black* became the accepted term in the decade of the 1970s. The organization of the NAACP was followed in 1911 by the National Urban League, and both of these organizations were in the forefront of the battle for more effective integration of American blacks.

Integration proved to be slow and difficult process, and in fact not all blacks agreed with the aims of the NAACP, since for much of its history the NAACP failed to touch the imagination of the masses. Blacks on the lower social and economic level, if they knew of the NAACP or similar organizations, were inclined to regard them as agencies of upper-class blacks or of liberal whites, who were not particularly aware of the economic necessities of remaining alive. Far more popular with the average black in the second decade of the twentieth century was the Universal Negro Improvement Association, founded by Marcus Garvey in 1914. Garvey exalted everything black, and insisted that black stood for strength and beauty, not inferiority. He asserted that Africans had a noble past of which Americans of African descent should be proud. In short, he had many of the same concepts of the "black is beautiful" movement of the 1960s and 1970s. Unable to see any hope for blacks in the United States, Garvey urged blacks to flee America and return to Africa, where they could build a country of their own. His appeal struck a responsive chord and his movement grew until it numbered in the millions. The Back to Africa movement ultimately collapsed, not because of black disillusionment with it, but because of Garvey's own personal failures as well as the antagonism of some powerful elements in the United States. Garvey was accused of using the mails to defraud in his attempt to raise money to run a steamship line to take blacks to Africa, and in 1925 he was sent to jail under a five-year sentence. When he was pardoned, he returned to his native Jamaica, and without him his movement rapidly declined.

The history of the American black in the twentieth century can, in part, be summarized as a conflict between the idea of DuBois and Garvey, with an occasional nod to the ideas of Booker T. Washington. One segment of the black community has pushed for integration, while another has emphasized black power and ties with Africa. Washington, though increasingly recognized for his important contribution, has little current following. In Washington's program, his advice to stay on the farm was most ignored, as is evident from census figures. In 1910, 73 percent of the black population were rural and overwhelmingly southern. By 1960, 73 percent were urban, and more blacks lived outside the South than in it.[14] This change has been emphasized through subsequent censuses. This means that, in one sense, the blacks are among the oldest immigrants, and, in another sense, they are also among the newest, since the change from the rural South to the urbanized industrialized cities has been so dramatic it was like going through a second immigration. In fact, it was the move into the urbanized industrial cities that ultimately gave the blacks enough political clout to force some basic changes in American policies towards them.

This movement, which had begun even before the Civil War (i.e., the Underground Railway) began to mushroom following the outbreak of World War I, had become a mass movement in the 1940s and 1950s, and is still taking place, although the movement is no longer from the south to the north and west as it once was. In the process of the migration, blacks came to have a politically potent voice in many urban centers, both North and South, and, as they became a political force and gained access to better education and some of the better-paying jobs, black demands for equality of opportunity increased. Cities as diverse as Gary (Indiana), Detroit, Cleveland, Washington, D.C., Atlanta, and Los Angeles have had black mayors, and state legislatures as well as Congress have strong black contingents. Nondiscriminatory provisions were required of defense industries in World War II, and this was followed by passage of state and national Fair Employment Practice Acts. The NAACP and some of the other civil rights and civil liberties groups had long looked to the courts to redress some of the most outrageous forms of discrimination against blacks, and, in the period from the end of World War II to today, the courts responded with a series of decisions declaring numerous laws unconstitutional—restrictive covenants in housing, segregated interstate transportations, separate but equal schools, segregated health facilities supported with federal monies; the list could go on. Declaring a law or practice unconstitutional and achieving equality were, unfortunately, often different things, and, beginning in the 1950s, a massive civil rights campaign led to more active enforcement of the constitutional guarantees of equality. In 1956, Martin Luther King, Jr. rose to fame and leadership through his role in the Montgomery, Alabama, bus boycott. Sit-in demonstrations at lunch counters led to the integration of many southern restaurants, and Congress itself through various Civil Rights Acts attempted to remove most of the remaining barriers against discrimination. The result was a period of turmoil and militancy by blacks as they awoke to the fact that much of the suffering they had endured in the past was no longer necessary. Change has not been easy for most Americans, and for many blacks the progress has seemed slow. The transition in power and status has been marked by riots in many ghettoes, as blacks rebelled at continuing forms of discrimination. These "race" riots differed from those in the past in that they were inspired and led by blacks protesting against their condition rather than directed against blacks by whites. Other minority groups, particularly the Spanish-speaking Americans, have also had their share of riots, as frustrations over the slow pace of change led to rage.

INEQUALITIES IN HEALTH AND HEALTH CARE

One of the areas in which the past history of discrimination, repression, and suspicion has most effectively left its mark upon the black of today is in the area of health care. Data on life expectancy that have been available since 1900 indicate that there has been a persistent gap between the expected length of life of the white and the nonwhite populations (until 1960, 94 percent of those classified as nonwhite were black; by 1978, only 85 percent were). Table 2 shows these life expectancies by decade. Although the gap has narrowed as the health of the total population has improved, there are still significant differences between the two groups. It is not only segregation and discrimination that have produced these differences in health but also poverty, lack of education, and the negative psychological responses that follow from these difficulties. If it were necessary to rank these variables, poverty would undoubtedly come first, but in a sense this is misleading, because poverty is inextricably intertwined with all forms of discrimination, each difficulty reinforcing the other. Nevertheless, when one uses the index of poverty originally developed by the Social Security Administration, 43.8 percent of the nation's nonwhite families (and 24.7 percent of the white families) fell below the poverty line in 1976 and received some

TABLE 2
LIFE EXPECTANCY AT BIRTH
FOR WHITE AND NONWHITE
POPULATIONS[15]

Year	White	Nonwhite
1900	47.6	33.0
1910	50.3	35.6
1920	54.9	45.3
1930	61.4	48.1
1940	64.2	53.1
1950	69.1	60.8
1960	70.6	63.6
1970	71.7	65.3
1977	73.8	68.8

kind of government assistance. Even after taking government assistance into account, 16.1 percent of the nonwhites were still classified as below the poverty level, compared to 7.3 percent of the whites. The 1979 figures were similar but are expected to rise with the Reagan cuts in assistance.[16] Since the aged make up a large proportion of the poor white group, poverty among young families is clearly more of a minority group phenomenon. These figures are important in assessing health care, because neglect of the current health needs of nonwhite children can and usually does have long term consequences for their health, even if as adults they are fortunate enough to escape the cycle of poverty.

Part of the explanation for the poverty of the nonwhite population is found in the lower educational level of the blacks, but the problem is much more complex than it appears on the surface. While job discrimination has lessened since the passage of state and federal legislation outlawing such practices, race remains an important factor in the kind of job one is likely to hold. Adding to the problem is the fact that the nature of industry in the United States has so changed during the last three to four decades that there is less of a demand for the unskilled worker. As industry has become more and more mechanized, or as the cybernetic revolution has gathered momentum, jobs for unskilled workers have become more and more difficult to obtain.

Even with education, black workers traditionally have faced numerous disadvantages. Many of the craft unions, traditionally the province of the highest-skilled and highest-paid workers, long denied admission to visible minority groups, and, though changes have taken place, the effect of these changes takes time. Moreover, the segregated educational system of the past gave black students an education of lower quality than that received by white counterparts who spent the same number of years in school. There are also more subtle kinds of discrimination: for example, the black workers may have been hired at the entry level but overlooked for advancement. It takes time, almost generations, for the remedial legislation and action to overcome past discrimination. The result has been a gap between the income of the white and black workers. The gap is narrowest between those blacks and whites who have less than an eighth grade education or a college or graduate degree (that is at the bottom and at the top of the scales). It is greatest between those who have attended or graduated from high school or who have attended a junior college.[17] Until recently, only a comparatively few blacks have graduated from college, and this has meant a greater concentration of blacks at the lower end of the wage scale. Inevitably, as jobs become difficult to find, the differential rate of unemployment increases, since it is the nonskilled individuals who are most likely to be laid off or unable to find a job. In 1979, for example, the unemployment rate for white workers was 6.2 percent, while the rate for black workers was 13.1 percent.[18] During the past decades, the ratio of unemployment between blacks and whites has varied, even reaching three times as much as for whites.[19] Probably the worst unemployment is among young people and, inevitably, there are thousands of young people in their twenties who, though finished with their schooling, have never held a job other than a temporary training job under the Office of Economic Opportunities. In 1978, for example, 13.5 percent of the white 16- to 19-year-olds hunting for work remained unemployed, while 34.4 percent of the black youths of the same group were unemployed. In the 20 to 24 age group, 7.6 percent of whites remained unemployed compared to 20 percent of the blacks. Cut off from the more skilled jobs by lack of education and by poor job preparation, blacks like other unskilled individuals have difficulty in finding work at all. It is the changing nature of employment opportunities that most clearly differentiates the current minority populations from the earlier European immigrants. Though the newly arrived European of a couple of generations ago also suffered from poverty, discrimination, and lack of schooling, they were usually able to find employment. Then, with hard work and a certain amount of luck, they, or more likely their children, were able to move up the occupational ladder. Increasingly, the bottom rung of the ladder has been missing.

Obviously, unemployed people or people whose incomes are below or near the poverty line cannot buy medical care on the open market. In the past, our health care delivery system was based upon the ability of individuals to pay for the care they received, and so the poor were cut off from much of modern medical development. Because health care is so crucially important to survival, the government, slowly and with considerable hesitation, has moved into the health care field, something that most of the advanced countries of the world did long before us.

HEALTH CARE

Before the government entered the field, private enterprise in the form of prepaid health insurance had entered the field of health care. However, as it developed it was distributed differentially. At the higher income levels, three-quarters of the families were insured, while at the lower levels only a third were covered.[20] This meant that large segments of the American population, including a significant percentage of blacks, relied either upon charity or welfare for health care. To justify this, Americans claimed that charity patients received outstanding medical care, and that the only people who really received decent medical treatment in this country were the very rich and the very poor. Unfortunately, statistics did not back up such popular insights, and the government in the form of Medicare and Medicaid has gradually taken over large segments of the health care industry.

Even with the government's entrance into the health insurance field, 75.0 percent of the population was covered by some form of private hospital insurance in 1976. Health insurance, however, paid for only one-quarter of all health care expenses in the fiscal year 1977. Direct expenditures by individuals counted for about one-third of all expenditures. The largest share of personal health care expenditures, some 40 percent, was paid by the government. One of the reasons for the private insurance sector remaining as strong as it does in percentage of coverage is that a significant number of people 65 and older who are covered by Medicare supplement their government insurance with private coverage. Even here, however, there is a race differential, with 56 percent of the whites over 65 having supplemental coverage and only 24 percent of the blacks and others.[21] The most troublesome statistic in 1977 was that 23 million people, 11 percent of the population, had no health coverage whatsoever and had to depend upon welfare or charity for assistance, although a very small percentage were simply too wealthy to be bothered with any kind of health insurance.

One effect of government intervention in medical care is demonstrated in the change in the number of physician visits. Between 1965 and 1967, white patients averaged 4.5 physician visits a year (most of which were non-hospital visits), while nonwhite patients averaged 3.1 visits a year. During the 1970s, physician visits for white persons remained relatively stable but increased for blacks and others, as efforts toward better care began to pay off. During the 1960s, individuals in families with higher incomes averaged more physician visits per year than those with lower incomes, but since 1970 this trend has reversed also. For example, from 1975 to 1976, people in the low-income families (less than $5,000 per year) reported 6.0 visits per person per year, compared with 4.9 visits reported by persons in high-income families ($15,000 or more per year). While this change may reflect a greater need for service, because of deficient health resulting from environmental facts and past inequities in receiving health care, another factor is the psychological barriers and lack of access among low-income families to early or preventive care. This often leads to a need for more physician visits for episodic illnesses.[22] Unfortunately, the increased number of physician visits also reflects the general health of the American public. People who assess their health to be poor or fair visit physicians almost three times as often as those in good health, 10.9 visits per person per year compared with 4.2. But self-assessment is the key, and though disabling illness, low income, and a lack of private health insurance tend to occur together, the people most likely to suffer from this combination do not always see themselves as ill.

A 1967 study that still has validity indicated that, when individuals were questioned as to whether anyone in their family had certain specific illnesses including arthritis, hypertension, heart trouble, ulcers, diabetes, or a vascular lesion, nonwhite patients were less likely to say yes than white patients were. Of the white patients, 51 percent reported that someone in their family had a specific chronic illness, but only 40 percent of the nonwhite individuals interviewed reported that a family member suffered from one of the conditions listed by the interviewers.[23] Since the evidence, including autopsy records, indicates that poor people actually have more illnesses than the affluent, the underreporting of chronic illnesses by minority patients seems to be due not only to a lack of sophistication but a lack of diagnosis. The poor black is undoubtedly aware that he or she has some kind of "misery" but cannot put the concise diagnostic label on it without the help of a physician. The black person probably does not even know that in many cases he or she could be cured or at least made more comfortable.

DISCRIMINATION

Perhaps as important as poverty in contributing to the inequalities of health care, as far as the blacks are concerned, are past and present practices of discrimination. When Gunnar Myrdal made his famous pioneering study of the Negro in America, completed in 1942, he reported widespread medical discrimination and segregation. Segregation existed not only in the South but also in the North, though it was more open in the South. Some southern hospitals treated both white and black patients, but segregated them in inadequate and inferior wards or refused to allow black physicians to treat their patients in such institutions. Some of the larger cities had all-black hospitals, which, of course, had black physicians on their staffs. In the North and in the West the patterns varied; in some states, hospitals were theoretically open to blacks on equal terms with whites, but in other states the courts had upheld the rights of the proprietors to prohibit or to segregate as they pleased.[24]

Not only was there discrimination in admissions, there was also discrimination in staffing.[25] Though both of these subjects will be discussed later in this book, it is important to emphasize the disastrous effect they had on medical care for blacks. A U.S. government survey of hospitals in 1963 found that blacks were still denied access or were segregated; in fact, many of the medical care facilities that received federal grants under the Hospital Survey and Construction Act of 1946 (popularly known as Hill-Burton) practiced discrimination, and, as late as 1962, a U.S. District Court found that private hospitals need not be subject to the equal protection clause of the Fourteenth Amendment.[26]

With the beginnings of Medicare in 1966, all participating hospitals were required to sign an affidavit of nondiscrimination, and some 92 percent of the nation's hospitals were certified as meeting this requirement. In large areas of the South, many hospitals simply refused to adopt the nondiscriminatory provision, and at least 200 hospitals stated that they would make no attempt to comply; this included all hospitals in blocks of counties in Mississippi, northern Louisiana, southern Alabama, southern Georgia, and eastern South Carolina and Virginia.[27] The U.S. government tended to ignore this noncompliance, until lawsuits by civil liberties and civil rights groups led the government to enforce its own regulations. As of this writing, the era of open segregation and discimination in hospital care is more or less ended, but subtle forms of discrimination continue to exist. Some hospital admissions officers still attempt to segregate patients, although the hospital lacks a particular section labeled "colored." The admissions officers admit the black patient and move him or her around if a white patient needs the bed next to the black, or they force the black patient to take a private room. Moreover, there are still white physicians who treat black patients much less favorably than they do whites.

FOLK MEDICINE

Folk medicine has remained important in the urban ghettoes and in the rural South. Of course, folk medicine is an aspect of any culture, but its importance varies among groups in society, depending upon income, education, and even discrimination. In an investigation of the process by which prospective patients arrive at the physician's door, Eliot Freidson found that most people went through a kind of lay referral system. That is, they asked the advice of friends and relatives and tried to deal with their symptoms themselves before calling a physician.[28] For well-educated professional persons, this period of self-treatment was usually relatively brief, but for people whose socioeconomic status was low or who felt estranged from the available medical practitioners because of cultural differences, the lay referral system was expanded. Such patients exhausted all the home remedies known to family members, friends, and even neighborhood unlicensed practitioners before they were forced to turn to a physician because of the continued seriousness of their illness.

As indicated earlier in this chapter, there has always been a black folk medicine presenting an amalgam of African traditions and the experiences of the black slave in the rural South.[29] Even the conjurer of slave days continues in the voodoo practitioners common among some of the poorer and less sophisticated blacks of today. In 1975, the *Journal of the American Medical Association* reported on the case of a 19-year-old black woman treated at Vanderbilt University Hospital who believed a hex put upon her by her mother-in-law caused her son to be stillborn, her husband to desert and divorce her, and for her to suffer from enteritis. Though the medical staff at the hospital believed their intervention saved the woman, the woman herself supplemented their medical treatment with a visit to a gypsy and to a Baptist minister who dealt in voodoo.[30] In the 1970s, many black newspapers carried classified advertisements from people offering to lift various spells and hexes.[31]

Some of the folk beliefs are purely magical, while others have been empirically tested over generations and seem, upon investigation, to be rather logical and reasonable kinds of treatments. Many seem rather harmless and the nurse or others dealing with the less sophisticated black patients sould probably be prepared to encounter such practices as putting a knife under the bed to cut the pain of labor and delivery, or a patient wearing a variety of amulets and charms to ward off disease. Some customs, however, pose greater difficulty, as do those subsumed under the term *pica,* the ingestion of normally considered inedible items, particularly during pregnancy. In the case of blacks, it often takes the form of geophagia, or in simple English, the eating of dirt or clay.[32] Clay eating was and is practiced in much of West Africa and the black slaves brought this custom with them. In the major cities of the South, clay can be purchased in large sacks or in many areas simply dug up from favorite clay banks. Blacks who moved north into the urban ghettoes often had clay mailed to them by their relatives, or if this was not available turned to eating laundry starch. The starch is high calorie; it's ingestion leads to the neglect of other more nutritious foods, obesity, deficiency diseases, and possibly poor fetal development. Since the custom has been handed down for generations, it is difficult to deal with unless it can be brought out in the open. A 1969 study of pregnant black patients in Cook County Hospital in Chicago found that 23.8 percent of the patients were willing to state that they ate starch during their pregnancy.[33] A rural study in Georgia done about the same time found that 55 percent of 200 randomly selected pregnant patients ate starch as well as other substances, such as coffee grounds, paraffin, dry milk of magnesia. Inevitably, toxemia was twice as frequent in the pica group as in the nonpica.[34] Some researchers have correlated the incidence of pica with lead poisoning in the ghetto. Where there is a family history of pica there is also a higher incidence of lead poisoning among children, since this results from eating or chewing on wood painted with the old lead-based paint.[35] Probably, the most effective way of dealing with pica is to counsel the patient, trying to give alternatives to starch eating and seeing that the patient has an adequate nutritional intake, as well as enough filling food so that they no longer crave starch.

Much of the folk medicine is also associated with empirical

procedures, such as massage, heat and baths for rheumatism, or the use of various herb teas and poultices for colds. These practices suggest a rich cultural heritage and should probably be supported by the nurse. They not only give comfort but help sustain patients through difficult times. The chief repository of folk remedies in the black community today, as in many other societies, is the older women who have gained their wisdom through long experience. In today's black community, the older woman may also have worked in a hospital, even though in a menial job, or perhaps just seems to have a knack or calling for such healing. The problem the health professional has is in updating such women's skills and knowledge without threatening them or forcing the patient to choose between modern medicine and traditional folklore. In a forced choice, there is a real danger that modern medicine would lose, or at the very least the patient's recovery might be delayed. Middle-class blacks, like middle-class whites, tend to have deserted the full range of folk remedies as more professional health services have become available to them. To the extent, however, that discriminatory practices operated in preventing access to adequate medical care, even some educated people are motivated to turn to folk practitioners for advice.

Because the genetic pool of blacks is different from those of people of European descent, blacks are also likely to suffer from somewhat different illnesses than whites. Sometimes this affects dietary intake. For example, a significant number of blacks, perhaps as many as 60 percent, are lactose intolerant. In some individuals, the actual drinking of milk results in unpleasant gastro-intestinal symptoms. The nurse has to be careful not to push milk upon a child who rejects it until she is certain that it will not unduly irritate the child's bowel. Since the decrease in milk intake might contribute to osteoporosis, alternative dietary supplements should be considered.[36] Blacks also are more likely to have sickle cell trait or actual anemia than whites; early testing for this deficiency should be instituted when it is suspected, with appropriate referrals for treatment or genetic counseling.

For those unaccustomed to dealing with blacks or other dark-skinned individuals, even simple nursing observations have to be altered. For example, one of the major problems among poor ghetto children is iron-deficiency anemia.[37] Yet, how does a nurse visually observe the pallor of anemia in a dark-skinned person? Such things as fever, rash, cyanosis, and other observations that many of us have learned to rely upon for clues are based upon persons with white skin. Color changes in both black adults and children are best observed where pigmentation for melanin, melanoid, and carotene is least:

sclera, conjuctiva, nail beds, lips, bucal mucosa, tongue, palms, and
soles. Pallor in the dark-skinned individual is observable by the absence of the underlying red tones that normally give the brown and
black skin its "glow" or "living color." The brown-skinned person
will therefore appear more yellowish brown, and the black-skinned
person will apear ashen gray. Admittedly, it takes an experienced eye
to identify the change, but those health care professionals who are
not acquainted with black patients can quickly learn the techniques.
Obviously, skin observation has to be supplemented by consultation
and other means of detection until the person acquires expertise.
Sometimes the best consultant is an experienced black mother who
can identify a "pale" appearance long before the health professional
can see it.

In part, because of the different genetic pool and hereditary immunity, blacks are also likely to suffer more from certain disease than
other groups. For example, the tuberculosis rate for blacks was until
recently nearly three times that of whites, although disproportionate
ratios have declined as more effective preventative measures and
treatment have lessened the general problem of tuberculosis. Sometimes it is not clear whether some disproportionate ratios are due to
different genetic inheritance or to the problems of living as a minority. For example, hypertension is higher among blacks than among
whites. This seems to have a genetic component, but high salt, high
carbohydrate diets, and stress are also implicated. Some other diseases are not so much genetically related as due to lack of effective
education or to ineffective health care delivery. Such diseases result
from lack of immunization against poliomyelitis and measles, poor
housing and sewage disposal, that serve as breeding grounds for
parasitic diseases, lack of flouridated community water supplies that
would prevent dental caries, and failure to give vision tests to children to correct myopia. Better prenatal care would also reduce the
infant and the perinatal mortality.[38] Clearly, many of the differences
are more associated with economic status than with race.

THE CULTURE OF POVERTY

Medical care for minorities is a complex problem, and it is not only
because of poverty and discrimination that there is a difference in
health between black and white Americans. Public health professionals often complain that poor people, particularly poor blacks, do
not take advantage of the preventive care that is available. The
complaint has validity as repeated studies have shown. People

whose socioeconomic status is low or who are nonwhite make less use of health facilities than other people, and the kind of service they are least likely to seek is preventive health care.[39] The reason for this low level of utilization of available health services seems to be at least partly psychological. Slavery, plus the generations of poverty and segregation, have left their mark upon blacks. This is not surprising because, even among minorities where discrimination is less of a factor, poverty can be debilitating to the spirit.

In attempts to explain further the reasons why some groups make less effective use of facilities than others, various methods of classifying the poor into groups have been developed. One of the simplest and most useful of these typologies is a dichotomy used by John Kosa.[40] Kosa suggested that there is an essential difference between acute and chronic poverty. By his definition, the acutely poor are those who have lived much of their life with an adequate income, at least by the standards of their society, but then either suddenly become unemployed or gradually become old and have to live in reduced circumstances. The acutely poor face severe problems of adjustment because they have to find ways of coping with their new status of being poor. They are more likely to attempt to find ways to modify their condition. On the other hand, the chronically poor have spent their whole lives in poverty or, as in the case of the black, poverty has often been a multigenerational phenomenon. The chronically poor, accustomed to poverty as they are, have developed a whole pattern of life for coping with their condition. This pattern, which the anthropologist Oscar Lewis called the *culture of poverty*, is passed on from one generation to another. Based on his studies in Mexico City, New York, and San Juan (Puerto Rico), Lewis argued that the culture of poverty transcends racial and national lines and that some of the traits that have been attributed to nationality groups are actually common to all people caught in this condition. The culture of poverty must of necessity exist inside of another more affluent culture, because the perception of being poor depends partly on knowing that there are others who are not poor. This culture is marked by low level of political power and participation in the decision-making aspects of the society. In the families he studied, Lewis also found a low marriage rate, a high rate of illegitimacy, and many families headed by women, all of which are also common characteristics among those American blacks whose socioeconomic status is low.

It is the psychological characteristics of the culture of poverty that seem to be most important for health care. Lewis found that fatalism, helplessness, dependence, and feelings of inferiority were common. He also found that the time orientation tends to be concentrated on the present rather than the future, as is the case with middle-class society. Getting through a day is enough of a problem without trying to also plan for the future.[41]

Others, mostly sociologists, have described the negative outlook of the people of the slums in terms of alienation; the poor feel cut off from power to control their own lives, and have no hope for the future improvement in their condition. With such an outlook, a future time orientation would be foolish, so most poor people try only to deal with the problems at hand. On the other hand, the middle-class orientation is linked to a system of deferred gratification because such planning has paid off, but the man who lives on the edge of starvation or disaster has never learned the value of deferring, so he does not save money or, in the case of health, does not seek preventive health care.

The importance of alienation in describing the negative outlook of the poor has been the subject of considerable empirical research. In one study, it was found that mothers who felt socially isolated and believed that they lacked the power to control their own lives or those of their children were less likely to bring their children into the well-baby clinics than mothers who felt less powerless and less isolated from the supports of friends and family.[42] In another study, it was found that the negative feelings of despair and alienation, as measured by the anomie scale constructed by Leo Srole, acted as barriers to mothers seeking prenatal care as well as immunizations for their children.[43] There is simple logic in these findings, since it would seem that the person who feels no control over what happens to him or her would not see the value in taking the necessary steps to obtain preventive health care; in his or her own mind, the person's health would be controlled by fate or other outside forces rather than by personal actions.

Following this line of reasoning, a comprehensive study of the psychological barriers to preventive health care was done by one of the authors (BB). During the winter and spring of 1970 to 1971, eight hundred mothers from the poor neighborhoods of East and South-Central Los Angeles were interviewed. Those with minority status, incomes below the poverty line, and meager education tended to have a much more negative outlook on life. They felt powerless, isolated, and hopeless. These feelings in turn were related to a low level of use of preventive health services for themselves and their children. This meant fewer check-ups, less dental care, fewer immunizations, and less prenatal care. However, the most significant correlations were with the various indices of effective family planning. Family planning seemed almost impossible for the alienated black or Mexican-American woman from a poverty neighborhood, even when services were available at a nearby clinic.[44]

Numerous previous studies have shown the correlation between effective family planning and socioeconomic status,[45] but alienation as a factor is just starting to be investigated.[46] Lee Rainwater pointed out that a sense of stability and trust in the future are essential preconditions for consistent family planning and, since these conditions are not present among the poor, effective long-range planning is rare.[47] Race also is a factor. Black women whose socioeconomic status is low have more difficulty with family planning than do white women at a comparable level. In spite of the fact that the black women desired a limited number of children, they ended up giving birth to more.[48] This emphasizes that, although poverty itself is important in creating the negative feelings that deter planning and preventive behavior, segregation and discrimination magnify the effects of poverty. In a study of housing patterns done earlier by an author of this book, it was found that segregation was a more important factor in creating feelings of alienation than simple poverty. Middle-class blacks were studied so that poverty was not a current factor in their lives, although many of them had been poor in the past. Central to the findings was the fact that experience with segregated schools and a segregated life-style was more strongly related to current feelings of powerlessness and hopelessness than past poverty. Unfortunately, these feelings of alienation then acted as barriers to integration, so that segregation and alienation seemed to relate to each other in a circular fashion.[49]

These findings do not necessarily contradict the idea that there is a culture of poverty transcending racial and national lines, but they do suggest that the experience of American blacks with discrimination of various sorts may have added to their feelings of fatalism, hopelessness, and powerlessness. Since such subjective factors act as barriers to preventive health care, it seems obvious that it is necessary to have a multifaceted program to cure the inequalities now existing between white and nonwhite citizens, in order to deal completely with the poor health of black Americans.

Obviously, preventive health care is more important to some kinds of illnesses than others. As yet, we can do little to prevent many of the degenerative processes associated with aging. However, an increasing number of contagious diseases can be prevented by immunization. In 1970, for example, there were several outbreaks of diphtheria in large urban areas that need not have occurred, if immunizations had been available to all, or if we could find a way of overcoming the powerlessness and hopelessness that keep the people of the ghettoes and barrios from bringing their children in for injections.

Perhaps the most obvious improvement would take place in the maternal mortality. In 1915, the mortality rate for nonwhite mothers of 105.6 per 1,000 births exceeded the rate for whites by 75 percent (60.0 per 1,000). Since that time, the overall maternal death rate has fallen because of improvements in the nature of hospitals and in medical and nursing knowledge. However, as the rates have fallen, the gap between white and nonwhite mothers has grown, until today it is 300 percent higher (26 per 100,000 live births for nonwhites, compared to 7.7 for whites).[50] To equalize the rates, the whole nature of the health care delivery system would have to be changed, although some statistical improvement undoubtedly could be made with the present system if ways could be found to encourage the nonwhite mother to seek more prenatal care.

One of the most obvious areas in which preventive medicine could be effectively applied is in the field of dentistry. Surprisingly, perhaps for hereditary reasons, blacks suffer less from dental caries than do white Americans. The first indication of this was found by R. W. Hyde in his study of draft recruits in World War II, although his results have since been replicated. Only Chinese Americans had fewer caries than American blacks.[51] Blacks as a group, however, visit dentists much less than most other groups in American society, largely because dentistry is so expensive and is associated with middle-class status. In a sociological study of attitudes toward illness, E. L. Koos divided his sample into three socioeconomic groups: (I) business and professionals; (II) skilled and semiskilled workers, and (III) unskilled workers. Almost 95 percent of the Class I households reported they had a family dentist, but only 12.5 percent of the Class III families had established such a relationship. In fact, 57 percent of the individuals in Class III and 9 percent of the individuals in Class II reported that they turned to dentists only to have a tooth extracted.[52] Koos' study is undoubtedly indicative of general attitudes toward dentists, and since so many blacks are trapped in the culture of poverty, they get very little preventive dental care. Additional evidence for this assumption comes from the fact that blacks have a much higher proportion of periodontal disease than whites, something that can be treated early by a dentist and often even prevented. In one study in which a scale ranging from zero to eight was used to rate the amount of periodontal disease, the white population was given a score of 1.1, while the black population was rated 1.6.[53]

CONCLUDING COMMENTS

In summary, it should be evident that the health problems faced by the large proportion of the black minority community remain monumental. In part, these difficulties can be understood through looking at the past history of the American black because this past has left its mark on today. Three variables seem most important in explaining the fact that mortality and morbidity rates are higher for blacks: poverty, discrimination, and the social-psychological barriers that tend to keep people from using the services that are available. All three of these factors interact and reinforce each other, just as poor health care interacts with and reinforces the other problems faced by black Americans.

REFERENCES

1. For a moving account of some of the difficulties faced by the migrants, read John Steinbeck's The Grapes of Wrath.
2. A popularized summary of some of these historical figures can be found in Lincoln, C. E. The Negro Pilgrimage in America. New York: Bantam Books, 1967, p. 9.
3. Frazier, E. F. Black Bourgeoisie. New York: Collier Books, 1962, pp. 15–16.
4. Frazier, E. F. The Negro Family in the United States. Chicago: University of Chicago Press, 1939.
5. Herskovits, M. J. The Myth of the Negro Past. Boston: Beacon Press, 1941, pp. 1 ff. Herskovits, M. J. The New World Negro (F. S. Herskovits, Ed.). Bloomington: Indiana University Press, 1966.
6. A good narrative description of this can be found in Alex Haley's Roots. Garden City: Doubleday, 1976. For a scholarly discussion, see Journal of Black Studies, 1980, 10, devoted to the Sea Island culture and edited by Keith Baird and Mary Twining.
7. Savitt, T. L. Medicine and Slavery. Urbana: University of Illinois, 1978, p. 161.
8. Ibid., p. 162.
9. Ibid. p. 164.
10. Ibid., p. 165.
11. Ibid., p. 180.
12. Ibid., p. 183.
13. For further amplification, see: Franklin, J. H. From Slavery to Freedom. New York: A. A. Knopf, 1967, pp. 324–43.
14. Taeuber, K. E. & Taeuber, A. F. Negroes in Cities. Chicago: Aldine Company, 1965, p. 14.

15. U.S. Bureau of Census. Statistical Abstract of U.S. 1979. Washington, D.C.: U.S. Government Printing Office, 1979, Table 100, p. 70.

16. Ibid., Table 757, p. 461. The poverty index was originally developed in 1964, modified in 1969, and is periodically updated to take in the effects of inflation. For an earlier discussion, see M. Orshansky, Who was Poor in 1966? Research and Statistics Note, No. 23. Washington, D.C.: U.S. Government Printing Office, 1967, Table 6. See also, How the Poor Will Be Hurt, *Newsweek*, March 23, 1981, pp. 23–24.

17. Blau, P. M. & Duncan, O.D. The American Occupational Structure. New York: Wiley, 1967, pp. 207–242. For more recent data, see the current Statistical Abstracts.

18. Statistical Abstract 1979, p. 396. For other data, see: U.S. Department of Labor. The Negro Family: The Case for National Action. Washington, D.C.: U.S. Government Printing Office, 1965, p. 66 passim.

19. Watts: Everything Has Changed—and Nothing. *Newsweek*, August 24, 1970, pp. 58–60. Bullock, P. Watts: The Aftermath. New York: Grove Press, 1969.

20. U.S. Department of Health, Education, and Welfare. Medical Care, Health Status and Family Income. U. S. Vital and Health Statistics, Public Health Publication No. 1000, Series 10, No. 9. Washington, D.C.: U.S. Government Printing Office, 1964, p. 6.

21. U.S. Department of Health, Education, and Welfare. Health, United States, 1978. (Hyattsville, Maryland: National Center for Health Statistics, 1978, DHEW Pub. No. (PHS) 78–1232, pp. 401–403.

22. Ibid., pp. 261–264.

23. U.S. Department of Health, Education, and Welfare. Differentials in Health Characteristics by Color. U.S. Vital and Health Statistics, July 1965 to June 1967, Public Health Publication No. 1000, Series, 10, No. 56. Washington, D.C.: U.S. Government Printing Office, 1969, p. 5.

24. Myrdal, G. with the assistance of R. Sterner & A. Rose. An American Dilemna: The Negro Problem and Modern Democracy. New York: Harper & Brothers, 1944, pp. 635–636.

25. For example, see: Bullough, V. & Bullough, B. What Color are Your Germs? Chicago: Committee to End Discrimination in Chicago Medical Institutions, 1955. The Untouchables. Chicago: Committee Against Discrimination and the Southern Conference on Education, 1955.

26. Civil Rights '63. Report of the U.S. Commission on Civil Rights. Washington, D.C.: U.S. Government Printing Office, 1963, pp. 133–134. See also: Nash, R. M. Compliance of Hospitals and Health Agencies With Title VI of the Civil Rights Act. *American Journal of Public Health*, 1968, *58*, 246–251.

27. Dorsen, N. Discrimination and Civil Rights. Boston: Little, Brown, 1969, p. 463, note 1.

28. Freidson, E. Client Control and Medical Practice. *American Journal of Sociology*, 1960, *65*, 374–382.

29. For a description of many of these, see: Puckett, N. N. Folk Beliefs of the

Southern Negro. Reprinted New York: Dover, 1969. Though a pioneering investigation when it was first published in 1926, this study would not meet today's standards of scholarship, because it jumps from one time period to another. Nevertheless, it does contain considerable information not readily available elsewhere.

30. Cappannori, S. C. et al. Voodoo in the General Hospital, A Case of Hexing and Regional Enteritis. *The Journal of the American Medical Association*, 1975, *232*, 938–940.

31. A sampling of some of these can be found in Martin, B. J. W. Ethnicity and Health Care: Afro-Americans. In Ethnicity and Health Care. New York: National League for Nursing, 1976, p. 53.

32. Halsted, J. Geophagia in Man: Its Nature and Nutritional Effects. *American Journal of Clinical Nutrition, 22*, No. 12, 1384–1393. Neumann, H. H. Pica—Symptom or Vestigial Instinct? *Pediatrics*, 1970, *46*, No. 3. Hertz, H. Notes on Clay and Starch Eating Among Negroes in a Southern Community. *Social Forces*, 1957, *25*, pp. 343–344.

33. Keith, L., Rosenberg, C., Brown, E. & Webster, A. Amylophagia During Pregnancy; A Second Look. *Chicago Medical School Quarterly*, 1969, *28*, 109.

34. O'Rourke, D. E. Quinn, J. G. Nicholson, J. O. & Gobson, H. H. Geophagia During Pregnancy. *Obstetrics and Gynecology*, 1967, *29*, 581.

35. Greenberg, M. et al. A Study of Pica in Relation to Lead Poisoning. *Pediatrics*, 1958, *22*, 756–760. Christian, J. R. Celevycz, B. S. & Andelman, S. L. A Three Year Study of Lead Poisoning in Chicago. *Epidemiology, American Journal of Public Health*, 1964, *54*, 1241–1245. See also: Health Programs: Slum Children Suffer Because of Low Funding. *Science*, 1971, *172*, 921–924.

36. For example, see: Hongladarom, G. C. & Russell, M. An Ethnic Difference—Lactose Intolerance. *Nursing Outlook*, 1976, *24*, No. 12, 764–765.

37. Gutelius, M. F. The Problem of Iron Deficiency Anemia in Preschool Negro Children. *American Journal of Public Health*, 1969, *59*, No. 2, 290–295.

38. See: Goldstein, M. S. Longevity and Health Status of the Negro American. *Journal of Negro Education*, 1963, *32*, 337–348. Kitagawa, E. M. & Hauser, P. M. Differential Mortality in the United States, A Study in Socioeconomic Epidemiology. Cambridge, Massachusetts: Harvard University Press, 1973.

39. Koos, E. L. The Health of Regionville. New York: Columbia University Press, 1954. James, G. Poverty and Public Health—New Outlooks: 1. Poverty as an Obstacle to Health Progress in Our Cities. *American Journal of Public Health*, 1965, *55*, 1757–1771. Deasy, L. C. Socio-Economic Status and Participation in the Poliomyelitis Vaccine Trial. *American Sociological Review*, 1956, *21*, 185–191. Matkins, E. L. Low-Income Negro Mothers—Their Decision to Seek Prenatal Care. *American Journal of Public Health*, 1968, *58*, 655–667. Milio, N. Values, Social Class and Community Health Services. *Nursing Research*, 1967, *16*, 26–31.

40. Kosa, J. The Nature of Poverty. In J. Kosa, A. Antonovsky, & I. K. Zola (Eds.), Poverty and Health: A Sociological Analysis, Cambridge, Massachusetts: Harvard University Press, A Commonwealth Fund Book, 1969, pp. 1–33.
41. Lewis, O. La Vida: A Puerto Rican Family in the Culture of Poverty. New York: Random House, 1965, pp. xlii–lii. Lewis, O. The Culture of Poverty. *Scientific American*, 1966, 19–25. There are those who object to the concept of the culture of poverty; for example, see: Valentine, C. A. Culture and Poverty: Critique and Counter Proposals. Chicago: University of Chicago Press, 1968.
42. Morris, N. M., Hatch, M. H. & Chipman, S. S. Alienation as a Deterrent to Well-Child Supervision. *American Journal of Public Health*, 1966, *56*, 1874–1882.
43. Nakagawa, H. Family Health Care Patterns and Anomie. An unpublished Ph.D. dissertation, University of California at Los Angeles, 1968.
44. Bullough, B. Poverty, Ethnic Identity and Preventive Health Care. *Journal of Health and Social Behavior*, 1972, *13*, 347–359. Bullough, B. The Measurement of Alienation as it Relates to Family Planning Behavior. *Proceedings WHEN Conference*, 1975, 41–52.
45. Whelpton, P. K. & Kiser, C. V. Social and Psychological Factors Affecting Fertility, Vol. V. New York: Milbank Memorial Fund, 1958. Westoff, C. F. Potter, Jr., R. G. Sagi, P. C. & Mishler, E. Family Growth in Metropolitan America. Princeton: Princeton University Press, 1961. Freedman, R., Whelpton, P. K. & Campbell, A. A. Family Planning, Sterility and Population Growth. New York: McGraw-Hill, 1959. Westoff, C. F. Potter, Jr., R. G. & Sagi, P. C. The Third Child. Princeton: Princeton University Press, 1963.
46. Groat, H. T. & Neal, A. G. Social Psychological Correlates of Urban Fertility. *American Sociological Review* 1967, *32*, 945–959.
47. Rainwater, L. And the Poor Get Children. Chicago: Quadrangle Books, 1960.
48. Campbell, A. A. Fertility and Family Planning Among Non-White Married Couples in the United States. *Eugenics Quarterly*, 1961, *12*, 124–131. Roach, J. L. Lewis, L. S. & Beauchamp, M. A. The Effects of Race and Socio-Economic Status on Family Planning. *Journal of Health and Social Behavior*, 1963, *4*, 40–45.
49. Bullough, B. Alienation in the Ghetto. *American Journal of Sociology*, 1967, *72*, 469–78. Bullough, B. *Social-Psychological Barriers to Housing Desegregation.* Los Angeles: University of California, Graduate School of Business Administration, 1969. Bullough, B. Alienation and School Segregation. *Integrated Education*, 1972, 29–35.
50. Anderson, E. H. & Lesser, A. J. Maternity Care in the United States: Gains and Gaps. *American Journal of Nursing*, 1966, *66*, *1539–1544*. *Recent figures are in Statistical Abstract 1979*, Table 108, p. 75.
51. Hyde, R. W. Socioeconomic Aspects of Dental Caries. *New England Journal of Medicine*, 1944, *230*, 506–510. More recent studies have verified

this finding. See: Pelton, W. J. Dunbar, J. B. McMillan, R. S. Moller, P. & Wolff, A. E. The Epidemiology of Oral Health. Cambridge: Harvard University Press, 1969, p. 9, Table 1.7.

52. Koos, E. L. op. cit. pp. 118–125.
53. Pelton, Dunbar, et al. op. cit., Table 2.7. See also: Selected Dental Findings in Adults by Age, Race and Sex, United States, 1960–1962. Vital and Health Statistics, U.S. Department of Health, Education, and Welfare, Public Health Publication No. 1000, Series 11, No. 7. Washington, D.C.: U.S. Government Printing Office, 1969. See also: U.S. Center for Health Statistics. Dental Visits: Volume and Interval Since Last Visit. Public Health Services, Series 10, No. 76. Rockville, Maryland: Center for Health Statistics, 1972, Table A.

4

The Spanish-Speaking Minority Groups

The fastest growing minority groups in the United States today are the Spanish-speaking peoples from various parts of the Western Hemisphere, particularly Mexico, Puerto Rico, and Cuba. Although characterized by a common language and grouped together for statistical purposes by their Spanish surnames, these three groups reflect quite different traditions. The largest of the nationality groups, and the one that has been in the United States the longest, is the Mexican Americans, or as some of the members of the group now term themselves, Chicanos.

MEXICAN AMERICANS

Most immigrants to the United States arrived by sea, but the Mexican Americans simply moved northward. In fact, many of them lived in the southwestern section of the United States before English-speaking pioneers moved westward and that section became part of this country. The closeness of the vast majority of Mexican Americans to their homeland and their unique treaty rights with the United States tend to set them apart from most other immigrants.

The Mexican-American War, fought between 1846 and 1848,

serves as the watershed for the history of Mexican Americans in the United States. Under the treaty of Guadalupe Hidalgo, executed on February 2, 1848, Mexico ceded a vast territory, including California, Arizona, New Mexico, Nevada, Utah, and much of Colorado, and also approved the prior annexation of Texas, previously a part of Mexico. The ceded lands represented one-half of the territory possessed by Mexico in 1821 when it had gained independence from Spain.

According to the provision of the treaty, all citizens of Mexico who decided to remain within the ceded territory were to become citizens of the United States. As a result, an estimated 75,000 Spanish-speaking people became U.S. citizens. The treaty also provided specific guarantees for the property and political rights of these Spanish-speaking Americans, who were given the right to retain their language, their religion, and their culture. No provision was made for the integration of the peoples as a group into U.S. society, although the treaty did contain a promise of early statehood for the area. California, which had about 7,500 Spanish-speaking inhabitants, was quickly admitted into the Union, as was Nevada, which had almost no Spanish-speaking residents. Texas, with some 5,000 Spanish Americans, was already a state. New Mexico, with its 60,000 former Mexican nationals, and Arizona, with approximately 1,000, were much slower to receive statehood. One reason for the delay was the fact that neither of these future states had many Anglo-American citizens, and U.S. politicians were reluctant to grant full civil rights to a people they considered to be largely illiterate and of an "alien" culture. The effect of this attitude toward the indigenous Mexican Americans was to retard assimilation and to encourage the survival of the Spanish cultural influence.

Though descendants of these Mexican nationals, along with later immigrants from Mexico, have all been classified as Spanish-speaking Americans, the term at best is a very ambiguous one, since Mexico itself was and is home to many different peoples. Citizens of Mexico can be descendants of European settlers (Spanish as well as others), or of the indigenous Indians, or any mixture thereof. In southwestern United States, people with Spanish surnames come from a variety of backgrounds. The mixed nature of this heritage is evident from the City of Los Angeles, which prides itself on its Spanish founders. Of these founders and their wives, two were Spaniards, two were blacks, nine were of mixed Negro-Spanish or Spanish-Indian backgrounds, nine were Indians, and one was Chinese. All, presumably except for the Chinese person, whose name is unknown, had Spanish names.

Today, the border between Mexico and the United States is about two thousand miles long, most of it desolate and sparsely populated. Until the Border Patrol of the U.S. Immigration Service was established in 1924, the border could be and was crossed in either direction with comparative ease. Moreover, much of northern Mexico is geographically separated from southern Mexico by deserts, which meant that the natural market and supply centers for much of the area were in the United States, particularly in those areas that had formerly been part of Mexico. There is also considerable geographic similarity between the southwestern United States and northern Mexico, so that Mexicans who moved north felt more or less at home. Inevitably, there has been considerable movement of Mexicans back and forth across the border, although no one knows for certain the total number of those who have crossed over. However, it is known that in the period before 1900 Mexican nationals played an important part in pioneering new techniques in the gold and silver mining industry in the Western and Pacific states, in the growth of the sugar beet industry, in the development of irrigation, and in the emergence of Texas as a leading cotton-growing state.

Generally speaking, however, the southwestern United States did not begin to grow very fast until the last decade of the nineteenth century. This growth has continued through most of the twentieth century because of the availability of cheap labor, consisting mostly of Mexicans who moved northward in large numbers. In the period between 1900 and 1930, it is estimated that 10 percent of the total population of Mexico, over a million migrants, crossed into the United States. For example, the Mexican population of Texas rose from 70,981 in 1910 to 683,681 in 1930. Mexican labor built the railroads, dug the irrigation ditches, picked the cotton, cleared the land, and ultimately built the highways opening up the Southwest. This meant that the massive wave of Mexican-American immigration coincided in large part with the mass exodus to this country of the Russian, Slavic, and Italian immigrants, but the Mexican Americans were never as isolated from their homeland as most other would-be citizens, since Mexico in most cases was never more than 150 miles away.

In fact, the overwhelming majority of the Mexican migrants settled down in a fan-shaped area stretching out from the Mexican border, up past Los Angeles, to Santa Barbara on the Pacific Ocean, and stretching eastward and southward through San Antonio to Corpus Christi on the Gulf of Mexico. Even today, most persons of Mexican descent live in this narrow belt of territory that includes parts of Texas, California, Arizona, New Mexico, and Colorado.

There has been a remarkable continuity of Mexican family life and customs in this area, in part because most Mexicans who have come north first moved in with relatives. Today, large numbers of Mexican Americans in the southwest United States have relatives across the border, which means there is considerable movement back and forth between the two countries. The extent and concentration of this Mexican migration has tended to make the border rather indistinguishable, with a heavy shading of Mexican Americans near the border that thins out as one travels north. This shading is on both sides of the border, since increasing numbers of Anglo-Americans have retired in Mexico or have winter homes in northern Mexico. Moreover, travel between Mexico and the United States is comparatively easy because the boundary is an imaginary line, marked only by a barbed wire fence, or an easily forded river that often changes its channel. The lack of effective natural border barriers has led to many problems, but it also has tended to lessen the hostility between Mexico and the United States. We do not have the kind of enmity that the Germans and the French who face each other across the Rhine have, but rather there is a sort of gradual fusion between two cultures and people, with the Spanish-speaking Americans in the Southwest providing a kind of organic union with the culture and civilization of Mexico.[1]

Immigration from Mexico has tended to be in spurts, depending in large part upon the economic conditions in the United States. Much of it has been through *contract labor*, a term used to describe imported workers whose freedom is restricted by the terms of contractual relations. Except in the case of skilled or professional workers, contract labor has been outlawed in the United States since 1885, though various legal ways have been found to circumvent the law. One of the largest loopholes appeared in the immigration law of 1917, which contained a provision allowing the Commissioner of Immigration and Naturalization to control and regulate the admission and return of otherwise inadmissible aliens applying for temporary admission. Though contract labor was still outlawed, this meant that large numbers of Mexican nationals could be imported into the United States, providing the consent of the Commissioner was obtained. During and following World War I, about 50,000 workers are known to have been recruited in Mexico, many of whom were sent to northern states as well as to the fields and industries of the Southwest. Some of the Mexicans who earlier had crossed the border into the United States were also recruited for work in northern states. In 1923, for example, the National Tube Company, an affiliate of U.S. Steel, brought 1,300 Mexicans from

Texas to work in its Lorain, Ohio, plant. In that same year, Bethlehem Steel imported 1,000 workers from Mexico to work in its plants in Pennsylvania. The Mexican colony in Detroit had its beginnings in 1918, when several hundred Mexicans were brought to work in the automobile industry as student workers, and others from Mexico soon followed.

However, the bulk of Mexicans who came north were recruited originally as farm laborers. The changing nature of farming in the United States, and the Depression of the 1930s created great difficulty. In fact, by 1937, machines had taken over 90 percent of the work involved in preparing, bedding, and cultivating the land to produce garden crops. This meant that farm labor became ever more seasonal, with the greatest demand coming at harvest time. As the Mexicans, many of whom now regarded themselves as Americans, lost their jobs, they attempted to organize and to strike. In the Southwest, there were a number of Mexican-led strikes that generally failed, because immigration authorities usually deported those workers who were not citizens, while others were intimidated by threats of violence. Moreover, in most of the strikes, Mexican workers stood alone, since they were not affiliated with the rest of organized labor. The result was a mass exodus of Mexicans from the United States to Mexico, often aided and encouraged by various governmental agencies. In February 1931, for example, the County of Los Angeles shipped a whole trainload of its residents back to Mexico at a cost of some $77,249.29. Authorities estimated that the county still saved $347,468.41 in relief money. In 1932, more than 11,000 Mexican nationals were repatriated from Los Angeles alone.[2]

With the advent of World War II, there was once again a demand for workers, and Mexico seemed to be an obvious source. In May 1942, the United States and Mexico agreed upon conditions under which Mexicans might be recruited to work in the United States. Imported workers were to be provided free transportation to and from their homes in Mexico, paid subsistence in route, were not to be used to displace other workers or to lower wages or salary rates, and given certain minimum working and living conditions. On September 29, 1942, the first shipment of 1,500 Mexican *braceros*, as they were called, arrived in Stockton, California. In 1945 alone, about 120,000 workers were recruited for agricultural employment in the United States, after which they were to return to Mexico. In addition, another 80,000 workers were imported from Mexico to work on maintaining railroad lines. The farm labor importation program came to an end in 1947, but there was still a demand for low-paid agricultural employees, and this demand led to human smuggling rings. To curtail this, in 1952 Congress reviewed and revised the wartime legislation to allow workers to be imported under temporary work permits or visas. In fairly rapid succession, nearly 500,000 workers were imported, the bulk of whom were from Mexico. Since that time there has been a gradual phasing out of most contract laborers, who were not only unpopular with organized labor but also with the domestic migratory farm workers who felt they were being used as strike breakers. Mexicans now enter legally as immigrants, under a general quota that covers all Western Hemisphere countries, obtain work permits for temporary stay, or slip across the border illegally. By far, the greatest number slip across the border illegally. In fact, there are so many that, rather than refer to them as illegal immigrants, we now use the term *undocumented aliens*. The new entrants from Mexico (or from other parts of Central or South America) quickly lose themselves in the large ghettoes of Spanish-speaking Americans, officially called *barrios*. Here they live a rather furtive and fearful existence, until they can get enough education or language skills to put themselves forward as Americans. Though officials know that large numbers of undocumented aliens exist, they have been reluctant to do much about it. In many of the largest cities of the Southwest, there are periodic sweeps through the barrios, designed to catch the illegals, but these sweeps usually involve as many native-born Americans as undocumented aliens so they increase antagonisms between government and the Spanish-speaking Americans. In certain areas of California, there are highway checks in which all cars are stopped, if only briefly, but since these are at officially designated areas, which most undocumented aliens avoid, they serve only to harass native-born Mexican Americans. Some states enact special discriminatory legislation. In 1975, Texas passed a law requiring all school children to prove citizenship or have legal entry permits before allowing them to enroll in public schools, but this discriminatory act was declared unconstitutional in 1980. Less blatant attempts at discrimination continue to exist.

Anyone who has visited the border between the United States and Mexico realizes that the United States could prevent much of the illegal crossing if it wanted to do so, although some of the measures would also make it more difficult for Americans to cross into Mexico. Fences in the Mexican border are usually in a bad state of repair, patrols are almost nonexistent, and economic opportunities so much better on the American side that it is not difficult to understand why so many cross illegally. The Canadian border is no more difficult to cross, and undoubtedly many people also cross from

Canada into the United States illegally, but the economic disparity between Canada and the United States is not as great as between Mexico and the United States.

In 1980, 14.6 or 6.4 percent of the population identified themselves as of Spanish origin. In the five states of the Southwest where the Spanish-speaking population is of Mexican origin, they are more than 10 percent of the population. Because of the change in the nature of agriculture, and the lessening demand for farm laborers, the majority of the Mexicans have come to settle in urban areas, with the result that Los Angeles is second only to Mexico City in its total Mexican population. Like the blacks, the Mexican Americans are also segregated within the urban complex, but in most of the cities of the Southwest the housing patterns are not quite so rigidly segregated as those of the blacks. In Los Angeles, for example, there are great barrios that border that city on the east, but there are also large numbers of Mexican Americans scattered throughout the city. Since many people with Spanish surnames have achieved positions of power and influence in the Southwest, discrimination against Mexican Americans tends to be far more subtle than that experienced by blacks. However, most members of the Mexican-American minority are still poor and face a language barrier. Although the immigrant cannot advance to a position of influence in the outside world without learning English, it is possible to live a lifetime in the larger barrios without becoming fluent in English. Many of the children from the barrios who go to school are bilingual, speaking Spanish at home and English at school. This tends to discourage all but the most dedicated students from continuing their schooling. Moreover, the fact that many of the Mexicans are in this country illegally makes the Mexican American worker more exploitable, because an unscrupulous employer can hire an illegal immigrant and use the threat of exposure over the immigrant or the immigrant's friends or relatives as a power tool in order to pay less than minimum wages or to avoid enforcing safety rules.

The peasant Mexican culture, from which most of the Mexican Americans are derived, also tends to work against easy assimilation into the Anglo-American middle-class culture. Since Mexico and the United States have, with a few exceptions, enjoyed fairly peaceful relationships for over a century, Mexicans have not felt they had to choose between their mother country and the United States, as many immigrant groups felt they had to do in either World War I or II. This has made it possible for large numbers of Mexican Americans to live together geographically in the United States but intellectually and emotionally in the local Mexican tradition. Moreover, at least in the period before World War I, Mexico was a very poor country, with society so organized that the sense of enterprise, thrift, and initiative highly valued by Americans was not encouraged. The patron system of land tenure in Mexico was not unlike the southern plantation system, which meant that the workers or peons were virtually powerless. In societies of this type, money is meaningless, trade is limited, and division of labor is either simple or almost nonexistent. In Mexico, native folk practices were interwoven with Catholic Church ritual. Inevitably, the Mexican villager with this background could rather easily become confused and demoralized in the American city. Unfortunately, these culturally conditioned traits have often been interpreted as racial or biological. The Mexican stereotype is usually one of extremes, either lawless and violent, or lacking in ambition and lazy. As a defense against these stereotypes and discrimination, in-group feeling has developed; on the other hand, those Mexicans who have managed to achieve in American society often cut themselves off from their countrymen by emphasizing that they are Spanish, instead of facing up to the cultural sterotype of being Mexican.

PUERTO RICANS

Puerto Rico was occupied by the United States in 1898 during the Spanish-American War and was ceded to this country as part of the treaty with Spain. Though the stated intention of the United States had been to provide revenues and civil government only on a temporary basis, annexation was soon followed by American investment, which revolutionized the production of sugar and changed the nature of farming on the island. In 1917, the Organic Act, sometimes called the Jones Act, admitted all Puerto Ricans to U.S. citizenship except those who petitioned to retain their former political status. Puerto Rico itself was recognized as an "organized but unincorporated territory." Jurisdiction over the territory was in the hands of the War Department until 1934, when it was transferred to the Interior Department, but it was not until 1947 that the Puerto Ricans could elect their own governor. In 1950, Congress passed legislation allowing Puerto Rico to become a Commonwealth, and in 1952 the Commonwealth of Puerto Rico was established, making Puerto Rico a self-governing political unit voluntarily associated with the United States whose inhabitants were U.S. citizens. Not all Puerto Ricans are happy with this status and many want independence, while others, perhaps a majority, want statehood.

United States annexation changed the economic organization of the island, while the introduction of U.S. medical techniques and sanitary improvements lowered the death rate. The result was a rapid growth in population that was not matched by an increase of jobs. The population of 953,243 in 1899 had grown to 2,210,703 by 1950 and 3.5 million by 1979. The island's current population density of more than 793 people per square mile makes it one of the most densely populated areas of the world. From 1901 to 1977, Puerto Rico's death rate dropped from 36.7 per 1,000 to a subnormal 6.0 per 1,000, a figure lower than that recorded in the United States. However, the birth rate declined at a much slower rate, from 43.2 in 1947 to 32.5 in 1960 to 22.5 in 1975. Though vast strides were made in economic progress, particularly in the last few decades, the median family income of $3,063 is still far below that of any U.S. state. Inevitably, large numbers of islanders migrated to the United States for work. During the 1950s, about 50,000 people a year left the island, a rate that has somewhat declined in recent years in part because many older people are now returning. Nontheless, there is still a consistent outpouring of residents into the United States.[4]

Before 1920, there were only an estimated 15,000 Puerto Ricans residing in the United States. However, once the Puerto Ricans were given citizenship, their status changed from immigrant to migrant, and the numbers rapidly increased. In the decade 1921–1930, some 52,774 settled on the mainland; in 1931–1940, 69,967; 1941–1950, 226,110; 1951–1960, 615,384. It is estimated that there are now more than one and a half million Puerto Ricans living in the United States, the majority of them in New York City.[5] Unlike early settlers, the Puerto Ricans came by air, and the comparative ease with which they can migrate has encouraged them to consider themselves only as temporary residents. Just as in the Southwest, there is also considerable two-way traffic between the island and the mainland.

Puerto Ricans are of mixed racial origin. The original Spanish conquest was so devastating that the Indian population was virtually wiped out. Most of the present inhabitants are descendants of the Spanish and their black slaves, with only a slight Indian mixture. In the 1960 census return, approximately 20 percent of the island population was classified as nonwhite. However, there is a wide variation in skin color among the population and, although there is no formal segregation or discrimination based upon skin color, there is informal prejudice against the darker members of society, particularly if their socioeconomic status is also low. Nonetheless, in New York City and other urban centers to which they have migrated, this comparative lack of prejudice and identity related to skin color has created considerable controversy between Puerto Ricans and blacks. Blacks expected the dark Puerto Ricans to give support to the civil rights and black-power movements, but in the past these people have been much more likely to identify with their light-skinned cousins from Puerto Rico than with American blacks.

In spite of intense efforts, Puerto Ricans still have low educational levels, are the newest migrants to the eastern cities, and also tend to be the poorest. They have inherited the most deteriorated slum areas, many moving into formerly black areas that the upwardly mobile blacks were happy to leave behind. The newly arrived workers also tend to find jobs as laborers or machine operators, which in New York usually means working in the garment industry. Although there are as yet few second-generation Puerto Ricans resident on the continent, some intergenerational upward mobility has been noted. A 1960 comparison of first- and second-generation migrants indicated that, while only 15 percent of the first-generation workers held white-collar jobs, 31 percent of the second-generation workers were in white-collar occupations. However, in spite of this statistical progress, the overwhelming majority of Puerto Ricans in this country hold very low-level jobs and are susceptible to being laid off as soon as the rate of employment rises.

CUBANS

Cuba was long closely tied economically to the United States, and in the past some analysts spoke of it as being essentially an economic dependency of the United States. The United States had originally become involved in the war with Spain largely as a result of Cuba's efforts to free itself, and, though we recognized the independence of Cuba, we were ceded a large naval base, Guantanamo Bay, in Cuba itself. The United States also reserved the right to intervene militarily in Cuba whenever it felt Cuban independence was threatened. American investment soon dominated Cuba, which in turn led to a considerable movement of Cubans to the United States. Even before the Spanish-American War, the cigar industry in Key West and Tampa had been founded by Cuban refugees. By 1960, the population of Cuban stock in the United States totalled 124,416 persons, of whom 116,354 were classified as white and 8,062 nonwhite. It is interesting to note that, although blacks comprised an estimated 25 percent of the Cuban population, only about 6.5 percent of the Cubans coming to the United States before the Castro takeover were classed as blacks. Most of the early Cuban immigrants settled in Florida and New York; New Jersey, Illinois, and California also had large numbers of Cubans.

The nature of this Cuban immigration changed radically when Fidel Castro overthrew the dictatorship of Fulgenico Batista at the beginning of 1959. Many of Batista's followers fled to the United States. Soon afterwards, Castro launched an intensive propaganda campaign, blaming many of the ills of his country on Americans. By the end of 1960, in retaliation for the United States' elimination of the Cuban sugar import quota, Castro nationalized United States' investments in Cuba—which amounted to more than one billion dollars. The United States broke diplomatic relations with Cuba at the beginning of 1961. An increasing number of Cubans sought refuge in the United States as Castro tightened his control on the country and adopted a program of encouraging those who did not agree with him to leave. There were regularly scheduled air flights from Cuba to Miami from the end of 1959 to October 1962, when they were discontinued during the missile crisis. A second large-scale exodus of Cubans began late in 1965, when the United States and Cuba agreed to allow special flights from Havana to Miami. A third wave arrived in 1980. As self-imposed political exiles, the Cubans were admitted under special refugee quotas. Most of them probably never intended to settle in the United States permanently, but rather planned to go back to Cuba as soon as Castro was overthrown. For a time, in fact, many of them were deeply involved in revolutionary activities designed to overthrow Castro. However, with the passage of time, more and more of them have begun to settle down and begin the process of becoming U.S. citizens. In the first great exodus from Cuba between 1959 and 1962, it is estimated that nearly a quarter of a million refugees arrived in the United States, with a high point of 3,000 a week at Miami airport just before the Cuban missile crisis.[6] The second wave of refugees was nearly as large, amounting to more than 100,000 people.

Although refugees in each of the three waves were forced to leave money and possessions behind them, the first two waves differed significantly from the third in educational level and job skills. The two earlier groups were drawn primarily from the middle and upper strata of society, with preparation in professional, business, clerical, or skilled occupations. For example, 25 percent of the refugees passing through the Miami Refugee Center between 1958 and 1963 were professionals of one sort or another. Another 12 percent were what could be regarded as managerial and executive persons. These people were better educated and far more sophisticated than the average

Cuban. Since 23 percent of the refugees in the first wave did not register at the Center, the professional and high-status occupational backgrounds of the refugees were probably even higher, since it is estimated that those who did not register were even more affluent and well-connected than those who did. Most of the refugees came from Havana or some other large city and so were more used to the urban conditions found in the United States and better prepared to move into the urban occupational structure.[7] Most Cubans also settled down in the Miami area, where their political influence was soon felt even if they were not citizens. The Cubans who came in the first waves of immigration were sophisticated and accustomed to using power and soon had an influential role in the affairs of Miami as well as other cities where they settled. Once the trauma of relocation was over, the vast majority of them were able to earn adequate or even high-level incomes and did not suffer from the long-term, poverty-related health problems. Undoubtedly, however, the loss in status was extremely painful, and the problems of adjusting to another language meant added burdens, but most of the Cubans adjusted fairly rapidly. Even though many professionals had to undergo new training or gain additional experience to qualify for U.S. licensure, and some—such as lawyers—had to find a new occupation because Cuban law has little in common with U.S. law, they still started with more basic education and more coping skills in the job market than the average Mexican or Puerto Rican migrant.

The refugees of the 1980 wave had less education and were more likely to be single and black than the earlier groups. Yet, a study done by the Immigration and Naturalizaton Service of the first 15,000 refugees in 1980 indicated that there was still a heavy concentration of skilled tradespersons. Fifty-five percent of the group had relatives in the United States, and this support system of past refugees undoubtedly proved helpful.[8] Still, the lower educational level, relative to earlier waves, will undoubtedly slow the integration into the job market.

The greatest health problems occurred in Florida as the refugees first landed. Control of epidemics is always a problem when large numbers of people are moved into temporary and crowded quarters, and this problem was complicated by the communication barriers. Eventually, Cuban nurses were hired as aides by the Miami health department until they qualified for U.S. licensure, and they proved remarkably effective in bridging the health information gap. Perhaps the most pressing problem was the more than 13,000 children who were not accompanied by parents. Most of these parents eventually did leave Cuba and re-established their families, but for a time the placement of the children and the problem of helping them to adjust to the loneliness and the new surroundings was an overwhelming task for the workers in Miami. It should be added that the federal government itself assumed a greater burden for these immigrants to U.S. shores than for any other group; in fact, up to 1967 the government had spent more than 200 million dollars in assisting Cubans to retrain and relocate, an average of about $1,000 per adult Cuban.[9] The 1980 relocation effort was even more expensive.

Other Spanish-speaking peoples have entered the United States both legally and illegally from Nicaragua, San Salvador, Guatemala, and most of the other countries of Central and South America. Although the various groups have in common the fact that they speak Spanish, ethnically and culturally they are quite different peoples. The remainder of this chapter will examine the health care of the Mexican Americans and the Puerto Ricans in this country.

HEALTH PROBLEMS OF MEXICAN AMERICANS

Since Mexican Americans are lumped together with other whites in official records, comparisons of their mortality and morbidity rates with those of other groups are difficult. However, it is not impossible. There have been some studies of mortality rates that use the Spanish surname as a category, and these studies suggest that Mexican Americans share the poverty-related health problems that are the main cause of poor health among blacks. A study of mortality rates conducted in Colorado indicated that the people with Spanish surnames were much more likely to die of rheumatic fever, pneumonia, and influenza than were members of the Anglo population. Since the timely administration of antibiotics for streptococcic infections can prevent rheumatic fever from ever developing, while the mortality rate for pneumonia and influenza can be lessened by early treatment, it seems obvious that these death rates are clearly related to a lack of adequate medical care.

The Colorado study also found that neonatal deaths were three times as high among the Spanish-surname group as among Anglos, reflecting not only less adequate conditions at and following delivery but also a lack of prenatal care, as well as the poor general nutrition and health of the mother. Fatal accidents were also a major cause of death among members of the Spanish-surname population; although lack of medical care may again be implicated here, the Colorado commission that sponsored the study believed that the use of old automobiles and unsafe equipment was the most important factor in explaining this finding.[10]

The City of San Antonio annually publishes statistics that allow comparisons to be made among Mexican-American, white, and non-white populations. In general, these tabulations support the findings of the Colorado study; respiratory diseases are a major cause of death and infant mortality rates are high. In addition, in San Antonio there is a noticeably high-fatality rate from diabetes among both nonwhite and Mexican-American populations. Although the fatality rate is again partly due to a lack of medical care, this is not the whole cause of the differential rate, because other studies have shown that the diabetes morbidity rate is also higher among these two ethnic groups than it is among the population in general.[11] More complete explanations for these differences await basic research into genetic factors and the effects of the high-starch diet that so often accompanies poverty.

It is important to note that Mexican Americans are much less likely to die of neoplasms, vascular diseases, and heart disease than other Americans. These diseases, commonly associated with aging, are much less common among all poverty populations, undoubtedly because of their earlier age of death from other causes. However, there is some indication that the life-styles associated with affluence may help cause heart and vascular diseases, and affluence is not yet a problem for the Mexican Americans as a group.

In working with the residents of the barrios, it appears that discrimination in health care delivery historically has not been so important to Spanish-speaking Americans as blacks, probably because discrimination has been overshadowed by problems associated with the language barriers and other aspects of the cultural differences between Mexican Americans and Anglos. The monolingual Spanish-speaking patient (like other non-English-speaking patients) finds a visit to an English-speaking physician or an American hospital frightening and often not particularly fruitful. Unless he or she takes a bilingual friend along as an interpreter, the exchange of information is apt to be meager, because until recently few health professionals in the Southwest were Spanish-speaking. The East Los Angeles Health Task Force, a community-based organization funded by the Office of Economic Opportunity, gathered information about the experiences of barrio residents when they confronted the Anglo health care system. Among the examples reported was that of a frightened old man watching as a young Anglo physician gave him penicillin although the old man believed, as did his excited family, that he was allergic to the drug. All tried to tell this to the physician, who did not understand them. There were numerous stories of patients who were taken to surgery who did not know they were going to be operated on, as well as tales about people who were merely being transferred from one ward or area to another and thought they were going to surgery. Matters of simple communication could be exaggerated into actions that were believed to have fearful consequences, yet even in the Los Angeles hospitals Spanish-speaking personnel were almost nonexistent. In fact, it was only after considerable agitation that the Health Task Force was able to convince Los Angeles County Hospital that more Spanish-speaking nurses' aides and attendants should be hired so that interpreters would be available not only to explain the hospital procedures to the patients but to assist in taking patients' histories. Health professionals who have been taught the importance of patient histories for treatment and diagnosis can begin to realize how inadequate much of the health care is when the patient cannot even describe subjective symptoms.

However, language is not the only barrier to effective communication. One of the difficulties is a cultural tradition that suggests that bad health, though unpleasant, is something that one endures. Men of the barrio tend to be particularly spartan in their attitude toward illness, and there is a belief that a man who admits to illness is not *macho* (i.e., tough and rugged). Sickliness somehow reflects moral and physical weakness. Often, a person who is ill is commended by friends and relatives for endurance. For example, a man with a high fever and accompanying pain who continues to work is admired because of his continued willingness to work. Women and children are allowed to show more weakness during illness than men. Some of this traditional acculturation is strengthened by the strains of wage earning in the United States, since a man unable to work is a man unable to support his family. For women who work outside the family, much of the same stoicism about pain is demonstrated.

Also complicating treatment is the traditional Mexican preoccupation with privacy, a preoccupation that demonstrates itself in the health setting in overpronounced modesty. Natural functions such as urinating, defecating, and bathing are considered one's private activities, not observed by others. This makes it difficult for Mexicans, even males, to visit a male physician who will probe, examine, and inspect bodily areas that Mexican Americans feel violate their privacy. Some of this feeling is true of patients of whatever culture, but it is accentuated in people raised in a Mexican cultural setting.

If the patient is hospitalized, other aspects of the culture also become significant. Many of the more recent migrants from Mexico feel that illness is a family affair, so the hospital is likely to be deluged with relatives, ranging from next of kin to far-distant second cousins. Hospital restrictions about visitors tend to make the sick patient feel harassed, distrustful, and frustrated, and it takes special empathy to be able to deal with the onslaught of visitors so that the patient will not feel slighted, the relatives unhappy, and the professional staff exhausted. The sick patients from the poorer sections of the barrio also have a low expectation of what can be done for them and often prove reluctant to ask for PRN medications without the nurse initiating the request. Generally, they have a feeling that they are getting more than they deserve or are fearful of being too much of a bother. Obviously, diet in the Anglo hospital is different from that to which many Mexican Americans are accustomed, and rather than complain many simply might not eat.[12]

PUERTO RICAN HEALTH

Puerto Ricans are as concentrated on the Eastern seaboard as Mexican Americans are in the Southwest, although both groups have also spread to all parts of the country. However, the climate of New York City is radically different from that of Puerto Rico, so that Puerto Ricans moving to New York must adjust to a more radical change in living conditions than the Mexican Americans in the Southwest. Since population in general is much more concentrated in the eastern part of the United States than in the western, and eastern cities are older than western, the migrants from Puerto Rico often find themselves in overcrowded and unsanitary areas. Because they are new migrants, the Puerto Ricans tend to settle in the most depressed housing areas, where their residences are often heavily infested with rats. For example, the New York City Department of Health reported an average of 500 cases of rat bites each year between 1947 and 1953 with an extremely high percentage of them among Puerto Rican families.[13]

Migration to the United States sometimes accentuates other health problems. For example, tuberculosis was long endemic in Puerto Rico and, until fairly recently, Puerto Rico had a higher death rate from tuberculosis than any country reporting health statistics. This susceptibility to tuberculosis tends to be increased in the United States by the poor, over crowded housing condition in which the migrants find themselves, as well as by deficient knowledge about health care and sanitation practices. Between 1949 and 1951, there were 474 reported cases of tuberculosis per 100,000 Puerto Rican residents.[14] Earlier (in the 1930s), Puerto Ricans living in New York had a higher mortality rate from tuberculosis than did those Puerto Ricans who remained on the island.[15] In a 1958 study of about 80 Puerto Rican families living in New York City, nine patients in six of the families were undergoing treatment for tuberculosis.[16] Since then, the incidence has declined but has remained higher than that of the general population.

Puerto Ricans also suffer from a variety of parasitic diseases, including dysentery; malaria; filariasis (caused by a small worm that lives in the lymphatics of the body and is spread by the mosquito); schistosomiasis mansoni (dependent upon a snail carrier), which attacks the liver; and hookworm (also found in the American South). The New York City Health Department has stated that the generally poor health conditions of large numbers of Puerto Ricans was largely due to the presence of these parasites.[17]

Influencing the general health of the Puerto Rican migrants is widespread malnutrition. The chief articles of food on the island for the poorer people are rice and beans, with beans serving as the main source of protein. Puerto Ricans eat few green or leafy vegetables, and only rarely do they use milk and eggs. Bread is also not generally used in all parts of the island. To this basic starch diet, the Puerto Rican adds cheap fats, usually lard or olive oil, in liberal quantities. Consequently, internal disorders are widespread. When the Puerto Rican is transplanted to New York, the deficiency in the diet is made even worse by the relative lack of sunshine.

The effect of migration upon health was demonstrated in a New York City study that found that 20 percent of a sample of 216 migrants were hospitalized within their first year after leaving Puerto Rico.[18] In the years following the first hospitalization, there tended to be a decline in recurring hospitalization. The reasons for this are not entirely clear. It might be that those suffering from chronic diseases prior to migration are apt to seek treatment soon after arrival; in fact, a few of them seem to have been sent north by their physicians or their families for treatment of a specific illness. The trauma of moving itself might also tend to aggravate long-standing illnesses. Separation from home and family can cause a painful adjustment as well as some practical difficulties. Since the family pattern in both Mexico and Puerto Rico tends to be extended, the individual can call on and expect help from many relatives in times of illness or other crises. Inevitably, moving to the United States breaks up some of these units and, although people may eventually re-establish the extended family pattern by helping relatives to move or by seeking out relatives who are already here, this often takes time, so that new migrants are forced to turn to clinics or hospitals for care that would have been available from relatives in their old environment.

The stress of moving is also further complicated by other family problems. Consensual unions are common in Puerto Rico,[19] but many of these unions are fairly stable so that they are for most practical purposes similar to the more formal union of marriage. However, under the impact of urbanization and migration, the informal arrangements tend to break down[20] and the single man and woman are left alone to cope with the new environment, or women are left as heads of households. For a woman who has grown up expecting help from all of her female relatives, as well as support from her husband, such a desertion can be overwhelming. For a man who has always been surrounded by relatives, the new-found freedom may spell loneliness.[21]

HEALTH CARE INSTITUTIONS

Inevitably the first- or second-generation Mexican American and the recent Puerto Rican immigrant faces the Anglo health care institutions with a certain amount of suspicion. One of the difficulties in treating tuberculosis among both of these groups has been the people's fear of the hospital; rather than be hospitalized, many people deny they have the disease until the case is very advanced.[22] Although physicians in Mexico have high standards, they are mainly confined to urban middle-class areas. The primary source of medical care in most Mexican villages and in the poorer sections of the cities is the folk medical practitioners whose knowledge is based upon an elaborate and well-developed system of beliefs acquired outside of any regular educational institution. Though upper-middle-class Mexican Americans, as well as the more Americanized person in the lower-income groups, have abandoned much of the folk medical practices, the newly arrived and the poor of the barrios usually favor the folk system over American scientific medicine. Often, they divide diseases into two categories, consulting a folk practitioner for the traditional diseases but an Anglo physician for "Anglo diseases." In an interview study of Mexican-American women living in a public housing project, it was found that the overwhelming majority knew about and used the folk system of diagnosis and therapy for at least part of their care.[23]

The major folk practitioner in the Mexican-American community is the *curandero* (*curandera*, in the case of a woman), who not only has acquired considerable empirical knowledge but also possesses the charismatic qualities associated with the more spiritual aspects of the role. A good *curandero* shows great warmth and concern for both the patient and his family. He offers advice, gives treatment, but asks for no fee. Special prayers are often a part of his therapy. If the treatment proves successful, the family is expected to give him an offering, but if he fails nothing is expected. This means that, because no fee will be forthcoming, the *curandero* will often refuse to treat a patient who from previous experience he knows he cannot cure or who he thinks has a bad prognosis. In these cases, the family turns to the Anglo physician or hospital. The implication of this is not lost upon the patient who tends to associate hospitalization and the American physician with a fear of death or serious disability, otherwise he could have been cured by the *curandero*.

The *curandero* is not the only folk practitioner; usually, before he is sought out, home remedies will have been tried and a neighborhood *señora* (older woman) will have been consulted. Actually, the line between the señora and the *curandera* is not a clear one, because older women usually start out helping their friends and family during times of illness and, if they gain a reputation for success, they then become known as healers. A male healer may start as a *sovador*, who specializes in giving massages, although from the beginning he may use the more general term of *curandero*. The *partera*, or midwife, is also an important practitioner in Mexico, but to a lesser extent in the United States, where hospital deliveries are more common.[24] The cultural acceptance of the *partera*, who is always a woman, still influences the attitudes of the Mexican-American woman, who has been accustomed to think that the female reproductive process should be a private matter between women. Male obstetricians, groups of medical students, and the matter-of-fact attitudes of the hospital and clinic personnel often prove to be traumatic in such cases. This tends to act as a further barrier to a woman's seeking prenatal care or accepting contraceptives.

The *curandero* also exists in the Puerto Rican community, although the role is not so well institutionalized. There are a variety of spiritualists in Spanish Harlem who trace their healing arts back to cults imported not only from Puerto Rico but also from other Caribbean islands.[25] These spiritualists emphasize healing through religious or medical ceremonies, potions, and amulets, rather than through empirical methods. There are also a variety of herbs and charms available that the layman can buy and use at home without consulting any practitioner. Although very often an older woman who has accumulated knowledge of these herbs and other home remedies will be consulted by her family or friends, she seldom takes this calling as an occupational role as her counterpart in the Mexican-Americn community might do.

Although there is a tradition of folk medicine in Cuba, the first two waves of immigrants to the United States were sufficiently affluent to have abandoned much of that tradition for professional care. The new wave of immigrants have lived for a generation with a fully subsidized socialized health care system (although at the level of essentials only).[26] Consequently, they too have moved away from the folk system to develop a pattern of seeking health care services from professionals. These factors make folk medicine less important in the Cuban-American culture than it is among the other Spanish-speaking minorities.

FOLK DISEASES

Some of the diseases recognized by the various folk practitioners are more or less the standard diagnoses recognized by the more scientific medical community. However, there are other kinds of illnesses that fit into an independent folk system of belief and practice, and it is for this group of diagnoses that the *curandero* is most likely to be consulted. Various researchers have worked out systems to classify or group these folk diseases. Margaret Clark, who did an indepth study of the health beliefs and practices of one Mexican-American community, could fit most of them into four categories: (1) diseases of hot and cold imbalance, (2) dislocations of internal organs, (3) illnesses of magical origin, and (4) illnesses of emotional origin.[27]

The hot and cold theory of illness has been traced back to ancient Greek theories that held that the healthy man was maintained in a balance between four humours (phlegm, blood, black bile, and yellow bile). Some of these humours were thought to be disproportionately hot, while others were cold; an imbalance between the various essences caused illness. This body of medical theory was brought to the new world by the sixteenth-century Spanish explorers and eventually diffused throughout Mexico. In the process, the theory was somewhat altered and the original idea of the four humours was reduced to a dichotomy between hot and cold.[28]

Illness is thought to be caused by a disequilibrium that can be the result of a dietary imbalance or exposure. Usually, a dietary regimen or herbs is prescribed to cure the imbalance. Whether a food used in this treatment is classified as hot or cold is not necessarily related to its actual temperature; for example, ice is considered hot because it burns the mouth. That such foods as chili peppers and onion are classified as hot seems quite logical, but the classification of tomatoes, citrus fruits, cucumbers, and chicken as cold is less apparent to the outsider, and the fact that white beans are considered hot while red beans are cold carries no clue to the uninitiated. It is apparent that the *curandero* must absorb a large body of knowledge in order to master the whole system. Because of the complexity of the system, the average individual usually does not know all of the classifications, and turns to the *curandero* for advice. Symptoms of imbalance include head colds, stomach upsets, and general malaise. Infants are thought to be particularly susceptible to "cold stomach," which means that dedicated believers in this system do not give cold foods, including citrus fruits, to their infants, in spite of the exhortations of public health nurses. Expectant mothers are often cautious about eating too many foods that are classified as hot, because it is believed this will cause their babies to have diaper rashes when they are born.

A common folk illness that is only tenuously related to the hot and cold theory is *empacho*. The symptoms of *empacho*, including swollen abdomen, diarrhea, vomiting, and fever, are attributed to a *bolita*, or small ball of food caught in the stomach. Sometimes massage or manipulation is used to dislodge the lump, although at other times a dietary regimen is prescribed as it is for ailments caused by a hot and cold imbalance. If the *curandero* decides a special diet is necessary, he will usually curtail the intake of cheese, bananas, eggs, and soft bread, because it is believed that these foods have a tendency to form a *bolita*.[29] At other times, a purgative is advised to clean out the stomach.[30]

Mollera ciada, or fallen fontanel, is the most common type of organ displacement. It is usually attributed to a too-sudden withdrawal of the nipple from the infant's mouth.[31] Symptoms of the ailment include diarrhea and vomiting. It is interesting that in folk medicine the cause and effect are often reversed from that of scientific medicine. In this case, the severe dehydration that accompanies infant diarrhea is taken as evidence for a depressed fontanel. Dehydration can be fatal, unless the diarrhea is checked and enough oral or parenteral fluids are given, but the folk practitioner does not realize this and the methods he tries are not really effective. He usually relies on topical remedies, or he may hold the infant up by his heels over a basin of water to try to get the fontanel to resume its normal appearance. The fact that *mollera ciada* is such a well-known ailment is evidence that severe diarrhea is still common among infants in the Mexican-American community and still a leading cause of the high infant mortality rate.[32]

A less common ailment attributed to a misplaced organ is that of infertility, which is sometimes explained as being due to a fallen uterus. Barrenness is a cause of great sadness, because marriage and family are such important aspects of the culture and women who are mothers are the most highly respected. Barrenness is also regarded as a threat to the male, since a man is measured by his *machismo*, or manliness, including the ability to produce children.[33] The *curandero* may attempt to treat the infertility with religious and magical cures and massage.

Diseases of purely magical origin include those attributed to the evil eye (*mal ojo*) and to bad air (*mal aire*). A folk belief in the evil eye as a cause of illness seems to be almost world-wide in scope, so that any health practitioner who is willing to step outside of the confines of the modern medical center and to communicate with people about their beliefs is likely to run into the concept of the evil eye. In Italy and other parts of Europe, religious medals may be worn to ward off the evil eye. In an unpublished study of hospitalized Egyptian infants done by the authors in 1966, it was found that approximately half of the mothers interviewed felt that their infants' illnesses had been caused by the "one with the evil eye." The women explained that the handsome, healthy male babies were the ones who were particularly vulnerable to this type of spell because they were the ones who were most likely to be the objects of envy from living persons, as well as from free-floating evil spirits. Similarly, the unsophisticated Mexican-Americn mother may believe that, when someone, particularly a woman, admires her infant but fails to touch him, the baby will develop symptoms of *mal ojo*, including fitful crying, wakefulness, diarrhea, vomiting, and fever. If the person who admires the child touches him, the spell will be broken and no illness occurs. Unfortunately, social workers and nurses are sometimes blamed for casting the spell because they unwittingly admire infants in this manner. Once the symptoms of *mal ojo* develop in either a child or an adult, the victim can be treated only by magical means.

Mal aire (bad air) as a cause of illness is not so well known throughout the world as the evil eye, although many peoples believe in vague types of airborne spirits that cause illness. Symptoms of *mal aire* can include facial paralysis, convulsions, or other frightening symptoms. The *curandero* may treat the disease with massage and counter-spells.

Bilis is more often a disease confined to adults. It is manifested by nervousness, emotional upset, and the physiological symptoms of the type psychologists and psychiatrists generally link with anxiety. Herbs and emotional support are used to treat it.[34]

Strong emotions and emotional trauma are recognized throughout Latin American as a cause of illness. The folk practitioners and the medical profession are actually in substantial agreement in this regard, although they do not use the same diagnostic labels. In the Southwest U.S., the two most common emotional illnesses are *susto* (fright) and *bilis* (anger). *Susto* is believed to occur most often in children, although no age is immune, because *susto* seems to be broadly defined to include much more than what we would call fright: almost any traumatic emotional illness can be the cause of *susto*. Ritual prayers are a common treatment of *susto*, sometimes combined with the use of herbal remedies. In such cases, the *curandero* may also try to manipulate the physical and psychological environment of the patient in order to lessen the emotional stress, although the patient undoubtedly would not explain his or her actions in these terms.

A good example of this type of creative manipulation is reported by Margaret Clark. She recounted the case of a young pregnant mother who became angry with her husband one night when he came home drunk. When she scolded him, he beat her and put her out of the house in the rain. The woman proceeded to walk to her mother's house a few blocks away, where she related her experiences; her relatives responded by becoming fearful that her unborn child would suffer from *susto* or "fright." Ordinarily, a woman in her culture would not have been justified in condemning her husband for beating her, since she had scolded and insulted him and therefore deserved the beating. However, because she was pregnant, she had recourse to a folk-defined disease, *susto;* thus, there was a possibility that her baby would be affected. She was given an outpouring of sympathy, and open criticism was directed against the unfeeling husband who had threatened the life of the unborn child. Community pressure forced him to repent, apologize to his wife, and promise that it would not happen again.[35] Imagine the situation if a more sophisticated relative had brought the young woman to the emergency room because her baby might suffer from *susto*, and the intake nurse did not know how to respond to such a complaint.

There is also a special folk diagnosis of an emotional illness, called *ataque*, that is recognized by the Puerto Ricans. It seems to be particularly widespread among lower-socioeconomic groups and represents a popular and conventional reaction to overwhelming catastrophe. Men and women appear to be equally susceptible. The episodes begin quite suddenly, usually without warning either to the spectators (a necessary part of the disease) or the patient. The patient sometimes utters a short cry or scream before sliding to the ground. Shortly after falling to the ground, or at the same time, the patient begins moving arms and legs in a kind of coordinated fashion. These movements seem purposeful and include beating the fists on the floor, striking out at persons nearby, or banging the head on the floor. Foaming at the mouth is common, but usually there is no incontinence or tongue biting as there would be in epilepsy. The attack usually ceases abruptly, with the individual resuming what he was doing before with little effect. During the *ataque*, no special change in pulse, blood pressure, or neurological signs have been noted by attending physicians. The *ataque* usually lasts for 5 to 10 minutes, but may go on for hours, and some have continued for four days.[36] *Ataques* may occur once in a lifetime or become a continuing pattern of reaction in particular individuals.

It is worthy of comment that, although there are accounts of successful collaboration between Western psychiatrists and Yorubu witch doctors in Nigeria, there does not seem to have been much collaboration between American health practitioners and Spanish folk healers. Anglo health workers tend either to ignore the folk beliefs and practices or try to "educate" their patients by deprecating the folk practitioners. Since available information suggests that the folk methods are often effective, it might well be that a creative cooperation between the two groups would improve the delivery of health services. The most obvious effectiveness of the folk practitioner seems to be in the field of mental illness. E. Gartly Jaco reported in 1959 that, in Texas, psychoses among the Spanish-surname population was less than among Anglos or among non-whites.[37] Since that time, there has been evidence that the incidence of mental illness among the younger Mexican-American population is rising, and it may be that Jaco's findings were somewhat biased, because there were few Mexican Americans in publicly supported facilities.[38] Still, all the evidence to date gives strength to the idea that the emotional support given both by the extended family and the folk practitioners is at least as effective if not more effective in preventing mental health problems than the help available to the rest of the population whose socioeconomic status is equally low and who lack such practitioners.

Cooperation could be even more helpful in attempting to eliminate the delays when folk medicine is clearly inadequate for saving lives, as is the case with infant diarrhea. If some sort of mutual agreement could be worked out, the professional health worker would not need to insist on wooing the patient away from the folk healer in all cases; moreover, mainstream medical practitioners could be more effective in the struggle to upgrade health if they could adopt some of the personal warmth and appearance of concern that the *curandero* has. All one needs to do is contrast the hospital admissions officer whose hand is out for cash or an insurance card before any treatment can be given with the *curandero* who says no payment is necessary unless he is successful. It is true that the *curandero* uses informal pressures to obtain his fees, but he is much more subtle and less demanding than the fee-for-service system that characterizes Anglo medicine.

Closer working relationships with the folk practitioners, knowledge about the culture, and understanding of the individual patient could help the health worker deliver more useful care. Often, the very definitions of health and illness differ between professional and patient. As indicated earlier, there is a widespread belief that, if a man is not emaciated or in pain and can perform his work role adequately, he is well and has no need for medical care.[39] The professional who holds a preventive orientation to illness may value health care for the well person in the form of immunizations and early treatment of illness before it is debilitating. Such workers would feel less frustrated if they realized that this difference in outlook exists to a certain extent among all poor people, because a preventive health outlook correlates with an ability to control the future, and poverty makes such control impossible. What the professional needs to do is make preventive services seem more reasonable to the patient by integrating them with the acute care that the patient realizes he or she needs. The practitioners would thus demonstrate that they are willing to do their share to bridge the existing gap between the health care professionals and the members of these Spanish-speaking subcultures.

Obviously, the most successful nurse or health professional at any level is the one who can adopt an open-minded approach to the problems of the patients she or he is dealing with. Folk concepts about health do not meet standards, nor do they always coincide with the insights gained by modern science, but within their framework, they are often logical and consistent and have to be dealt with. To try to ignore folk concepts is to handicap the healing process of the patient.

REFERENCES

1. McWilliams, C. North From Mexico: The Spanish-Speaking People of the United States. Reprinted, New York: Greenwood Press, 1968, p. 62.
2. Ibid., p. 193.
3. Galarza, E., Gallegos, H. & Samora, J. Mexican-Americans in the Southwest. Santa Barbara: McNally & Loftin, in cooperation with the Anti-Defamation League of B'Nai B'rith, 1969, p. 4. Median Age in U.S. Increases to 30, Highest Since 1950. L.A. Times-Washington Post, May 25, 1981.
4. See: Lewis, O. La Vida: A Puerto Rican Family in the Culture of Poverty. New York: Random House, 1965, pp. xi–xiii. For updates on statistics, see: U.S. Bureau of the Census. Statistical Abstract of the United States: 1979. Washington, D.C.: U.S. Government Printing Office, 1979, section 32, pp. 873–889.
5. Senior, C. Our Citizens from the Caribbean. New York: McGraw Hill, 1965, p. 71. Senior, C. The Puerto Ricans. Chicago: Quandrangle Books, 1965, p. 38. Statistical Abstract: 1979. Table 37, p. 34.
6. Fagen, R., Brody, R.A. & O'Leary, T. J. Cubans in Exile: Disaffection and the Revolution. Stanford: Stanford University Press, 1968, pp. 17 ff.
7. For a study of the first wave of Cubans, see Fagen, R. R., Brody, R. A., & O'Leary, T. J. Cubans in Exile: Disaffection and the Revolution. Stanford: Stanford University Press, 1968, especially chapters 1 and 2, pp. 1–28.
8. For the more recent immigrants, see the various news reports. Newsweek (May 26, 1980) had a good discussion of the Cuban refugees, pp. 24–28.
9. For a discussion of some of the problems, see Cuba's Children in Exile: The Story of the Unaccompanied Cuban Refugee Children's Program. Children's Bureau of the U.S. Department of Health, Education, and Welfare, 1967. Also, Cuban Refugee Problem. A report of the hearings before the Subcommittee to Investigate Problems Connected with Refugees and Escapees, Committee on the Judiciary, U. S. Senate, in three parts. Washington, D.C.: U.S. Government Printing Office, 1966. Also, Those Amazing Cuban Emigrés. Fortune, 1966, 74, 144–149.
10. Moustafa, A. T. & Weiss, G. Health Status and Practices of Mexican Americans. Mexican-American Study Project, Advance Report II. Los Angeles: University of California, 1968, pp. 5–6.
11. Ibid., pp. 7–11.
12. See: Clark, M. Health in the Mexican-American Culture. Berkeley: University of California Press, 1970, pp. 194–206. See also: Gonzalez, H. H. Health Care Needs of the Mexican-American. In Ethnicity and Health Care. New York: National League for Nursing, 1976, pp. 21–28.
13. Dworkis, M. B., (Ed.) The Impact of Puerto Rican Migration on Governmental Services in New York City. New York: New York University Press, 1957, p. 46.
14. Ibid., pp. 46–47.
15. Chenault, L. R. The Puerto Rican Migrant in New York City. New York: Columbia University Press, 1938, p. 115.

16. Berle, B. B. Eighty Puerto Rican Families in New York City: Health and Disease Studied in Context. New York: Columbia University Press, 1958, p. 151.
17. Chenault. op. cit., p. 122.
18. Berle. op. cit., p. 122.
19. Goode, W. Illegitimacy in the Caribbean Social Structure. *American Sociological Review*, 1960, *25*, 21–30.
20. Ibid. Otterbein, K. Caribbean Family. *American Anthropologist*, 1965, *67*, 66–79.
21. For an overview of the Puerto Ricans in New York, see: Wakefield, D. Island in the Sun. New York: Houghton Mifflin, 1959.
22. Berle. op. cit., p. 156.
23. Martinez, C. & Martin, H. W. Folk Diseases Among Urban Mexican-Americans. *Journal of the American Medical Association, 1966, 196*, 147–150.
24. Ruble, A. J. Across the Tracks: Mexican Americans in a Texas City. Austin: University of Texas Press, 1966, pp. 175–193, Saunders, L. Cultural Differences and Medical Care: The Case of the Spanish-Speaking People of the Southwest. New York: Russell Sage Foundation, 1954, pp. 160–164.
25. Wakefield. op. cit., pp. 49–84.
26. For a discussion of more recent developments in Cuban medicine, see: Danielson, R. Cuban Medicine. New Brunswick, N.J.: Transaction Books, 1979. The mass exodus of Cuban professionals forced a recasting of Cuban medical practice. Danielson examines both pre-Castro and post-Castro medicine.
27. Clark. op. cit., pp. 164–183.
28. Foster, G. M. Relationships Between Spanish and Spanish-American Folk Medicine *Journal of American Folklore*, 1953, *66*, 201–217. See also: Ingham, J. M. On Mexican Folk Medicine. *American Anthropologist*, 1970, *72*, 76–87.
29. Clark. op. cit., pp. 163–217.
30. Saunders. op. cit., p. 147.
31. Martinez & Martin. op. cit., pp. 147–150.
32. Baca, J. Some Health Beliefs of the Spanish Speaking. *American Journal of Nursing*, 1969, *69*, 2172–2176.
33. For example, see: Lewis, O. The Children of Sanchez. New York: Vintage Books, 1961.
34. Clark. op. cit., pp. 163–217.
35. Ibid., pp. 198–199.
36. Berle. op. cit., p. 159.
37. Jaco, E. G. Mental Health of the Spanish-American in Texas. In M. Opler (Ed.), *Culture and Mental Health: Cross Cultural Studies* New York: Macmillan, 1959, pp. 467–584.
38. Moustafa and Weiss. op. cit., pp. 31–35.
39. Schulman, S. & Smith, A. M. The Concept of Health Among Spanish Speaking Villagers of New Mexico and Colorado. *Journal of Health and Human Behavior*, 1963, *4*, 226–234.

5

Native Americans

In 1964, it was estimated that between 10 and 16 million residents had some Indian ancestor, or in more technical terms had an ancestor who might be classified as an indigenous native American.[1] This worked out to a ratio ranging from one in every eighteen persons to one in every eleven; today, the ratio is closer to one in ten or one in nine, as Americans intermarry with each other and the proportion with Indian ancestors increases, even as the ancestor becomes further and further removed. However, most of these Americans would never be classified as Indians by the United States Census, since by definition an Indian is a person who resides either on a reservation (trust land) or whose name appears on a "tribal roll." Less than half of the Indians classified by the Census are "pure blooded" and the majority have one-half, one-quarter, one-eighth, or even lesser amounts of Indian ancestry.

Such a definition of who is an Indian is not a historical one, and in the recent past there was a tendency to classify any European married to an Indian or to people of mixed Indian ancestry as Indian, much as the present tendency is to classify anyone with any kind of black ancestor as black. In 1977, 648,700 individuals classified as Indians by the government lived under some kind of control of the Bureau of Indian Affairs. These individuals furnish the basic subject matter of this chapter.

Ignored in both the census and historical definitions are vast numbers of Indians. Perhaps the largest group is found among the Spanish-speaking Americans, large numbers who in Mexico were classified as Indians and who in fact are more or less pure-blooded descendants of the pre-Spanish residents of that country. In Mexico, any Indian who moves away from his tribal village and adopts the customs and language of Mexico ceases to be regarded as an Indian, something that large numbers of Indians have done, although great numbers still remain in their native villages. Also ignored are large numbers of Indians with black ancestors who are classed as black by the government, even though they have more Indian ancestry than black.

Confusion over just who is an Indian is compounded by past policies of the United States Bureau of Indian Affairs, which, in 1954, admitted that it could not really make an adequate definition of just who an Indian is or was.[2] As a result, the term *Indian* in various government reports can mean a racial grouping, a legal concept, a sociocultural group, or a caste. Today, the largest centers of Indian population (as defined by the census) in the United States are Arizona and Oklahoma, with more than 95,000 Indians; New Mexico, with approximately 72,000; Alaska, with some 50,000 Indians and Eskimos; California, 91,000; North Carolina, 45,000; South Dakota, 32,000; New York, 28,000; Montana, 27,000; Washington, 33,000; and Minnesota, 23,000 persons classified as Indians. Tribal lands amount to nearly 40 million acres, with an additional 12 million acres in allotted land. Individual reservations range in size from one acre (Strawberry Valley Rancheria in Yuba County, California) to 15 million acres (the Navaho reservation in Arizona, New Mexico, and Utah, which is about the size of the state of West Virginia). The eastern states in particular have small communities of Indians, like the Pequots in Connecticut, Shinnecocks on Long Island in New York, the Tuscarora and Seneca in Buffalo, and the Mattaponys in Virginia, who have almost blended into surrounding American society but still maintain their unity and their own cohesive settlements and, in some cases, enjoy recognition as Indians by the government of the states in which they live.[3]

Prior to the coming of the European settlers to these shores, it has been estimated that there were about 600,000 Indians within the 48 mainland states, which means that, by government count, there are now as many reservation Indians as there were indigenous Americans 300 years ago. For a time in the last part of the nineteenth century, it seemed as if the Indian would disappear altogether. Many tribal gatherings did disappear, but, due in part to a change in government policy, the Indian managed to survive and even in some cases, such as the Navaho, to increase. In spite of Hollywood stereotypes, the native American Indians were not uniform in physical appearance and their stature and skin tones varied as much as those of the European settlers, although all had black hair, brown eyes, and some shade of brown skin. The Winnebagos were noted for their large heads; the Utes for their squat, powerful frames; the Crows for their height. These physical variations, coupled with the hundreds of different dialects belonging to some six major language groups, indicate the diversity of the Indian heritage. Culturally, they also differed. The Chippewa rode a birchbark canoe, the Chickasaw in a dugout; the Sac slept in a bark wigwam, the Kiowa in a skin tepee, and the Pueblo in a stone apartment house. The Seminole hunted with a blowgun, the Sioux with a bow. In summary, the American Indians differed as much or more from one another as the English did from the Russians or the French from the Egyptians. In fact one of the difficulties present day Indians have in organizing more effectively is the traditional hostilities and suspicions that continue to exist between certain tribal groupings.

Contact with the oncoming European settlers radically changed the nature of Indian life and, although all took something from the new culture, some were better able to adjust than others. However, all came to depend upon the Europeans, whether they wanted to or not. The acquisition of metal tools and utensils, firearms, horses, and sheep greatly simplified life for the Indians. Sheep made a new way of life for a few tribes, such as the Navaho, but it was the horse that had the greatest impact, and on the plains Indians it created a genuine revolution. For example, the Nez Pearcé changed from their old subsistence of fishing, root digging, and hunting small animals, to trailing the buffalo herds. The Navahos went so far as to deny their prehorse history by stating that, if "there were no horses, there were no Navahos." Some of the Indians, such as the Iroquois and the Apaches, adopted the European weapons with devastating effect on their Indian neighbors, driving them from choice hunting grounds, seizing their property, and enslaving and killing them. The European penetration forced a wholesale restructuring of Indian political alliances and territorial control, and increasingly the Europeans were the only source for supplies and goods that Indians could not manufacture themselves. Because some of the Indians looked to the French settlers for supplies and others to the British, the wars in Europe had repercussions for the Indians, and the European wars quickly became Indian wars in colonial America. Even if the Indians had all been friendly, which they were not, there would have been Indian wars, because of conditions beyond the control of the Indians. Once the United States was founded, the Indians continued to fight, if only to save their homelands. The American settlers were involved in about 37 Indian wars, as they attempted to remove the Indians from the path of their intended settlement.

European explorers and settlers also brought diseases with them that sometimes almost annihilated tribes and scattered the panic stricken survivors. Among the major division of the species homo sapiens, the American Indians, with the possible exception of the Australian aborigine, had the dangerous privilege of having the longest isolation from the rest of mankind. Almost none of the diseases that are first-rank killers are native to the Americas. Instead, they were brought to these shores; not only did the fatal diseases of the Old World kill more effectively in the New, but some comparatively benign diseases of the Old World turned killer in the New. With little exaggeration, a German missionary in 1699 reported that

> ... the Indians die so easily that the bare look and smell of a Spaniard causes them to give up the ghost.[4]

The most spectacular periods of mortality occurred during the first hundred years of contact with the Europeans and Africans. Tuberculosis, syphilis, smallpox, and measles were the principal diseases given to the Indians by the European settlers, although it is possible that syphilis had existed in more quiescent forms before.[5] The Pilgrims regarded it as a sign of divine intervention that some disease, probably smallpox left by visiting sailors, had decimated the Indian population of eastern Massachusetts shortly before their arrival. One of the few tribes whose strength remained unimpaired by the plague, the Pequots, attempted to resist the movement of European settlers into the Connecticut valley in the so-called Pequot War of 1637. During this engagement, a small party of whites surrounded the Pequot stronghold during the night, fired it, and killed or burned to death about 500 Indians, while losing only two men of their party. Increase Mather, a New England minister, called upon his congregation to thank God for allowing the settlers to send so many "heathen souls to hell." The surviving remnants of the tribe were sold into slavery.[6]

The forerunner of the reservation system can be dated to King Philip's War (1675 to 1676), a European war with American repercussions, and which the English settlers won largely because the bulk of the Indians supported them. In the aftermath of the war, both hostile and friendly Indians were required to live in specified villages, denied arms and ammunition, and prevented from meeting in assembly. Kept in semi-isolation, cut off from their old ways of making a living, the New England Indians entered a period of rapid decline, as European diseases and customs undermined their old way of life and were difficult to adjust to.

As Americans moved West, they continued to set aside certain western areas as Indian territory, usually the lands they considered least desirable. By 1840, survivors of most of the Eastern tribes had been removed to the West. This practice soon proved a failure, largely because Americans themselves continued to move West, coveting the very territory they a few years before had granted in perpetuity to the Indians. The great Sioux chief Spotted Tail became so discouraged with the continual government relocation schemes that he rather plaintively questioned why the "Great Father" did not "put his red children on wheels, so he can move them as he will?"[7]

In the last part of the nineteenth century, there was growing agitation for change in Indian policy, as many came to realize that we were in effect exterminating Indians. One of the most infleuntial forces for change was a book by Helen Hunt Jackson, whose novel *Ramona* had made her famous. Thus, she had a ready audience when, in 1881, she published *A Century of Dishonor*, an eloquent, impassioned, and biased plea to right the wrongs being done to the Indians by the perfidious policies of the United States government.[8] Like any human problem, however, there was no easy solution. Even friends of the Indians disagreed on the best way to achieve an equitable solution without sacrificing what they felt were the justified needs of an expanding United States. At first, the United States acted as if the Indian nations or tribes were independent foreign powers and made treaties with them. To counter the growing opposition to regarding Indians as independent subjects, Congress in 1871 stipulated that Indians were no longer citizens of foreign nations. Unfortunately, Congress did not take the next logical step and make Indians citizens of the United States. Still, the Congressional action did result in some benefits: for example, the appropriation of the first sums specifically marked for Indian eduction; but in return the government made it clear that internal tribal matters could be the subject of national legislation.

Even well-intentioned legislation often proved disastrous. Many advocates of better treatment felt that the only way the Indians could progress was to remove them from the reservation or from their old tribal groupings, both of which were regarded as keeping

Indians in their old ways. Unfortunately, this same kind of recommendation was also favored by groups hostile to the Indians and who coveted Indian land, which they were unable to buy as long as the tribe itself controlled it. Both groups came together to support the Dawes General Allotment Act of 1887, designed to encourage the growth of private enterprise among the Indians. Each adult Indian was to receive 160 acres and each child 80 acres from the tribal lands; the remaining lands were to be sold. Recognizing that most Indians still had no concept of private property, the legislation provided that the allotted lands would be held in trust for 25 years by the government, after which the individual Indian would be granted outright ownership and could sell the land if he wished to do so. The effect upon the Indian was disastrous. As one authority has written, the Dawes Act ". . . may not have civilized the Indian, but it definitely corrupted most of the white men who had any contact with it."[9] Between 1887 and 1934, the Indians lost 86 million of the 138 million acres held by them when the legislation was enacted. Though a small minority of Indians did well by the Dawes Act, and there were several "oil Indians" who made great money through their control of land, for every Indian whose allotment proved to contain oil, there were a score who were reduced to charity. In retrospect, the Dawes Act was extremely unwise and failed to take into account reality; most Indians traditionally had been hunters and gatherers and could not or would not be transformed into farmers overnight. The result was a generation of landless Indians with no vocational training and almost total demoralization.

Only a little more successful was the whole concept behind the development of Indian schools. Again, the motivation was rapid assimilation of Indians into the American mainstream, although the cupidity so evident in allotting Indians lands was not a factor this time. By 1899, more than $2,500,000 was being expended annually on 148 boarding schools and 225 day schools, with almost 20,000 children in attendance. Most of these schools were far removed from the reservation, since the educational authorities of the day were in agreement that a complete break with the home environment was essential if the Indians were to become effective citizens. In theory, attendance was voluntary, which meant that recruiting students was always a problem. Often, the students enrolled at the distant boarding schools were orphans or from families so low in the tribal heirarchy they were unable to resist administrative pressure. Indian parents were generally reluctant to lose their children for months, and death rates among the students were abnormally high. Moreover, many of the skills the Indians were taught in the school had no application to the type of life they would lead when they returned home. This meant that students who did not adapt to the routine at school were miserable while they were there, but those who did adapt successfully were miserable when they returned home to their families.[10]

The same kind of basic misunderstanding characterized some of the other attempts to force Indians to assimilate. For a time, the Bureau of Indian Affairs ordered reservation officials to slash food and clothing rations on the assumption that this would force the Indians to support themselves. Instead, most of the Indians did what their people traditionally had done—shared what little they had and went hungry together. Officials in Washington also ordered all male Indians to have their hair cut, even though some tribesmen believed that long hair had supernatural significance. On at least one reservation, refractory Indians were shackled so that the hair cutting could be carried out.

Reasons for the continual misunderstanding of Indian psychology are difficult to come by. It could be that Americans regarded Indians with considerable hostility, and, though this hostility might have been a cover-up for deeper feelings of guilt over the maltreatment and exploitation of the Indian, it could not help but be reflected in official policies. Adding to this was the popular stereotype that Indian culture was homogenous, which meant that policies all too frequently failed to consider the differences in customs that existed between the tribes. Even though the civil servants who worked for the Bureau of Indian Affairs were often well-educated people, with college or even graduate training, they were usually not trained to understand or work in a culture other than their own.[11] Somehow, in spite of the American misunderstanding, the Indians managed to survive, but their living conditions never approached that of their European neighbors.

In examining the Indian past, it seems that the hostility to the Indian often increased with proximity, and those most tolerant were those who had little day-to-day contact. This is most evident in the prohibitions against voting. In 1924, as acknowledgement of American gratitude for the Indians who had served in World War I, the Snyder Act finally conferred citizenship upon all Indians who requested it. Two states with large Indian populations, Arizona and New Mexico, refused to allow Indians to vote, until finally, in 1948, the Courts ordered them to do so. However, the Snyder Act seemed to mark an official change in the federal government's attitude. It was followed two years later by a special study of the Indian under the direction of Lewis Meriam, who proposed a sweeping list of reforms including a halt to allotment of land, which the report argued had impoverished and demoralized the Indians. The full effect of the Meriam recommendations was not felt until the election of Franklin D. Roosevelt, who appointed John Collier as Commissioner of Indian Affairs in 1933.

Collier felt that, rather than working for the immediate integration of Indians into American society, which was the avowed aim of United States policy since 1887, the integrity of the tribe should be supported. He believed in the concept of local community organization and supported the tribal leaders, even to the point of allocating resources through them rather than to individuals. He, as well as others, argued that the "clan instinct" was dominant among Indians and that tribal operation of assets was a more natural way of administering property than the traditional American concept of private property. He believed that it was only through the tribal system that the Indians could develop self-reliance.[12] The result of his efforts and the recommendations of the Meriam survey was the Wheeler Howard Act of 1934, better known as the Indian Reorganization Act. The Act was an admission that assimilation of the Indian was still far off, although assimilation remained the policy of the United States.

Since the retirement of Collier in 1945, the official policy of the various governmental agencies dealing with Indians has tended to vacillate between one that supports the cultural integrity of the tribal unit and one that encourages integration of Indians into the mainstream of American life. Actually, there are problems inherent in both points of view, as evidenced by similar arguments that took place in black communities over black separatism and the preservation of the ghetto culture versus integration. The older policy of encouraging integration sounds reasonable to most Americans, but it tended to place a low value on Indian culture and threw the Indian on to the marketplace ill-equipped to deal with the demands of American life. White officials often treated traditional Indian values and customs with disdain, so the values did not survive well away from the reservation. The result was not only to erect a barrier to effective communication between the Indian and the non-Indian but also in the process to foster feelings of inferiority among the Indians. In effect, assimilation proved demoralizing to the vast majority of Indians.

The difficulty with preserving the cultural integrity of the tribal unit, however, is simply that reservation life in modern American society is an anomaly that makes surviving difficult for the Indian. There is no way to earn an adequate living on most reservations.

Unemployment rates as high as 33 percent are not uncommon, and among some tribes the only employed persons are those who work for a governmental agency or for the tribe itself. Even on those reservations with high employment, underemployment is the norm. Farming on most reservations is at best marginal, if partly because so many reservations were selected by the government because of their poor soil and lack of water. It is estimated that less than 7 percent of all Indian-held land is suitable for farming.[13] Yet, reservations are much too crowded to sustain a hunting or food-gathering economy. Under the tribal policy, the individual who decides to leave the reservation must face the fact that the government's policy is to support the tribal unit instead of the individual. This means that the Indian must not only leave behind family and friends, but also his or her share of community-owned property. Moreover, the various governmental assistance programs for Indians, including health services, are available only to reservation residents. Since the tribal way of life among most of the Indian cultures is a communal one that stresses cooperation rather than competition, the nonreservation Indian is also faced with a whole set of capitalistic norms, which tends to make moving from the reservation even more traumatic.

HEALTH AND HEALTH SERVICES

Nowhere are the difficulties of American policy toward the Indians more evident than in the delivery of health services. Although Americans tended to discourage and denigrate the Indian medicine man and herbalist, these two were usually the only "medical professionals" available to the Indian until this century. Occasionally, civilian or military physicians visited reservations to give medical care, but it was not until 1908 that the Bureau of Indian Affairs appointed the first Chief Medical Supervisor. More effective concern was demonstrated in 1910, when Congress appropriated funds to combat the spread of trachoma, an infectious granular conjunctivitis that causes eye damage and even blindness when it is allowed to progress to a chronic state. Trachoma is rarely seen among affluent populations, although it is still endemic in large parts of the Near East and Orient, as well as in other areas where poverty and lack of facilities for personal hygiene exist. A survey of Indians made after Congress appropriated the money disclosed that 23 percent of the reservation population had trachoma, with the highest incidence among Oklahoma Indians; 69 percent of the people examined had symptoms of the disease. Also showing a high rate of infection were the children in the off-reservation boarding schools,[14] another sign of the difficulties inherent in American policies toward the Indians. Trachoma remained a serious health problem among Indians until the advent of the sulfonamides, but even then its eradication was slowed by the lack of adequate health care. Today, the disease is regarded as under control on the reservations, although the residual eye damage left by the earlier ravages of the disease is still reflected in the high rates of blindness among the older Indian population.

The findings of trachoma among Indians proved shocking to authorities, and adding further fuel to demand for a change was a survey by the Marine Hospital Health Service in 1913, which revealed the appalling health conditions under which the Indians lived, including the lack of even minimal types of medical care.[15] However, making findings and acting effectively to deal with them are two different things. Change came only gradually. In 1924, a health division was created within the Bureau of Indian Affairs, and in that same year Public Health nurses were officially hired. By 1939, however, there were still only 110 Public Health nurses in the service. Dental services had been inaugurated in 1913, but by 1925 there were only seven traveling dentists to cover all the reservations. District medical officers were appointed in 1926 and officers of the Public Health Service Commissioned Corps were detailed to the Indian Bureau, but never in very large numbers. The investigation of Indian affairs commenced by Lewis Meriam in 1926 found Indian health conditions little improved over what they had been in th 1913 report.[16] Many of those active in Health Service felt that the best solution was to transfer the health program to the Public Health Service. Agitation for such a transfer had begun as early as 1919, but this was not finally accomplished until the enactment legislation was passed in 1954. Actual transfer took place in 1955, and this has proven to be an extremely important step in upgrading health services. As part of the transfer program, the Public Health Service made a comprehensive survey of Indian health problems. The report stated that, though the government had long been interested in health services for Indians,

> ...the American Indian is still the victim of an appalling amount of sickness. The health facilities are either non-existent in some areas, or for the most part obsolescent and in need of repair; personnel housing is lacking or inadequate; workloads have been such as to test the patience and endurance of professional staff. This all points to a gross lack of resources equal to the present load of sickness and accumulated neglect.[17]

One of the groups most deficient in health services in 1955 was the Alaskan natives, a category that included not only the Indians of the southern coastal regions and the interior but the Eskimos farther north and the Aleuts who lived in the Aleutian islands as well as on the coast of Alaska. Neither of these last two groups are Indians, but the problem of the Alaskan natives emphasized the problems that the Indians had. Though the vast distances and the hostile climate in Alaska impose great difficulties, the report pointed out that in 1954 there were only 600 beds available for patients in the six hospitals that admitted natives, even though there were 2,452 new tuberculosis cases reported in that year in addition to all other types of illness requiring hospitalization.[18]

With the incorporation of Indian health services into the Public Health Service, appropriations for Indian medical care expanded rapidly. Observers of the Congressional scene, as well as the supporters of the transfer, believed that a major reason for the increase in funds was that Congress no longer had to appropriate money specifically for Indian health services, an act that apparently still had considerable political opposition. Instead, Congress could appropriate funds for general public health; therefore, the section on Indian health did not receive the same hostile scrutiny and publicity that a separate appropriation would. Whatever the cause, the appropriations rose from $35 million in 1956,[19] to $109 million in 1969,[20] and they continue to rise. By 1970, the Indian Health Service was operating 51 hospitals, 77 health centers, and more than 300 health stations and field clinics, and it had contracted with various state and community health facilities to serve 410,000 individuals on some 250 reservations or native villages (as is the case with Alaskan natives).[21] The number served has since risen, along with the number of facilities both on reservations and under contract.[22]

Compare this to the situation when Elinor D. Gregg began nursing on a South Dakota reservation in 1922. She was the only graduate nurse for some 6,000 Indians, and she and one physician cared for the health needs of the Indians, including a 20-bed hospital. When she went to the reservation, tuberculosis was the major cause of death, but, because hospital facilities were limited and Indian custom opposed the isolation of patients, tuberculosis was almost totally ignored by people in authority. Instead, she reported, the general theory was that, in any case, most "Indians would ultimately die of epidemic diseases," whether tuberculosis, measles, or whooping cough.[23]

In 1924, Gregg became the first Supervisor of the new Public Health Nursing department in the Medical Division of the Indian

Bureau. In this capacity, she traveled around the country. Though she was generally impressed with the dedication of the nurses and physicians, she found working conditions almost intolerable. One of her visits was to the Navaho reservation at Fort Defiance in New Mexico, where there was a 40-bed hospital.

> The day I visited, there was a conglomeration of cases in the women's ward that shocked my nursing sensibilities. A delirious woman lay on a mattress on the floor because she was afraid of bedsteads. She had an open abcess over the spine, so wide and deep that the vertebrae was laid bare. There was a mother and a baby, the mother with puerperal insanity, and in the far corner was a child with diptheria. Two children with pneumonia following measles were there as well as a newly delivered mother and baby, a typhoid fever case, and a tubercular meningitis baby.[24]

In retrospect, the improvements in Indian health care have been remarkable, but great needs still remain. For example, a 1980 report by the University of Nevada team set up to encourage health careers among the 10,000 Indians on Nevada tribal rolls recounted the success of their three-week preceptorship summer course designed to encourage American Indians and others to enter the field of Indian health care. Though the teams were somewhat successful in this endeavor, the report included a statement that the screening clinics in many of the Nevada Indian communities were the only time during the year that health services were provided on the reservation.[25]

Even the best health care delivery system, however, cannot fully overcome the long-term effects of poverty and malnutrition and the stress of rapid social change. In 1979, life expectancy for Indians was estimated at 65.1, which meant that the death rate of Indians was as high or higher than that of any other minority ethnic group.[26] For notifiable diseases, such as amebic and bacillary dysentery, gonorrhea, hepatitis, measles, mumps, syphilis, tuberculosis, the incidence for native Americans is much higher than for any other group in the United States.[27] However, the nature of improvement can be seen in such things as the infant mortality rate, which fell from 62.5 per 1,000 in 1955, to 32.2 in 1967, to 20.1 in 1971, much lower than the black infant death rate.[28]

The death rate reflects not only the conditions of poverty but also the stress on the cultural group. For example, fatal accidents are significantly higher among Indians than among other groups, and this disproportion has tended to increase rather than decrease.

Though the accident statistics reflect such factors as unsafe vehicles, poor housing, and unsafe working conditions, they also indicate a much more serious problem, the difficulty Indians have in adjusting to a dominant culture different from their own. Further evidence of this problem comes from the suicide rate, the homicide rate, and deaths from cirrhosis of the liver, all of which are more common among reservation Indians than among other Americans, sometimes as much as four times as common.[29]

In sociological terms, the Indians might be described as living under the conditions of *anomie,* a concept developed by Emile Durkheim at the beginning of this century. Though Durkheim made his generalizations on the basis of rapid social changes created by industrialization, they could also apply to any society undergoing rapid social change that causes old norms to lose their saliency without their being immediately replaced with functional new rules. According to Durkheim, during this period of adjustment, people are either so unsure of themselves or so torn between conflicting sets of norms that social pathology such as suicide is common.[30]

Reasons for feelings of *anomie* can be illustrated by the classical case of Ishi, a Yahi Indian from northern California. Following the California gold rush of 1849, the Yahi had come into such conflict with settlers in the area around Mount Lassen that, by the end of the nineteenth century, it was believed that all the Yahi had been killed by vigilantes and ranchers. In 1911, however, a Yahi survivor, a wild-looking terrified man of about fifty years of age, was found near the town of Oroville. Starving and exhausted, he had come down from the hills to give himself up, expecting to be killed by whites, a fate he had prepared for by burning his hair off close to his head, a sign of mourning. Instead of being killed, the man was taken up by anthropologists at the University of California, where he lived until he died in 1916. Since he would not tell anyone his name, he came to be known as Ishi, "man," in his language. The story of Ishi was not fully told until 1960, when Theodora Kroeber, the wife of the distinguished anthropologist A. L. Kroeber, wrote down the experiences of herself and her husband with Ishi.[31] As the story was reconstructed, Ishi had been one of only twelve Yahi left in 1870, after a massacre had killed more than 60 people. The twelve had taken to hiding in the hills, but by 1894 only five persons remained alive, and they survived by hunting, fishing, and raiding cabins. In 1909, settlers tracked and raided the camp of the surviving Yahi. Only Ishi and his mother survived the raid and she soon died. Alone and minus his supplies, tools, and weapons, which the raiders had taken as souvenirs, Ishi lived in the hills, hungry and grieving, until in desperation he surrendered. Understandably, vast numbers of Indians felt overwhelmed by the technologically superior American society.

All kinds of stressors come into play when two competing populations, different in outlook and technologically unequal encounter each other. The extent of stress imposed by the conflicting life-styles is not always predictable, if only because it varies from group to group. Anthropologists have developed various terms to describe the types and degrees of contact between two life-styles, which are helpful in trying to understand the differences in Indian adjustment, since stresses vary according to the nature of contact. One type of contact is called *diffusion*, the process of a people borrowing an idea or a piece of equipment or a type of food from another people and incorporating it into their way of life. People often borrow attractive or prestigious traits without acquiring the resources to minimize the health risks. To take a non-Indian example, some of the tribespeople of New Guinea adopted the blankets and fitted clothing of the Westerners but not the custom of washing or cleaning them. This gave a new home to the mites that caused scabies since they thrived in these garments. The initial result of contact with the Western life-style was greater health problems for the New Guinea tribespeople than existed before.

Another type of contact is termed *acculturation*. This implies intense and continuous contact between two previously autonomous cultural traditions, with extensive changes in one or both systems. Large numbers of Indians have become acculturated, but the exchange has usually been one-sided. *Assimilation*, a third type of contact, occurs when one group changes so completely that it becomes fully integrated into the dominant society or when two groups merge into a new cultural system. Most immigrants to the United States have eventually assimilated into American society; other than the fact that our last names are often recognizably Italian or Polish or German or Japanese, for example, we have more in common as Americans than we have with the countries or peoples from which we come.

When racial or class barriers to assimilation deter total changes in life-style, or when people become disillusioned and frustrated in their attempt to accommodate to a powerful foreign culture, an effective coping mechanism has been to revitalize old systems in slightly new forms. In fact, this can be a stage in the assimilation process, since at each level of contact and acculturation some individuals look to traditional ritual or political mechanisms to regain a sense of control, to revitalize their culture, and to attempt to restore

equilibrium. A classic example of this is the Peyote ceremony incorporated into the Native American Church, which enabled many Indians, particularly those associated with the Great Plains tribes, to
retain much of their old culture although in a new form (i.e., one
more acceptable to American culture).[32] It seems particularly important in any process of cultural exchange that the less technologically
efficient culture is not entirely submerged. In a positive sense, the
rise of Indian consciousness, an assertion by Indians that their own
heritage is something about which they can be proud, should result
in a more effective health care delivery system, since the Indians
will not only be the recipients but will have an effective voice in its
planning and a significant role in its delivery.

Examining the concept of anomie in relation to the different
types of cultural contact, it seems clear why the extent of anomie
varies from group to group. Many Indians, including most of those
who still live east of the Mississippi River, had already accepted
European customs before the advent of the reservation era so tht
their time of greatest trauma was behind them. But in some of the
western tribes, the problem of transition remains acute. Some individuals, particularly the older Indians, are still well-adjusted to the
old traditions, but others, particularly young adults, are caught in
an identity crisis, unable to find a satisfactory life-style either as
traditionally oriented Indians or as members of the mainstream of
American society.[33] If they stay on the reservation, they are caught
in a crippling web of poverty, unemployment, and dependency on
welfare. If they leave the reservation to find employment, the available jobs are often seasonal, low-paying, or hazardous; in the case of
forest-fire fighting, which the western tribesmen perform, it is all
three. The feelings of ambivalence and hopelessness that follow
from this seemingly impossible situation are expressed in various
other ways besides suicide.[34] Although most Indian children now get
some education, the drop-out rate is so high that few Indians
achieve the level of education necessary for skilled employment in
today's world.[35]

Traditionally, alcoholism has been a severe problem among Indians, and, for long periods in Americn history, it was against the law
to sell alcohol to Indians. The 1953 repeal of this prohibition was an
important reform in that it removed one more vestige of white pater-
nalism, but this did not by any means solve the drinking problem.[36]
Either because of a carry-over from the time when drinking was
forbidden and alcohol was consumed rapidly to avoid apprehension,
or because alcohol helps drown one's problems, large numbers of
Indians still consume liquor so rapidly and in such great quantity

that drunkenness inevitably follows. The inebriated Indians are then killed by trains, automobiles, or even by their companions.[37] If they survive their drinking bout, they are often thrown into jail where they can easily develop pneumonia; if they survive this crisis as well, large numbers ultimately die of cirrhosis of the liver.

Another health problem that continues to plague the Indians is tuberculosis. In the 1913 health survey, it was found that only the relatively assimilated Indian populations of New York and Michigan had low tuberculosis rates. On the western reservations, it was not unusual to find 20 percent of a tribe afflicted, and, among the Paiutes of the Pyramid Lake Region in Nevada, some 33 percent had the disease. Since this survey was made before such diagnostic tools as x-ray or the tuberculin tests were available and depended only upon a physical examination, the true incidence may well have been higher than the figures reported.[38] In spite of the advances made in recent years, the mortality rate for tuberculosis is still several times as high for Indians as for the general population. When the age-adjusted rate was used to compensate for the relatively youthful age of the Indian population (because of the lower longevity rates), the tuberculosis rate in 1969 was found to be eight times as high as that of the general population.[39] Because tuberculosis has been such a serious menace to Indian survival, there were some experts in the early part of the twentieth century who believed that Indians had some special genetic susceptibility to the disease. This idea has now been discarded and current research suggests that the high incidence is more closely related to poverty and inadequate living conditions than to other factors.[40]

Among the Navaho, the largest of the modern Indian tribes, tuberculosis was a major cause of death and suffering until the last few years. It is estimated that, in the period following World War II, tuberculosis in some form or another affected one out of every ten Navahos. The situation was so bad that mobile case findings and roentgenographic surveys were abandoned, because there were not enough facilities available to hospitalize the known cases. When Isoniazid was developed in 1952, the early field trials of the drug were undertaken on the reservation simply because there were so many cases regarded as medically hopeless. Physicians from Cornell University treated 30 cases of miliary tuberculosis, a form considered fatal because infection is rapidly spread throughout the body via the bloodstream. Some 28 of the patients were saved, which meant that, if the drug could cure such severe cases, it would be even more effective against other forms of tuberculosis.

Elsewhere in this book, we have criticized the tendency of members of the medical establishment to use either poverty-stricken or minority populations as testing grounds to perfect individual skills or try out new therapies that are later used on middle-class patients. The experimental use of Isoniazid should be differentiated from this type of experimentation since, while the Navahos were the research subjects, they were also among the worst sufferers from the disease and the follow-through treatment was concentrated on the very group that most needed it, the Indians themselves. It is not drug experimentation that we condemn, but the use of subjects who as a group do not receive any major benefits from the experimentation.

With the development of Isoniazid and similar drugs, the technology was available for the control of tuberculosis. The entrance of the Public Health Service into the field after 1955 made the necessary medical services available, and within a few years the disease was brought to its present level of control. The fact that tuberculosis still remains such a serious problem seems to emphasize again that adequate medical care cannot solve all the problems and that low socioeconomic status and cultural and geographic barriers still act as effective deterrents to good health.

Both poverty and geographic barriers also seem to be implicated in the infant mortality resulting for the most part from pneumonia or diarrhea. Infant diarrhea can usually be treated successfully, if steps are taken soon enough to restore the fluid and electrolyte balance. The physical isolation of many reservation residents and the uncertain condition of their vehicles often cause the family to put off the trip to the hospital until it is too late. Moreover, crowded living quarters and lack of sanitation help communicable diseases to spread, and an inadequate diet predisposes to illness. If the Indian population is to be a healthy one, problems associated with poverty and isolation must be solved.

INDIAN MEDICAL TRADITIONS

Elinor D. Gregg, whose book about her work among the Indians has been mentioned earlier in this chapter, describes briefly the efforts of the Indian office under John Collier to teach professionals working with Indians about Indian culture by sending them to meetings of the American Anthropological Association in 1934.[41] The late date of official concern about indigenous customs and beliefs by those professionals dealing with Indians every day only serves to accentuate the accumulated barriers to bringing effective health care to the American Indians.

The problem is further complicated by the fact that Indian folk beliefs about health are as varied as the number of Indian groupings, and there are over 300 tribal groupings in the United States, each with its own language, religion, folkways, mores, and patterns of interpersonal relationships. What proves effective among one group of Indians might not be so effective among another group.[42] Generally, however, before contact with Western medical and health practices, the Indian tended to attribute the inexplicable ailments that beset mankind to the anger of the gods or malevolent spirits. Medicine as such was not only a herb or a drug, but also some supernatural article or agency that might aid in curing a disease. Most tribes usually had special persons known as medicine men, who were organized into societies in some tribes and practiced as individuals in others.

Among the Navahos, the most populous of American tribes, the so-called "hand trembler" is an important person. He receives his name from the fact that the diagnosis is made through the intervention of the deities, who take over the diagnostician's hand as he draws a picture interpreting the cause of illness. When the drawing is completed, the hand trembler informs the patient what his or her diagnosis is and recommends the action to correct the situation. Standard treatments include medications, sweat baths, bedrest, isolation, diet, exercise, and other types of therapy common to good nursing and medical practice everywhere, although the nature of such treatment is given a peculiarly Navaho flavor. Contemporary Navahos often combine both the traditional tribal medicine and modern medicine. For example, a Navaho who is acutely injured in an automobile accident will go to a hospital, but a patient scheduled for delicate surgery may first go to a medicine man for a treatment to ensure the success of the impending surgery.[43] Even in the hospital, there are often rituals associated with illness that might be carried out. For example, a grandmother might sprinkle cornmeal around an ill child's bed, and, though in some instances a family member might allow the cornmeal to be removed instantly, in other instances it should be left for a longer period of time. Whatever the circumstances, the cornmeal should be preserved when it is swept up.

Many Indian patients possess an item that they believe has special curative powers. In a hospital setting, this item might be hung on the bed or placed on the bedside stand. Sometimes the patient insists on wearing it. Usually, such items consist of herbs or mixtures in a small cloth bag. Some of the contents are pungently odoriferous. The *American Journal of Nursing* reported a case where nurses, acutely aware that just such a bag had an offensive odor, removed it and the necklace to which it was attached from the patient's body, before a family visit was scheduled, and placed it away from the bedside, along with other personal items. When family members visited, the elderly patient told them of the incident. Believing that breaking such a tribal taboo by the nurses would cause the death of the patient, the distraught relatives confronted the nurse, who chided them for thinking such a "silly" thing. Silly though it might have been, the patient became critically ill within a few hours and died within a few days.[44] Whether the woman would have died is beside the point. Both the patient and the family believed she would not have died if the nurse had been acculturated to Indian beliefs.

Like most Indians, the Indians of the Southwest are family oriented, so the sick patient is often visited by vast numbers of people. To have many relatives come to the hospital is both comforting and important to the Indian patient and visitation rules are difficult to enforce. Another difficulty, or at least apparent difficulty, in dealing with Indian health is that so few American Indians are future oriented. This is a general problem with most people of low socioeconomic status and inevitably leads to frustration among professionals in the health care delivery system. The problem for the professional is to fit the preventive practice into the rituals and customs of the various Indian groups that are believed to ensure good health. The sprinkling of cornmeal mentioned above could be tied in with more effective preventive measures, and so perhaps could the use of the charm bag. However, fitting these traditional customs into effective preventive health care is difficult. To these statements, a caution should be added: namely, that not all Indians are the same, not even members of the same tribe. They range from individuals uneducated in Anglo ways, poor, speaking their own language almost exclusively, to persons well-educated in both their own and Anglo cultures. The health professional has to judge where on the continuum of sophistication the patient is located.[45]

The point to emphasize is that the two systems, tribal and traditional versus modern American and scientific, need not be antagonistic. It simply takes a sophisticated health care professional to overcome the barriers. The task probably would be easier if there were more Indian health professionals, but until recently almost all such individuals were hired at the lowest levels of the health care hierarchy. In fact, until anthropologists were finally able to convince the professionals in the Indian service of the importance of the Indian medicine man, medical workers opposed traditional health practices; such opposition served only to make the Indians suspicious of the white health worker and discouraged many from trying to enter the field.

Even as recently as 1945, the medicine man among the Navaho had a preferred status over the physician, and, if there was a conflict between the two, scientific medicine lost out. Among the Pueblo Indians, the councils often still retain control over day-to-day actions to the extent that permission must be granted by the Council before a mother can allow a public health official to inoculate a child. Recognition of the importance of Indian customs by modern health workers has cut down some of the hostility between the Indian and Western medicine systems, and this hostility has further decreased, as more effective attempts have been made to use Indians in more creative ways as health educators, home health aides, and other types of health workers. Still, as late as 1972, there were only 42 American physicians, 500 nurses, 5 dentists, 4 Ph.D. social scientists, and 5 Ph.D. physical scientists among those classified as *Indian* by the census.[46] Since that time, more Indians have entered the professions, but the best bet for rapid improvement from our perspective would be to upgrade the most numerous group, nurses, into nurse practitioners. On the western reservations, where the great distances and the isolation of the people work against effective health care, the nurse practitioner or, alternatively, the physician's assistant seems to be the most effective type of health worker, particularly if they have strong roots among the people. It should be added that, if the Indian is to care for himself, health workers of all types have to be encouraged to set their sights at becoming professional, a task complicated by the fact that, until recently, many of the professional schools barred Indians from admission. Obviously, there will be a shortage of indigenous health workers for a long time.

Non-Indians also have an important role in improving health care but primarily for those able to see things from an Indian perspective as well as their own. For example, among the Navaho, the crucial factor in changing long-term suspicion into favorable support has been the success of Western medicine in treating tuberculosis. Until this happened, Western medicine was only able to offer palliative therapy, which was not too different or any more effective than what the medicine man could offer; besides, the medicine man kept the person at home instead of sending him or her to the hospital to die. In fact, Western medicine found itself in a circuitous web. Indians often turned to Western medicine only when the medicine man had given up on treatment, and then the sick Indian was taken to a hospital where he or she did indeed die. It was only when Indians could see that Western medicine was actually doing some good that they began to believe it had some merit. Now, although the medicine man is still important, he is considered an alternative or religious approach to healing that does not preclude the use of Western therapy.[47]

Though the Indian health seems to be getting better today, it is still too early to indicate that problems are really under control. Much of the advance in the 1960s and early 1970s was due to the fact that young physicians took the Indian Health Service as an alternative to the Armed Forces in the medical draft. This tended to increase the number of physicians available, even though many of them lacked the necessary skills to accomplish what was needed. As draft calls receded, the number of available physicians also receded, and the Public Health Service now must rely more and more on indigenous professionals. Even if they are successful and have the funds to carry through, there will be difficulty, because the Indians are so widely dispersed—at least in the western states—that a physician who works among the Indians is able to accomplish much less than a physician would in a more concentrated urban center.[48]

Decreases in Indian mortality figures are also dependent upon decreasing malnutrition, improving sanitation, and raising the level of employment. Health care in itself is not enough. Obviously, the Indians of today are much better off than they were just a few years ago, at least as far as general health standards are concerned, but they still have a long way to go to meet the standards of the more affluent Americans. Cultural conflict is still a problem, and the anomie and feelings of hopelessness created by this conflict are still evident. In the long run, the only effective way to overcome the remaining health problems is to deal with base causes, starting with the problem of poverty.

REFERENCES

1. Forbes, J. D. (Ed.). The Indian in America's Past. Englewood Cliffs, N.J.: Prentice Hall, 1964, pp. 3–4.
2. See the testimony of Leonard M. Hill, Sacramento Area Director, Bureau of Indian Affairs, as reported in the Progress Report to the Legislature by the Senate Interim Committee on Indian Affairs. Sacramento: California State Senate, 1955, pp. 241–242, 407–408.
3. Josephy, Jr., A. M. The Indian Heritage of America. New York: Alfred A. Knopf, 1969, pp. 359–360. U.S. Bureau of Census. Statistical Abstract of the United States, 1979. Washington, D.C.: U.S. Government Printing Office, 1979, pp. 35–36.

4. Crosby, A. W. The Columbian Exchange: Biological and Cultural Consequences of 1492. Westport, Conn.: Greenwood Publishing, 1972, p. 37.

5. See: Bullough, V. & Bullough, B. Sin, Sickness, and Sanity. New York: New American Library, 1977, pp. 140–148.

6. Hagan, W. T. American Indians. Chicago: University of Chicago, 1961, p. 13.

7. Ibid., p. 121.

8. See: Jackson, H. M. H. A Century of Dishonor (new edition edited by A. F. Rolle). Reprinted, New York: Harper and Row, 1965.

9. Hagan. op. cit., p. 146.

10. Ibid., pp. 134–135.

11. Fey, H. E. & McNickle, D. Indians and Other Americans: Two Ways of Life. New York: Harper & Brothers, 1959, p. 195.

12. Hagan. op. cit., p. 156.

13. Health Service for American Indians. Prepared by the Office of Surgeon General, U.S. Department of Health, Education, and Welfare, Public Health Service Publication No. 531. Washington, D.C.: U.S. Government Printing Office, 1957, p. 28.

14. Ibid., Appendix C, pp. 261–262.

15. Kraus, B. S. Indian Health in Arizona. Tucson: University of Arizona Press, 1954, p. 4.

16. For a summary of the report, see: Health Service for American Indians. Appendix C., Report II, pp. 264–269.

17. Ibid., p. vii.

18. Division of Indian Health, Program Analysis and Special Studies Branch. Eskimos, Indians and Aleuts of Alaska. Part of U.S. Department of Health, Education, and Welfare Report on Indians on Federal Reservations. Washington, D.C.: U.S. Government Printing Office, 1963, pp. 7–8.

19. Health Service for American Indians. p. 98.

20. Indian Health Service. To the First Americans: The Third Annual Report on the Indian Health Program of the U.S. Public Health Service. Washington, D.C.: U.S. Government Printing Office, 1969, p. 13.

21. U.S. Department of Health, Education, and Welfare. Nursing Careers Among the American Indians. Public Health Service, 1970, p. 1.

22. U.S. Division of Indian Health. Indians on Federal Reservations in the United States, Phoenix Area: Arizona, California, Nevada, Utah. U.S. Department of Health, Education, and Welfare, Public Health Service Publication No. 615, Part 6 (January 1961), p. 32.

23. Gregg, E. D. The Indians and the Nurse. Norman, Oklahoma: University of Oklahoma Press, 1965, passim. The quotation is from p. 38.

24. Ibid., p. 104.

25. Baldwin, Jr., D. C., Baldwin, M. A., Edinberg, M. A., & Rowley, B. D. A Model for Recruitment and Service—the University of Nevada's Summer Preceptorships in Indian Communities. Public Health Reports, 1980, 95, 19–22.

26. Senator & Mrs. Fred R. Harris. Indian Health. In Sources: A Blue Cross Report of Health Problems of the Poor. Chicago: Blue Cross Association, 1968, pp. 38–43. This article gave a figure of 63.5 for 1965. The 1979 figure represents the best estimate of the U.S. Office of Indian Affairs and is based upon data from the 25 states with the largest Indian population (personal communication).

27. Minority Health Chart Book. Prepared for the 102nd Annual Meeting of the American Public Health Association by the APA staff, under USPHS/DHEW, Contract No. HRA 106–174, p. 59.28.

28. Ibid., p. 36. Indian Health Services. Trends and Services, 1969 Edition. U.S. Department of Health, Education, and Welfare. Washington D.C.: U.S. Government Printing Office, 1969, p. 8.

29. Trends and Services, p. 25. Minority Health Chart Book, p. 29. See also: Indian Health Service. Suicide Among the American Indians. U.S. Public Health Service Publication No. 1903. Washington, D.C.: U.S. Government Printing Office, 1967. Health Problems of U.S. and North American Indian Populations. N.Y.: MSS Information Corp., 1972.

30. Durkheim, E. Suicide: A Study in Sociology. Translated from the French by J. A. Spaulding & G. Simpson. Glencoe, Ill.: The Free Press, 1951.

31. Kroeber, T. Ishi in Two Worlds. Berkeley: University of California Press, 1961.

32. For a discussion of these concepts in a health setting, see: McElroy, A. & Townsend, P. K. Medical Anthropology in Ecological Perspective. North Scituate, Mass.: Duxbury Press, 1979, pp. 334–338, & passim.

33. Bongarts, R. Who Am I? The Indian Sickness. *The Nation* (April 27, 1970), pp. 496–498.

34. Suicide Among the American Indians. Public Health Service Publication No. 1903. Washington, D.C.: U.S. Government Printing Office, 1969.

35. Aurbach, H. A. The Status of American Indian Education. University Park: Pennsylvania State University, 1970. Bryde, J. F. The Indian Student: A Study of Scholastic Failure and Personality Conflict. Second edition, Pine Ridge, S.D.: n.p., 1970. Peterson, S. A. How Well are Indian Children Educated? Washington, D.C.: U.S. Indian Service, 1948. See also: U.S. Congress, Report of Senate Special Subcommittee on Indian Education. Indian Education: A National Tragedy, A National Challenge. Washington, D.C.: U.S. Government Printing Office, 1969.

36. Adair, J., & Deuschle, K. W. The People's Health: Medicine and Anthropology in a Navaho Community. New York: Appleton, 1970. Also, Harris. op. cit.

37. Personal communication from Pamela Brink, based upon her studies of Paiute Reservation life.

38. Health Service for American Indians. Appendix C, p. 262.

39. Trends and Services. 1969 edition, pp. 16–18.

40. Townsend, J. G. Indian Health—Past, Present, and Future. In O. La-

Farge (Ed.), The Changing Indian. Norman, Oklahoma: University of Oklahoma Press, 1942, pp. 28–41.

41. Gregg. op. cit., pp. 142–44.
42. See: Stone, E. Medicine Among the American Indians. Reprinted New York: Hafner Publishing Company, 1962. Vogel, V. American Indian Medicine. Norman, Oklahoma: University of Oklahoma Press, 1970.
43. Joe, J., Gallerito, C. & Pino, J. Cultural Health Traditions: American Indian Perspectives. In M. F. Branch & P. P. Paxton (Eds), Providing Safe Nursing Care for Ethnic People of Color. New York: Appleton 1976, pp. 87–88.
44. Primeaux, M. Caring for the Indian Patient. *American Journal of Nursing*, 1977, 77, 91–96.
45. Kniep-Hardy, M. & Burkhardt, M. A. Nursing the Navajo. *American Journal of Nursing*, 1977, 77, 95–96.
46. Wood, R. American Indian and Health. Ethnicity and Health Care. New York: National League for Nursing, 1976, pp. 29–35.
47. Adair, J. & Deuschle, K. W. op. cit., pp. 1–13, 21.
48. See Public Health Reports. Cited above.

6

New Immigrants and Old Traditions

In recent years, the term *transcultural nursing*, originated by Madeline Leininger, has called attention to the cultural variables that are crucial but often overlooked aspects of patient care.[1] The term should not be restricted to nursing but should be expanded to include all aspects of health care.

There are at least three crucial elements in successful transcultural health care. The first is a basic knowledge about the culture of the patient. This book attempts to supply some of that knowledge, although no book can replace listening to the patient and having him or her tell about customs and beliefs. Moreover, talking to the patient is more personal and far more interesting, and it helps involve the patient in making decisions.

The second element involved is an individual assessment of the patient from the cultural standpoint. The health care provider needs to know not only that the patient is Mexican American or Indian but also whether he or she is first, second, or third generation, since the mix of old and new varies by generation. There are also great individual differences among persons in minority cultures, just as there are in the mainstream Anglo culture. Many Mexican Americans have gone to college and hold highly sophisticated jobs. Obviously, they have different attitudes than the uneducated new undocumented alien. To treat one in the same way as the other is an insult.

116

The third element in successful transcultural health care is to apply the broad knowledge base and the individual assessment to the health care problems at hand. A treatment strategy congruent with the patient's own beliefs simply has a better chance of success. Deeply engrained cultural beliefs about the efficacy of herbal teas in the curative process have to be taken into account rather than repressed. Dehydration can be cured with tea as well as with coca cola. Medication with tea may be as efficacious as medication with water. For some people, prayer may work better than surgery alone, while any attempt to utilize prayer on others would be laughed at. The important point to be incorporated into health care knowledge is that treatments that violate strongly held beliefs should not be carried out without coming to terms with those beliefs. The consideration of the cultural variable is crucial.

So far, three major ethnic/racial groupings have been examined: Blacks, Spanish-speaking Americans, and Indians. Although these are the largest minority group members and the most significant in terms of health care, the United States is an extremely diversified country and is becoming more polyglot each year. Though everyone in the United States is descended from immigrants—even the Indians—there have been periods of greater or lesser restriction on the number and source of immigrants. Vast numbers still want to come to the United States and, to date, four million people apply every year. During the 1970s, an average of one million people per year entered this country, at least one-third of them illegally.

The motivations for coming to the United States remain much the same as they always were. The Irish came in 1845 to 1849 because the potato blight caused mass starvation in Ireland just as the Haitians came to the United States in 1980 because they were also threatened with starvation. Germans came in great numbers as a result of the political fallout after the failure of the German Revolution of 1848, and large numbers of today's immigrants also are here because of political difficulties in their homeland. Undoubtedly, the majority come, as they always have, because they regard the United States as the land of opportunity. Whatever the reason, they come almost in flood tides and, during the Congressional hearings on the problems of Cuban and Haitian refugees in 1980, Texas Congressman Sam Hall, Jr., plaintively demanded to know, "How long is this country going to be the recipient of people from all over the earth? . . . When is this going to end?"[2]

As long as they continue to come, the immigrants will pose new types of challenges for health care, although these challenges vary from area to area. Today's immigrants, as did yesterday's, often settle initially where other immigrants from their country have settled. Increasing numbers of Arab-speaking peoples have settled in the Detroit area; there is a large Samoan community near Long Beach, California; a "Korea town" exists not far from City Hall in Los Angeles; a Tai Dam community from North Vietnam in Des Moines, Iowa; Hmong tribesmen from Laos in Selma, Alabama; Cubans in Miami, Florida; Armenians in Fresno, California; Jamaicans and Trinidadians in New York City; French Canadians in Maine, Vermont, and throughout New England; Ukranians in Chicago; Poles in Buffalo; and Iranians everywhere. In fiscal year 1980, the State Department estimated that the United States had received 168,000 refugees from Indochina (Vietnam, Laos, Cambodia), 117,000 from Cuba, 50,000 from the Soviet Union and Eastern Europe, and 15,000 from other areas. In addition, there were the regular immigrants who come under quota, some 272,600 every year, no more than 20,000 from any one country, chosen according to a system of preferences based on family connections and job skills. There is still a third category, close relatives of U.S citizens who are admitted without quota, and these numbered 125,000 in 1978. Yearly summaries differ but, in 1978, the result was an official admission through one of these categories of 92,367 immigrants from Mexico, 88,543 from Vietnam, 37,216 from the Philippines, 29,754 from Cuba, 39,288 from Korea, 21,315 from Taiwan, 20,753 from India, 19,458 from the Dominican Republic, 19,265 from Jamaica, 14,245 from the United Kingdom (England, Scotland, Wales, and Northern Ireland), and lesser amounts from other countries.[3] Some immigrants adjust better than others, but even the best qualified have severe obstacles to overcome.

Many of the immigrants from the Philippines, Korea, Taiwan, and elsewhere are nurses, admitted because of their special job skills, and recruited by West coast hospitals where there is a nursing shortage. The nurses work on temporary licenses until they have passed their state board examinations, but significant numbers never pass, in part because of the language difficulties. They work under considerable pressure since, once settled, the nurses serve as key persons for bringing other members of their families to the U.S. Similarly, large numbers of interns come into this country under the same job skill opening from all parts of the world. Often, these new immigrants take the examinations for licensure several times, and in recent years there have been several major cheating scandals involving various foreign trained professionals, as they grow more and more desperate in their effort to pass the examinations. At the same time, there is also growing pressure to abolish the exams as culturally biased, which they are, but since these foreign trained practitioners are essentially treating Americans, members of some state boards of nursing argued they need to be able to deal with American ways of thinking. As the failure rate rose, there was a demand for a screening test for immigrants in the professional groups before they could be recruited. Screening has tended to cut down some of the more unqualified. As the stricter entry standards are applied, the pass rate will probably begin to match that enjoyed by American trained professionals. To meet these rising U.S. standards, many foreign nursing schools are teaching from U.S. texts, even giving courses in U.S. law, diet, and so forth.

The nurse and physician professionals who immigrate usually have jobs awaiting them when they arrive. Other immigrants are not so lucky, although the type of support they receive varies from group to group. Even people with considerable organized support have difficulty, as the 70,000 Russians of Jewish background who have immigrated to the United States since 1969 would demonstrate. In a sense, these are a highly selected group of immigrants, skilled in a trade or profession, but the Russian ways they were accustomed to differ from those in the United States. As *Newsweek* reported in 1980:

> Russians exult in their new freedom, but it is hard for them to get the knack of independence. They have never learned to look for jobs and apartments on their own. . . . Most of the Russians eventually find work here, but it often is a struggle. They have no concept of upward mobility. So they will turn down a job if they suspect it isn't as good as the one they held in Russia; once a cabdriver, always a cabdriver is their experience. To the Americans who work with them, they seem hypersensitive to class and status. Immigrants who were professionals in Russia often expect to receive bigger living allowances than manual workers.[4]

In any immigrant group, children, adolescents, and young adults are the most rapidly socialized, but this adds to the problems of adjustment for many of the adults. They complain that the young do not know their place, that they do not respect the old customs, that everything is out of control. Almost every parent says this, but the problem is far more exaggerated for the new immigrants. Americans television and schooling are very assimilating experiences, and the influence of both are all pervasive, particularly on the young.

HEALTH CARE

In spite of the fact that this is the last part of the twentieth century, immigrants face many of the same kinds of health problems that earlier generations of immigrants did. First, large numbers come from radically different cultural settings, with radically different notions of what constitutes sickness and health. Second, even if there is not this kind of health barrier, there is usually a language barrier, with communication carried out through an interpreter. Without an interpreter, care can only be minimal and restricted to emergency situations. Third, problems arise from the different diets of the immirants. Kim Chi is a standard of Korean diet, but to the non-Korean it might seem as an odoriferous mess of spoiled cabbage. Fourth, vast differences in life-style exist, including such things as child rearing, response to illness and stress, and any number of similar aspects of life. Fifth, different genetic inheritances cause problems; for example, some Orientals have the same kind of lactose intolerance as many black Americans, and certain populations have greater susceptibility to certain diseases. The listing could go on. Obviously, the most effective health care takes into account the cultural and genetic background of the patient. Customs of some of the new immigrant groups are discussed in this chapter.

CHINESE TRADITION

Many immigrants from Indochina, China, and Japan have been deeply influenced by Chinese concepts of health and medicine, just as Western-oriented people have been influenced by Greek, Roman, or medieval concepts in their attitudes. The essential principles of Chinese medicine were laid down several thousand years ago, based upon the concept of yin and yang. *Yang* represents the male, positive energy in nature that produces light, warmth, and fullness. *Yin* represents the female, negative energy in nature, the force of darkness, cold, and emptiness. The inside of the body is yin; the surface of the body is yang; the front part of the body is yin, the back is yang; yin is in the liver, heart, spleen, lungs, and kidneys; yang is in the gallbladder, stomach, large intestine, small intestine, and the *warmer*, a term difficult to define but interpreted by some modern scholars as the lymphathic system.[5]

The diseases of the winter and spring are localized in the yin area, those of summer and fall in the yang. The pulse is controlled by both yin and yang, although yin wants to turn inside and yang seeks to thrust outside. The aura of the yang nourishes the mind, simultaneously influencing the muscles. If it does not succeed in opening and closing the pores properly, coldness sets in, swelling occurs, ulcers penetrate into the flesh, the blood vessels are weakened, and the patient is full of anxiety and fears. If the aura in the blood vessels is not brought into harmony with the condition of the flesh, ulcers and tumors result, perspiration is inhibited, the body begins to waste away, and the *hollow points* (the terms used in acupuncture) close up. Eventually, the patient dies from this overaccumulation. The solution is to relieve the compression. Conversely, if the yin essence becomes too strong, the patient perspires incessantly and appears nervous and apprehensive. In time, if nothing is done the patient becomes rebellious and dies of overloading.

Those who do not achieve a balance between yin and yang in their own bodies die; only when the yin and yang auras are sound and sane, living in peaceful interaction, can the body and mind be in proper order and life go on. Thus, the key to good health is keeping the body in a balance. One way of doing so is to use the hollow points for acupuncture, which requires skill and ability. There are nine needles, each with a specific purpose, and 365 points on the skin to which acupuncture can be applied. Acupuncture is regarded as a cold treatment and is used mainly in diseases where there is an excess of yang; when there is an excess of yin, moxibustion is performed. This involves heating pulverized wormwood and applying this concoction over certain specific meridians, the network extending out from the hollow points of the skin where acupuncture is performed. Herbs are also important in Chinese medicine. One of the most valuable herbs in the Chinese pharmacology is ginseng root, which is supposed to be harvested at midnight during a full moon.[6]

In recent years, the concepts of traditional Chinese medicine have been overlaid with ideas and practices drawn from Western medicine. Still, the Chinese, both in China and elsewhere, retain much of the traditional ideas and practices. For example, acupuncture is still believed to have therapeutic value and, since the 1970s, there has been considerable experimentation with it as a pain reliever in the West. Some aspects of Western medicine have been more effectively incorporated into Chinese practices than others; this means that certain accepted Western medical practices are more likely to upset both the new immigrants and the older, less sophisticated residents who retain much of the old customs of China or Japan or elsewhere. Since Chinese traditional medicine avoids such intrusive techniques as drawing of blood, and a diagnosis is usually made without the kind of workup involved in Western medicine, many immigrants are often reluctant to undergo the intrusive surgical and diagnostic procedures.[7]

TRADITIONS OF INDIA

Another alternative medical system was brought over by the Hindus and other immigrants from India, 20,000 of whom arrived in 1978. Generally, the Indian immigrants are better educated and have long been accustomed to speaking English, compared with the Vietnam or other Indochina refugees. English control of India, which ended only after World War II, also gave India a strong base for Western medicine. Still, as any traveler to India will note, there are many indigenous medical practitioners and some of their ideas have also influenced immigrants to the United States. Traditional Indian medicine relies heavily upon a wide ranging pharmacopeia. Ingredients for remedies come from almost every natural substance available, and mastery of these substances' medicinal properties is the key to an effective medical practitioner.

Taste is an important part of the treatment, since each taste is also believed to have special properties; sweet increases phlegm, appeases hunger and thirst, and causes flatulence, worms, and goiter; acid increases salivation and appetite, improves digestion, and causes heartburn; salt purifies the blood and stimulates digestion, but in excess gives headache and causes convulsions; pungent provokes the appetite and lessens corpulence; bitter stimulates the appetite and clears the complexion; astringent augments the action of any of the above, if taken with them. Within each of these categories, there are also hot and cold, heavy and light, sticky and dry, energizing and sluggish, stationary and fluid, soft and hard, clear and slimy, smooth and rough, coarse and subtle, and dense and liquid qualities that have special effect. Hindus regard the cow as sacred so they do not eat beef. Vast numbers are vegetarians. Inevitably, the study of medicines is more important than the study of diseases, and the traditional healer deals with symptoms and ignores the disease.[8]

One Hindu group that has received great attention in the United States is not so much an immigrant group but a religious one to which native Americans have converted. The Society for Krishna Consciousness has prosletyzed heavily among college groups, and, in almost every American city in the United States, they can be seen chanting, dancing, and swaying to the drumbeat of their mantra.

The founder of the U.S. sect of Krishna Consciousness was Swami A. C. Bhak-Bhaktivendanta, who arrived in the United States in 1965 at the age of 70. Bhaktivendanta demanded that his followers observe four rules of conduct: (1) no eating of meat, fish, or eggs; (2) no illicit sex; (3) no intoxicants; and (4) no gambling. Krishna Consciousness teaches that the body is ruled by passion and the soul by serentiy; therefore, an attempt should be made to liberate the soul from the body (by chanting "Hare Krishna"). Krishna liberation is a liberation from oneself, and this attitude can obviously bar a person from acknowledging that a health problem exists. Krishna life-style is strictly regulated, with certain things being done at certain times, and illness should not interfere with these activities. Krishna devotees do seek professional health care when they feel they are truly ill; however, even in the hospital, they try to keep up their chanting, devotions, and ablutions, and some of this is not understood by the health professional unaccustomed to such activities and unprepared for them.

ISLAMIC TRADITION

Traditional Islamic medicine is more like Western medicine than either Hindu or Chinese medicine, since the Muslims, like the Europeans, looked to the Greek writers for their sources. In fact, much of the surviving knowledge of Greek medicine came to us through Arabic editions, and Islamic writers, such as Avicenna, were utilized as basic medical texts in Western medical schools until almost the beginning of the nineteenth century. Arab immigrants to the United States are both Muslim and Christian. Lebanese and Syrian Christians are spread throughout the United States, and there are Coptic (Egyptian Christian) communities in Los Angeles, Washington, D.C., New York City, and other places. Christian Arabs share the same religious holidays and dietary customs with Greek and other Eastern Orthodox Christians, although they have different patriarchs (or popes) and their services are in different languages. But, some of their attitudes toward illness and health are Arabic, much the same as their Muslim countrymen.

As a group, Muslims, whether Arab or non-Arab, have more in common with Orthodox Jews than with Orthodox Christians. For example, Muslims are opposed to eating pork and have many of the same dietary restrictions that Jews do. In addition, alcohol is forbidden, except for medicinal purposes. Like some of the unsophisticated Jews, the Arab Muslims believe in the existence of the evil eye.

Unsophisticated Arab parents often keep their children encrusted with filth so that they will not attract the attention of the evil eye. Stating publicly, as health professionals might do, that a particular Arab child is a beautiful child, is inviting the attention of the evil eye and almost putting a curse upon the child. A child cannot be too dirty or ragged, however, because evil spirits, called *Jinn* (hence, the Genie of Aladdin's lamp), are attracted to the ill, the weak, and the aged and cause illness, sickness, and accidents.

To help overcome the evil spirits and fight off illness, the Muslim often recites passages from the Koran and calls out *bismillah a-rahman a-rahim* ("In the name of God the merciful, the compassionate") for help. Charms are also used to ward off the evil eye or evil spirits, and health professionals have to be careful not to lose them. Though these customs complicate health care, Muslims also are interested in health care and are more willing to seek preventive care than some other immigrant groups. Many Muslim customs, such as ritual cleaning and bathing and taking preventive measures to ward off evil spirits, help counteract some roadblocks raised by the problem of the evil eye or evil spirits.[9]

Although there are many immigrants from Islamic countries, probably the most ubiquitous Muslim group in U.S. society is that founded by the black American, Elijah Muhammad. For a time, this movement was separate from the mainstream of Islam and was instead a black supremacist, anti-white group.[10] After the death of Elijah Muhammad, the black Muslims entered more into the mainstream of Islam and, in recent years, have sought to recruit whites as well as blacks to their membership. A particularly difficult time for many Muslims is the month-long fast associated with Ramadam, and, since the Muslims use a lunar rather than a solar calendar, the fast is not at the same time every year. No food or drink is to be taken from sunup to sundown. In the summer, such abstenance is difficult and can cause dehydration. Although the sick, the aged, and the very young are exempted from the fast, many patients in hospitals try to observe the tenets of their religion, and the professional has to be prepared to deal with this. Sometimes a religious official from a particular Islamic sect can help the patient to adjust to his or her condition.

FILIPINO-AMERICAN TRADITION

The Filipino heritage is diversified. Based primarily upon Malayan culture, it has been influenced by Chinese, Arabic, Indian, Spanish, and American beliefs and represents a combination of different traditions—from the sophisticated beliefs of the health practitioner who comes to the United States to the traditional health notions of the less sophisticated immigrant. For the less sophisticated, belief in supernatural causes of disease is widespread, and individuals protect themselves from this by talismans, amulets, and prayer, or resort to folk healers.

Underlying Filipino-American folk beliefs are three basic concepts: flushing, heating, and protection. Flushing keeps the body free from debris; heating maintains a balanced internal temperature, and protection guards the body from outside influences. Flushing is more than simple purging of the body, since it also involves rubbing the skin with lemons, the special care taken during menstruation, and the limitation of activites after giving birth. For example, women are not supposed to read after giving birth because it will strain their eyes and, if they persist, cause them to go blind. Heat involves not only local application but rubbing and massage. Protection is providing a gatekeeping system against the invasion of both natural and supernatural forces into the body.[11]

Even immigrants well-adjusted to Western medicine, like the Filipinos, carry a set of traditional attitudes with them that affect their outlook on health care. People from Oriental cultural backgrounds are often silent and compliant, but this does not mean that they are not in pain. Patients with Middle Eastern backgrounds often vocalize their pain, punctuating any conversation with a kind of moaning that is distracting until one becomes accustomed to it. Often, they moan not so much to indicate pain as to express the fact that they feel poorly; this is permissible and encouraged in many Middle Eastern cultures. Undoubtedly, the range of responses in the new immigrant patient is similar to the variety of responses encountered in a traditional patient mix, with the stoic at one extreme, who not only suffers silently but refuses to ask for medication or relief, to the chronic complainer at the other extreme, who complains at every opportunity and makes the members of the health care team miserable because there seems to be no basic reason for the complaint.[12]

GYPSY TRADITION

Some cultural groups pose particular health-care problems. One such group, found in all parts of the United States, is the gypsies. Gypsies came to the United States primarily in the period before

World War I, but as a general rule they have remained far less integrated than other groups that arrived at the same time. Just who should be counted as a gypsy is debatable, but a working definition might be a person or group that accepts nomadism as a way of life; follows one or more of the traditional gypsy occupations, such as fortune telling, music and other entertainment, animal healing, metal work, begging and poaching, and doctoring, both medical and magical; and usually speaks the Romany language of the gypsy. As a group, gypsies have a characteristic tribal structure, with four main tribes and extended family groups in each tribe called "vitsas." Each "vitsa," ranging in size from 25 to 50 people, has a chief or king whose responsibilities include directing the people's economic opportunities, hiring lawyers to represent them, and protecting their interests economically, politically, and socially.

Gypsy culture traces the source of disease to demons, the evil eye, breaking taboos, and the fear of disease itself. Cutting one's fingernails on Tuesday or Friday is unlucky and might cause illness. Many gypsy treatments involve symbolic transference of disease to another person or object. Like many of the other groups in the poverty culture, the gypsy attitude towards health care seems different, depending on the nature of the crisis. Generally, gypsies turn to the hospitals and Western medicine for a crisis; when serious illness does strike, they demand the best specialists and are willing to pay any price. Preventive and follow-up care is not used very much. When a gypsy is hospitalized, the entire tribe descends upon a hospital, since they believe the sick individual needs much support to become well and the number of relatives present indicates the amount of support the individual is receiving. Medicine is for curing, not preventing disease, so serious problems such as diabetes or high blood pressure go undetected until far advanced. Two other characteristics seem to give health care professionals some difficulty. Gypsies generally have a high degree of vanity about their personal appearance, particularly facial features, and are reluctant, for example, to use eye glasses or hearing aids, which detract from their concept of what constitutes a good appearance. There is also a great deal of modesty about the female genitalia (but not about breasts). Women are extremely reluctant to expose themselves to male health professionals. Most gypsies carry amulets or other protection against the evil eye. Early in her career as a nurse, one of the authors of this book accidentally lost a medal attached to a gypsy infant and, in the ensuing uproar, learned an early lesson in the importance of transcultural health care: gypsies believe special precautions have to be taken with children. For example, one of the more common methods of offering protection against the evil eye is to tie a red string around the wrist of the child. Removing that, even accidentally, might in gypsy eyes endanger the child.

Gypsies often detest official records and are reluctant to identify themselves as gypsies or give information to non-gypsies. They often use assumed names and may not give truthful answers to non-gypsies, in order to protect their anonymity and culture. However, once they find a health professional they can trust, they rely upon that person for all kinds of service. A recent researcher on gypsies summed up their attitudes in the following quotation:

> He is a strange man, this modern Gypsy, so basically honest that he would not even steal a box of matches, yet he exists to beat the system which is out to beat him; a chameleon, master linguist, Jekyll and Hyde character, half occidental and half oriental. You know nothing about him, he knows much about you. Always on the prowl, he looks for that one loophole in the staid and super sophisticated society around him that will enable him to make a fast buck. . . . He is invisible and has many weapons. You have one name but he has two; one you will never know and one he is always changing. . . . one day soon he will hit the jackpot and be off to another city with his family, while you remain, as you will always remain, as a part of that monument to the time when your ancestors and his, once united, came to the crossroads of human evolution. Yours chose to give up their personal freedom while his retained their freedom as nomads.[13]

RELIGION

Probably the dominant factor influencing the health care beliefs of vast numbers of native-born Americans is not their ethnic background or their racial composition but their religious beliefs. In spite of the pluralistic and secular nature of much of U.S. society, religion is a crucial part in patient well-being. When most hospitals were run under religious auspices, the religious support system was conspicuously present, sometimes overwhelmingly so in the eyes of the non-believer or the atheistic and humanistic minority (which also needs consideration). As the cost of hospital care has escalated, religious hospitals have been secularized; though many still have a nominal religious sponsorship, their religious roots are not always so apparent.

This increasing secularization of health care has thrown those patients who look to religion as a source of comfort in the face of pain, illness, or death at the mercy of the health professionals. And for many, religion is all important, much more so than the health professionals. For example, a 1979 study of breast cancer patients by Connie Bertholf found that, in her sample of 139, prayer was a major coping mechanism for 20 percent of the group.[14] Though chaplains are affiliated with most hospitals, the diversity of American religious beliefs makes it impossible for any one professional person to satisfy the needs of all the hospitalized patients. Thus, the health professional, particularly the nurse, has to make certain that patients have the quiet time they might need for prayer; it is also up to the nurse to find a member of the proper clergy, if a patient expresses a need. Many religious groups believe and teach that special spiritual assistance is necessary during illness. Some groups, such as the Greek Orthodox and the Roman Catholics, give Holy Communion to those who desire it; some, such as the Lutherans, Mormons, and Roman Catholics, believe in a special anointing of the sick. Many Baptist groups practice the "laying on of hands," as do Armenians, Christians, Nazarenes, and others.

Many religious people wear special symbols of their religion. Mentioned earlier in this chapter was the gypsy child's special relic that caused trouble to one of the authors of this book, but this custom is not confined to gypsies. Many Catholics insist upon taking a special saint's medal into the operating room with them. People of various Orthodox Christian groups feel it is important to wear a cross. Mormons wear a special undergarment that a few insist on wearing in the hospital, and some, when being given a bath, desperately try to keep a portion of it at least touching their body. A few insist on keeping an arm or a leg in their garments when they go to surgery.

Religious beliefs are also an important factor in diets, perhaps even more important than ethnic origins. For example, Mormons will not drink coffee or tea; Seventh Day Adventists not only abstain from coffee and tea but are often vegetarians, as are other large segments of the American population. Orthodox Jews, as well as many who belong to Conservative temples, insist upon kosher food. Keeping kosher implies not only avoiding pork, pork products, and shellfish but also in not mixing meat and milk products, killing animals in a special way, and even using special methods of preparation. Many Jews who are members of Reform congregations or who belong to no organized Jewish group at all find it difficult to eat pork. As indicated above, Muslims also refuse to eat pork. Many religious groups advocate special diets during the year. Most Christian groups do some fasting during Lent, while Muslims fast from sunup to sundown during Ramadam.

Though hospitals rarely schedule surgery on such traditional holidays as Christmas or New Years, they often ignore the religious needs of their patients for surgical or diagnostic procedures. For example, Orthodox Jews observe the Sabbath from sundown Friday to sundown Saturday, while Muslims worship on Fridays, and most Christians on Sunday. Members of these groups often resist surgical procedures on these days, except in cases of emergency. Religious beliefs also affect how both the professional and the patient look upon such things as abortion (Catholics oppose), contraceptives and family planning, autopsies (Orthodox Jews oppose), blood transfusions (Jehovah's Witnesses oppose), circumcision (in the case of Orthodox Jews, to be done by the Rabbi on the eighth day, and opposed by other religious groups). Death and dying is also a time when religion enters the picture. Among most Orthodox Jews, the human remains are ritually washed by the family or specifically designated members, and burial takes place as soon as possible, usually the same day. Muslims have a carefully prescribed procedure for washing and shrouding the dead, similar in many respects to that of the Jews. No body part should be removed and the final ritual should be performed by relatives or friends. Buddhists often engage in chanting at the patient's bedside soon after death has been announced. With Hindus, the priest ties a thread around the neck or wrist to signify a blessing, the family then washes the body, and it is cremated. Among the Parsi (Zoroastrians), the dead person is neither buried nor cremated but left exposed for the elements and the birds to dispose of. Last rites are administered by Catholics, Episcopalians, various Orthodox Christian churches, the Armenian Church, and others. Some allow last rites to be given by a lay person, even a nonmember, while others insist that they be given by a cleric.

Another area where religious practices influence patient care is in childbirth. For Roman Catholics, infant baptism is mandatory and especially urgent if the prognosis is not favorable. According to Catholic dogma, baptism can be given by any person, even a non-Christian, providing the person is motivated by a desire to help the patient. When there is not time to call a priest and no Catholic is present, the infant (or even an aborted fetus) should be baptized by sprinkling water upon it and repeating, "I baptize thee in the name of the Father, the Son, and the Holy Ghost." Orthodox churches also believe in infant baptism but wait until the infant is slightly older and then baptize by immersion. Sometimes an "air" baptism is allowed. Episcopalians have much the same attitude as Catholics on infant baptism, but aborted fetuses and stillborns are not baptized. Other religious groups are opposed to infant baptism and would be upset if a nurse or other health professional attempted to baptize an infant.

Some religious groups have strong traditions of folk medicine. A good example of this is the Old Order Amish, most of whom live in Pennsylvania, Ohio, and Indiana. They are descended from sixteenth-century Anabaptists who emigrated to the United States in the eighteenth century. Their religion is heavily based upon the Bible. For example, their clothes have no buttons because buttons are not mentioned in the Bible, they also refuse to drive automobiles because automobiles were invented after the time of Jesus. The Amish rules of discipline also prevent members from securing higher education; thus, they have no physicians among their members. As far as medicine is concerned, the Amish adopt a sort of dual path. For critical, incapacitating illnesses, such as appendicitis, infections, and broken bones, scientific modes of healing are accepted. For chronic, noninca-pacitating malfunctions or for treatments not responding to scientific modes of healing, the Amish turn to folk treatments. Folk medicine includes both natural cures, such as herbs, plants, minerals, and animal substances, and occult elements, such as charms and seeking supernatural forms of support.

A common practice among the Amish is *Brauche* or *Braucherei,* a German term that can best be translated as "sympathy healing." In English, the word has often been rendered as powwowing because of its similarity to some of the practices of the Indian medicine man. *Brauche* is usually performed by one of the older Amish members, and the patient does not always need to be present when the incantations are performed, but he or she must believe in the practice in order to experience healing. During the *Brauche,* certain verses or charms are repeated silently. It is performed for hemorrhaging, toothache, burns, scalds, the common cold, bed wetting, mortification, sores in the mouth, and warts. It is also used to treat "livergrown" in infants, which is believed to be caused by too sudden exposure to the outside atmosphere or being shaken up by a buggy drive. The symptoms are similar to what is usually diagnosed as colic.[15]

While the Old Order Amish supplement the physician with their folk beliefs, some religious groups are more actively opposed to modern medical practices. For example, Christian Scientists deny the existence of health crises. Sickness, sin, and death are errors of the human mind that can be eliminated by altering thoughts; drugs and medicine are not needed. Since Christian Science leaves the ultimate decision of health care up to the individual, there is disagreement among members about whether to go to the hospital. Some members refuse all medical treatments, while others, in times of great pain or stress, will turn to the hospital or other institutions. Often, those who do seek scientific medicine feel guilt and anguish over their failure to cure themselves, a psychological state that has to be taken into account by the health professional. Generally, Christian Scientists do not use drugs or blood transfusions, accept vaccines only when required to do so by law, and do not seek biopsies or have physical examinations. When they need spiritual and mental reinforcement for problems that the medical community would call "illness," they turn to Christian Science practitioners.

Unorthodox practitioners are more common among some religious groups than others. Chiropractors, naturopaths, and spiritualists are used by differing groups, and some of these unorthodox healers, such as chiropractors and Christian Science practitioners, are recognized by insurance agencies as well as by Medicare and Medicaid.[16]

In sum, health care is more than simply a knowledge of the physical causes of a disease, it also requires a knowledge of the sociological, psychological, cultural, and historical setting from which the patient comes. Because the United States is so diverse, this remains a major task for the American health care professional.

REFERENCES

1. Leininger, M. M. Nursing and Anthropology: Two Worlds to Blend. New York: Wiley, 1970.
2. *Newsweek*, July 7, 1980, p. 24.
3. Ibid., pp. 24–30.
4. Ibid., p. 30.
5. For a discussion of the warmer, see: Hübotter, F. Chinesisch-Tibetische Pharmakologie. Ulm, Germany: K. F. Haug, 1957. For a general discussion of Chinese medicine, see: Wallnöfer, H. & von Rottauscher, A. Chinese Folk Medicine (translated by M. Palmedo). New York: Crown Publishers, 1965, pp. 10–12. Needham, J. assisted by W. Ling. Science and Civilization in China, Vol. 2. Cambridge, England: University Press, 1956, passim. One of the key sources is: Veith, I. (Ed.). The Yellow Emperor's Classic of Internal Medicine. Berkeley: University of California Press, 1972.
6. Wallnöfer and von Rottauscher. op. cit., passim. Mann, F. Acupuncture: The Ancient Chinese Art of Healing. New York: Vintage Books, 1972. Leong, L. Acupuncture. New York: Signet, 1974. For a general listing of herbs, see: Shih-Chen, L. Chinese Medicinal Herbs. (translated by F. P. Smith & G. A. Stuart) San Francisco: Georgetown Press, 1973.
7. See: Li, F. P. et al. Health Care for the Chinese Community in Boston. *American Journal of Public Health*, April 1972, pp. 536–537.

8. A good outline of Hindu medical beliefs can be found in Walker, B. The Hindu World: An Encyclopedic Survey of Hinduism, 2 vols. New York: Praeger, 1968, II, pp. 56–58. References are included.

9. For a description of health care in an Arab community in the U.S., see: Chilungu, S. W. A Study of Health and Cultural Variants in an Industrial Community. Unpublished Ph.D. dissertation, State University of New York, Buffalo, 1974.

10. See: Lincoln, C. E. The Black Muslims in America. Boston: Beacon Press, 1961.

11. For example, see: McKenzie, J. L. & Chrisman, N. J. Healing Herbs, Gods, and Magic: Folk Beliefs Among Filipino-Americans. Nursing Outlook, 1977, 25, 326–329.

12. For example, see some of the research on reaction to pain: Blaylock, J. (Ed.). The Psychological and Cultural Influences on the Reaction to Pain. Nursing Forum, VII, No. 3, 1968. Zborowski, M. Cultural Components in Responses to Pain. Journal of Social Issues, August 1952, pp. 21–25. Davitz, L. J. Sameshima, Y. Davitz, J. Suffering as Viewed in Six Different Cultures. American Journal of Nursing, 1976, 76, 1296–1297.

13. Lee, R. The Gypsies in Canada—An Ethnological Study. Journal of the Gypsy Lore Society, 1967, 66, 38–51, and 1968, 67, pp. 12–28. The quotation is from p. 38. There is a vast literature on gypsy beliefs and health customs. Hand, W. D. Passing Through: Folk Medical Magic and Symbolism. Proceedings of the American Philosophical Society, 1968, 112, 379–401. Anderson, G. & Tighe, B. Gypsy Culture and Health Care. American Journal of Nursing, 1973, 73, 282–285. Nemeth, D. J. Nomad Gypsies in Los Angeles: Patterns of Livelihood. Unpublished master's thesis, San Fernando Valley State College, Northridge, 1970. Vesey, B. & Fitzgerald, F. Gypsy Medicine. Journal of the Gypsy Lore Society, 1944, 23, 21–33. Clebert, J. The Gypsies. Baltimore: Penguin Books, 1963. Boles, D. & Boles, J. The Gypsies' Doctor in Georgia. Journal of the Gypsy Lore Society, 1959, 38, 55–63.

14. Berthol, C. Prayer as a Coping Mechanism Among Mastectomy Patients. Unpublished master's thesis, California State University, Long Beach, California, 1979.

15. Hostetler, J. A. Folk Medicine and Sympath Healing Among the Amish. In W. D. Hand (Ed.). American Folk Medicine: A Symposium. Berkeley-Los Angeles: University of California Press, 1976, pp. 249–258.

16. Much of this is based upon our own personal experiences. A helpful chart is included in Spector, R. Cultural Diversity in Health and Illness. New York: Appleton-Century-Crofts, 1979, pp. 114–123. The chart was taken from Nursing Update, July 1975. However, we should add that our own observations and research do not always agree with those on the chart. We believe there is a wider divergence than is indicated on the chart among differing segments of the religious community in the U.S. Also helpful are the various publications of W. D. Hand, whose collection of healing practices is cited above.

7

Poverty and Hunger Transcend Racial Lines

Generally, Americans assume that only members of minority groups are likely to be poor. Many people, even those from poverty backgrounds, do not seem to realize the extent of poverty in the United States or its implications for the health of the nation. The president of a Los Angeles area chapter of the National Association for the Advancement of Colored People, a sincere and thoughtful man, stated:

> I really do not understand how a white person can be poor. In the town I grew up in the whites had everything. They went to the brick school and they owned all of the stores. They lived in the best houses and had all the advantages. It seems impossible that a white person would be poor unless he is lazy or stupid.

For this reason, if for no other, it seems essential to state that in twentieth-century United States, it is still possible to be white and poor without being lazy or stupid. Poverty transcends racial lines.

White poverty exists for many of the same reasons that it exists among the various nonwhite minority groups: insufficient education, lack of employment opportunities or chances for advancement, too many children, poor geographic location, age, as well as the cycle of poverty itself, which creates feelings of powerlessness and hopelessness and makes success difficult.

Poverty too often can be a way of life, something that Oscar Lewis described as the "culture of poverty." For Lewis, a *culture* implies a pattern of beliefs, feeling, and behavior, all of which are interdependent. By combining the concept of culture with that of poverty, he wanted to emphasize that there is a life-style often associated with long-term impoverishment that makes adjustment to hardship possible. Once established, it is difficult to overcome. Lewis wrote that

> ... poverty in modern nations is not only a statement of economic deprivation, of disorganization or of the absence of something. It is also something positive in the sense that it has a structure, a rationale and defense mechanism without which the poor could hardly carry on. In short, it is a way of life, remarkably stable and persistent, passed down from generation to generation along family lines. The culture of poverty has its own modalities and destructive social and psychological consequences.[1]

Understanding the existence of a culture of poverty leads to the realization that overcoming poverty is not a simple matter of giving the poor more short-term economic opportunities. Instead, it is a long hard process, since it takes years to break down the suspicions and hostilities inherent in generations of poverty. Whether the United States is willing to devote the long-term commitment of resources to overcome poverty is not always clear, since the short-term results are so easy to criticize. A good example of this was the proclamation of President Lyndon B. Johnson in 1964 of a war on poverty. Johnson went on the rather naive assumption that a nation that could forge new frontiers in outer space ought to be able to deal with serious domestic problems such as poverty. The key to the Johnson War on Poverty was federal planning and a new symphony of programs orchestrated to solve the problems of the poor. The result of the Johnson programs, which were in part dismantled by President Richard M. Nixon, was not the harmonious cooperation envisioned by Johnson but a cacaphony of conflicting soloists. Both supporters of the poverty program and more hostile critics found much to criticize. There were also successes. In 1974, a decade after the war on poverty had been declared, the Institute for Research on Poverty sponsored a conference to evaluate the success of the poverty program. Conference speakers concluded that, among the great successes of the program, was Medicare and Medicaid. When combined with more effective health care delivery, these programs helped bring about some of the improvements in the U.S health picture demonstrated by the statistics presented in various sections of this book. Another success of the War on Poverty was the effort to make legal services available to the poor. On the other hand, one major failure of the War on Poverty was the inability to increase the incomes of the poor from other than governmental sources.[2]

More debatable was the claim by the conference participants that the War on Poverty had increased the political participation of previously excluded citizens. This was a critical factor, since it was regarded as a key to overcoming the alienation so debilitating to those caught in the culture of poverty. Alienation is a concept developed by social scientists to describe several different values. Melvin Seeman, a sociologist active in formulating theories of alienation, listed five related attitudes: powerlessness, meaninglessness, normlessness, social isolation, and self-estrangement.[3] By encouraging the support of the poor in planning and organization, it was hoped that they would begin to feel a sense of power that would help propel them from the poverty cycle. However, this was not necessarily the case. Probably the most devastating criticism of this aspect of the poverty program came from Daniel P. Moynihan, one of the Johnson administration officials involved in drafting the poverty legislation, later an official in the Nixon administration, and, to date, a U.S. Senator from New York. Moynihan was particularly critical of the claim that the War on Poverty increased political participation through the development of inner-city community action agencies, a major element in involving the poor.[4]

By the end of 1966, the federal government had made more than 900 grants to establish or plan Community Action Programs (C.A.P.) in over 1,000 counties. All of the 50 largest cities were involved in such programs. Moynihan charged that the immediate beneficiaries of many of these programs were not the poor but the poverty professionals, many of them from minority groups, who were given executive, technical, and professional positions in the program. Saul Alinsky, one of the pioneer community organizers, put the matter more bluntly, saying that there was a "vast network of sergeants drawing general's pay" in the poverty program.[5]

These are rather harsh terms to describe the "poverty" professionals, but the essential problem was not so much the existence of this group, but that the programs were both too big and too small. They were far too large for unsophisticated managers to handle, especially when various organizing and competing groups fought for control, and far too small to accomplish what they were supposed to accomplish. Moynihan went even further to claim:

It may be that the poor are never "ready" to assume power in an advanced society; the exercise of power in an effective manner is an ability acquired through apprenticeship and seasoning. Thrust on an individual or a group, the results are often painful to observe, and when what in fact is conveyed is not power, but a kind of playacting at power, the results can be absurd. The device of holding elections among the poor to choose representatives for CAP governing boards made the program look absurd. The turnouts in effect declared that the poor weren't interested: in Philadelphia 2.7 percent; Los Angeles 0.7 percent; Boston 2.4 percent; Cleveland 4.2 percent; Kansas City, Mo., 5.0 percent.[6]

However, Moynihan might well have had a too simplistic notion of what to expect from the CAPs. He speculated that perhaps the CAPs did give rise to new leadership and, if the issue of blackness is separated from the problem of poverty, this is undoubtedly true. A 1977 survey of 210 elected black officials, mayors, aldermen, city councilmen and state representatives found that about 20 percent of the group had been involved with CAP in one way or another, many for nearly four years.[7] Though many might have been the sergeants doing the generals' jobs, as Alinsky charged, they did help create opportunities for blacks to gain leadership. Probably a lesser number of Mexican Americans also emerged in leadership positions. If any of these people who emerged from poverty continue to battle for the poverty stricken, the CAPs cannot entirely be labeled a failure.

Obviously, the War on Poverty was a failure in the sense that it did not eliminate poverty, but no time-limited program could. It did lessen the impact of poverty on large segments of society. The difficulty with Moynihan, as well as some of the less responsible critics of the federal poverty programs,[8] is the tendency to exaggerate. For example, Moynihan was highly critical of the "social science" upon which the community action program was based, but then, as he points out, it was not really based upon objective analytical studies but upon a few untested theories. The planners of the War on Poverty simply ignored all data and hypotheses that did not conform to their own. This led Moynihan to conclude that social science is at its weakest when it offers theories of individual or collective behavior that raise the possibility of bringing about mass behavioral change by controlling certain input. There is considerable truth in this generalization, but we think the problem was that the political process dictated certain approaches that were bound to fail. Unfortunately it is now entirely possible that both the effective and ineffective poverty programs will be dismantled during the decade of the eighties simply because they do not conform to the ideological stance of the administration in power. The problems of poverty will, however, remain or even worsen.

Poverty is not simply something that will be solved tomorrow. This multi-headed hydra is extremely difficult to combat and is not solvable by the same technical expertise that sent us to the moon. The easiest poverty group to deal with in terms of public programs, including health care, is the one whose poverty is short term, or seen as something to escape. This has been the vision of vast hordes of immigrants. Many people whose income was once adequate can fall below the poverty line in their later years, either because illness drains their resources or retirement causes a drop in their income. Even individuals able to save or invest during their most productive years experience difficulty, because inflation devalued their possessions and investments. There are also some aged persons who, though very much in need of assistance, are given no welfare aid. Through ignorance, some of these people have never applied; welfare departments do not usually seek out possible recipients. Others have attempted to get some assistance but were turned down because they could not prove their age or because they encountered some other technicality. However, the percent of old people in poverty levels is less than ever before, and the Johnson program and its successors have made the lot of the old person comparatively much better than that for the young. In spite of the increase in the number of people over 65, total numbers of those in poverty dropped from 35.2 million in 1959, to 24.6 million in 1970, to 14.1 million at the beginning of 1977, and the number is still dropping.[9] In 1966, two out of five households defined as consisting of one aged person or elderly couple fell below the poverty line, compared with one in seven in other types of households. In 1977, approximately one out of every seven persons over 65 was at or below the poverty level, compared with one out of every eight persons under 65.[10]

One of the reasons for the success in lessening the impact of poverty on the aged is that the programs for the aged cut across all social groups. Medicare is available to all people on Social Security, and Social Security is regarded not as welfare but as an earned right; thus, the aged poor are not put in the welfare class, although they are lumped with all old people. Being aged in our society still carries some stigma, but the fact that the aged are grouped together regardless of their previous social and economic background weakens some of the effects of alienation. Moreover, as a society, we expect older people to be somewhat more dependent either upon their families or upon social institutions than we do for those who are young adults or middle aged, so there is less stigma in looking for support. As a result, a significant portion of the aged population in the United States live at a much higher standard than they did when they were younger. Their major fear now is not so much economic as it is a physical assault, illness and disease, and the debilities associated with aging.

RURAL POOR

Poverty is both urban and rural. Based on percentages, the largest group of poor is found in rural America. In 1977, approximately 14 percent of the people in nonmetropolitan areas were classed as living below the poverty level, slightly under ten million. On the other hand, approximately 10.5 percent of the people in metropolitan areas were classed as living in poverty, approximately 15 million. The rural poor constitutes 40 percent of the nation's poor, although only about 27 percent of the total population is rural. Rural poor differ racially and ethnically from urban poor. In 1977, some 7,151,000 of the 9,861,000 rural poor classed as living at or below poverty levels were white, which means that, while the urban poor compose a mosaic of ethnic identities, the rural poor are predominantly poor white from old American families.[11]

One reason for such large numbers of rural poor is the technological changes that made their occupational skills worthless. In the twentieth century, perhaps the most revolutionary change has been in the nature of agriculture. Some statistics indicate the change. In 1822, it took 50 to 60 work hours to raise 20 bushels of wheat; by 1890, this total had dropped to 8 to 10; and by 1930, to 3 to 4 work hours. The rate has continued to drop until it takes fewer people to raise more wheat than ever before, both in percentages and in absolute numbers. In the United States, the number of farm workers continues to drop from 18.7 percent of the population in 1940, to 7.4 percent in 1960, to 3 percent in 1978. This percentage includes not only farmers and farm workers but also unpaid family workers.[12] During this time, the basic farm unit has changed from the small farmer or tenant farmer to the big business with specialized money crops. Those farmers who have survived the change have tremendous sums of money invested in equipment, land, and know-how.

While in the long run revolutions can be beneficial, they are usually brought about with tremendous human suffering. The agricultural revolution is no exception to the general rule, and, though many people have left farming voluntarily, many others have been forced off the land by depression, lack of investment capital, bankruptcy, and inability to make a living. Many still live on farms that are no longer viable economically, although they scratch out a living. Within the past half century, the small American farmer has led an ever more precarious existence, and vast numbers have left the farms. Since many of the farmers and farm workers were unskilled when they left the farm, they were eligible only for the lowest paying jobs in the cities. Some migrated great distances to find farm work. Large numbers of residents of Texas, Oklahoma, and Arkansas, whose economic plight was worsened by the "dust bowl" of the 1930s, migrated to California in search of jobs in the fruit and vegetable fields. As mentioned in an earlier chapter, John Steinbeck's *The Grapes of Wrath* painted a classic picture of this displaced group, as it slowly worked its way westward. Even today, more than half of the people born in such states as Arkansas no longer live there.

As the size of farms and the amount of equipment and investment necessary to operate them increases, farmers continue to face difficulties. The small farmer either has to expand radically to justify his investment in equipment or sell out to even larger owners. Some still hang on, trying to supplement their farm wages with a job in the nearby town, but such jobs are increasingly difficult to obtain, as the small town itself is hit by the changing nature of agriculture. Small-town merchants, businessmen, tradesmen, and others have perhaps undergone as radical a change as the farmer as the United States becomes increasingly urbanized. The extent of their dilemma is evidenced from the fact that most of the rural poor do not actually live on farms but in the small towns and villages. Job opportunities in the rural towns are scarce and becoming scarcer; eventually, many of these people will be forced to migrate to major metropolitan areas, without the grub stake that the sale of farm land might have given them. Unfortunately, large numbers of the rural poor are handicapped in seeking jobs when they do move to the city because of their low educational level, which, in 1968, averaged only about 8.8 years of schooling.[13] The educational level, has risen markedly since then but is still not up to urban standards.

Still another factor that has handicapped the farmer in the struggle against poverty is family size. Though it is true that high birth rates tend to correlate with low educational and income levels, there is also a cultural lag involved as far as rural Americans are concerned. Before the era of the mechanized farm, a large family was an economic asset, since so many hands were needed to carry out the work on the farm. Although the trend of birth rate is downward, rural families are still somewhat larger than urban ones.[14]

Rural poverty exists everywhere in the United States, but there are groups of people who face a more desperate situation than others, such as the residents of southern Appalachia, most of whom are white, the southern farmers outside Appalachia, many of whom are black, and the migrant farm workers throughout the country, who tend to have mixed ethnic identities. Although Mexican-American farm laborers are predominant in the western states, in other areas of the country this is not the case.

APPALACHIA

In terms of economic difficulties, one of the most troubled regions is southern Appalachia. This area can serve as a mirror for other troubled areas. Variously defined, it includes parts of Alabama, Georgia, Tennessee, North Carolina, Virginia, Kentucky, and West Virginia. Some surveys also include parts of Pennsylvania, Maryland, South Carolina, and New York, which are on the fringe of the area. However, the hard core covers 190 counties and is about 600 miles long and nearly 250 miles across at its widest point. It encompasses approximately 80,000 square miles and, in the 1960 census, contained 5,672,178 people. The region was identified as a problem area first in the 1930s, when the U.S. Department of Agriculture concluded that the area held the highest concentration of low-income farms in the country; moreover, the density of farm population was much greater than in the richest agricultural areas of the Middle West, but without any real major cash crop. Included in the Appalachian area, the Cumberland Plateau area stood out as the lowest income group in U.S. agriculture in the mid-1930s, with a gross income per farm inhabitant of less than $150 in most of the counties. Six counties had more than half their population on relief during the Depression. A study made in the 1930s concluded that 350,000 people should leave the region's agriculture, and that 60,000 should leave mining—this *before* the current radical changes in farming. In this region, through its public programs, the Depression actually raised living standards for many families who previously had lacked contact with the American standard of living. The region remained one with a high rate of relief and a low basis for economic security. Self-employment and a deficit of large-scale industry left many occupations uncovered by social security, thus placing a double burden on welfare agencies. In addition, residential requirements for aid, which have only recently been modified, served to immobilize many workers and their families in problem areas.[15]

Although Appalchia is now becoming less isolated and more industrialized than it once was, parts of the area still lag behind the rest of the nation. The small Appalachian farmers, perhaps the last of the "rugged individualists," live on subsistence farms that grow only a few staples, so they cannot afford to cut back production to benefit from the federal government's crop subsidies program. They need to plant all of their land in order to have enough yield to feed their families, yet the overuse of the soil has in the long run decreased that production, so their situation is a deteriorating one. The small coal mining enterprises also continue to fail. A decade or so ago, they failed because other types of fuel replaced coal; now, when there is increased demand for coal, the enterprises continue to fail because the small owners cannot raise the capital to modernize the mines. Because of this depressed economic situation, the residents of Appalachia receive more outside relief from government, church, and private agencies in proportion to their contribution than any other area of comparable size in the nation.[16] Complicating the poverty are the very factors that once helped survival in the region—a dogged independence, a suspicion of outsiders, and a low value for education—all of which now serve to perpetuate the poverty of the area. When Appalachians migrate to cities outside of the area, these same qualities often act as barriers to their success and acceptance in the urban environment.[17]

Still, migration seems to be one way of solving the area's problems. During the ten years between 1950 and 1960, the Southern Appalachia Region lost more than one million persons, a number equal to a fifth of the total population in 1950. As a result, the 1960 census revealed a population decrease in the region for the first time since the region was settled.[18] Population continues to decline, although not as rapidly. The problem is complicated by the fact that migrant population is made up primarily of young adults between 18 and 34 years of age; this means that the number of persons in dependent ages, particularly those under 15 and over 65, remain comparatively high. Adding to the problem is the fact that often the most ambitious people have left.

A good example is the case of Clean Eagle, West Virginia, which finally ceased to exist in 1980. When Clean Eagle was flourishing in the 1920s, it and similar company towns housed over 300,000 miners and their families. Though the mine that had given the town its name shut down early in the 1950s, many people remained in the town on land and in houses owned by the coal company. Tenants paid rent of $40 per month for four-room houses, many with no indoor toilets. Finally, in 1980, the land development company that bought the town decided it would cost more to repair the houses than to tear them down and get at the coal underlying the property with the new techniques that made mining once again feasible. When it finally closed down, most of those who remained were the old, the widowed, and the poor with large families.[19]

Migrants from the rural areas of Appalachia have gone to cities in the south, such as Atlanta or Birmingham, but many of those in the northern part of the area have drifted northward into Baltimore, Washington, D.C., Cincinnati, Cleveland, Chicago, Dayton, Detroit, and other major cities. Although Appalachian people are descended from families who have lived in the United States for hundreds of years and could popularly be termed *WASPS* (white, Anglo-Saxon Protestants*), in large northern urban areas they are treated as a minority group. There are Appalachian enclaves in the slums that border the black and Puerto Rican settlements and replace the Italians and Poles who are moving to the suburbs. The talk and folk wisdom are from "down home," rather than from a foreign country, but the poverty, underemployment, big families, inadequate housing, and discouragement is the same as it is in the slum areas where ethnic minority groups live.

One problem facing many of the rural poor, and rural people in general, is the lack of qualified health professionals. Though this is a problem in cities, since the health facilities are not always located where the poor can reach them, it is a particular problem in areas where population is widely dispersed. Inevitably, the poor of any group fall back upon their own meager resources; nowhere has this been more true than in Appalachia, where physicians and other health professionals traditionally have been scarce.

In the 1940s, a folklore specialist wrote that the "backwoods country" swarmed with "yarb doctors," "rubbin' doctors," and "nature doctors" who had never studied medicine, many of them unable to read or write. Though professionals such as the public health nurses who went into the Kentucky hills on horseback have lessened the isolation of the hill people, there is still a strong carryover of some of the old attitudes. Like many unsophisticated people, the sick in Appalachia seem to feel that the efficacy of the treatment varies directly with its unpleasantness: bitter tea is always best, and the more a poultice hurts, the better they like it. Folk medicine in

---

*Actually, most Appalachians are descendants of Scots-Irish ancestors and technically not Anglo-Saxons, but the term WASP has an elastic interpretation. Clearly, Appalachians are white and Protestant.

Appalachia also relies heavily on herbs, motivated by the belief that God made a remedy for every ailment. Kerosene and coal oil are also widely used, both externally and internally.

Some of the folk wisdom has to be overcome in order to deal with patients effectively. Generally, in the past there has been a great suspicion of surgery. This hostility carries over to fear of hypodermic needles and to intravenous administration of medications. Many of the hill people are also great believers in the signs of the zodiac. Certain treatments should be performed at certain times, while necessary treatment might be delayed because the signs are not right.

Sometimes folk treatment is drastic. A patient suffering from what he called "locked bowels" was brought to a newly established physician in one of the hill communities. The physician felt the patient would soon die but recommended he be taken to the hospital at once. Instead, the relatives knocked the patient unconscious, because they believed that unconsciousness allowed the internal organs to relax and thus might dispose of the obstruction. The physician who saw this action thought the relatives were murdering the patient and left, but the relatives continued to "treat" the patient by "cupping" him with fruit jars that they clamped againt his abdomen. After the patient died, the physician tried to get the county official to place manslaughter charges against the bereaved family, but the county officials refused, knowing of the folk customs.

Sometimes when an infant does not grow and function properly, it is diagnosed as having "liver-growed," that is, the liver somehow became attached to the body wall. In such cases, a stout old woman grasps the baby's left hand and right foot and twists them together behind its back, then does the same with the right hand and left foot. She puils hard, and the child cries, but it is believed to be the only effective treatment. The more difficult it is to bring the hands and feet together, the more certain it is that the child is "liver-growed." Though this treatment probably is not too harmful, many infants died of nephritis, caused by dosing them with turpentine.[20] Gradually, as the people grow more sophisticated, many of these practices are abandoned, but they still survive among large segments of the population.

MIGRANT FARM WORKERS

More widely dispersed is another form of rural poverty: namely, that of the farm wage worker, many of whom are migrant workers.

As the number and nature of farms have declined, so has the number of migratory workers. In the past and still today, most of the paid farm workers were nonmigratory workers who lived in the community and supplemented their income during rush times in the agricultural cycle. However, large numbers of them were migratory workers, with about 300,000 still so classified in 1977. In 1977, the average daily salary for the migratory workers was $20 for those 20 years of age or older, and $13.63 for those 19 or under.[21]

There are three major streams of migratory workers. One group spends the winter in Florida and Georgia harvesting winter crops, then moves northward through the Atlantic states in the summer and returns late in the fall; a second group moves northward from Texas and spreads out through the Central states; while a third stream is centered in California and the Pacific states. Since the workers usually travel as a family or in small groups, there are large variations in case histories of individuals and families. They indicate quite different patterns prompted by hope, rumor, and sometimes even accurate job information or contracts. Though many of the migrant workers are members of ethnic minority groups, large numbers are white.

Some casual observers of the migrant workers have claimed that farm migrancy exists because of the seasonal labor requirements of agriculture and that the people become migrants because they like the life. Neither of these generalizations seems valid on investigation in most cases, although a few crops do demand intense attention for only one or two weeks. Investigators have found that the majority of U.S.-born migrant farm workers seem to be victims of either occupational displacement, racial discrimination, illiteracy, poor health, or accidents, and they have turned to farm labor to survive. In effect, seasonal farm work in the past has provided an opportunity for those who are not qualified for or are not accepted in the more desirable occupations.

Although on the lowest rung of the economic ladder and the most in need, migratory farm workers were excluded from the protection of major national and state statutes dealing with working and living conditions, until the last few years. They were not covered by unemployment insurance, had no right to organize, lacked protection of minimum wage guarantees, and had little say about their working conditions. They also had little political power, because few were able to meet the residence requirements for voting, and the lack of guarantee for them to organize meant that they lacked the protection group efforts might have given them. Their economic difficulties are complicated by the fact that they travel as a family unit, and this means that their children also suffer. To eke out a living, everyone who is able to work, including children, go to the fields, although many states now prevent those under 14 from working. Little supervision is given to the children while the mother is in the field, and the accident rate among these children is high. Schooling for children of migratory workers is inadequate, because long periods of time are spent on the road and distances between jobs are great. Housing is mainly improvised, and medical care in the past has been mostly nonexistent. Education, child care, health, and sanitation are difficult enough under migratory conditions, but, when this is compounded by the uncertainty of employment and by real poverty, the results are too often deplorable.

HEALTH PROBLEMS OF THE POOR

Most of the health problems associated with poverty have been mentioned before, because they are the same kind of problems faced by minority group members, most of whom are also poor. Whatever their ethnic identity, the members of the poverty population are much more likely to die of contagious diseases than the general population, and, because they die younger, they are less likely to die of malignant neoplasms and cardiovascular diseases. Naturally, maternal and infant mortality rates are higher for the poverty group. Poverty itself is not listed on the death certificate, because poverty is not an illness; instead, it has to be classed as a major contributing factor in many deaths. Some of the reasons are obvious. With our present health care system, a lack of funds acts as a barrier to adequate medical care, which means that untreated or improperly treated illness is more common among the poor and that major health crises are more likely to occur. Overcrowded living conditions and lack of sanitary facilities are major contributors to the spread of infectious diseases. However, one aspect of poverty and health that has not been so widely publicized is the correlation between poverty and malnutrition.

In 1964, the Social Security Administration developed a poverty index in terms of money income and such factors as family size, sex and age of the family head, number of children under age 18, and whether or not people were farm or nonfarm residents. In 1977, poverty level for a family of four (both farm and nonfarm) was $6,191. Definitions of poverty level have varied with inflation, and in 1960 it was $3,022. By 1977 standards, nearly 25 million people were in families at or below poverty level, a figure equal to 11.6

percent of the total population. If the number of people at poverty level is calculated without income supplement programs, then the total number has remained at or near 25 million since 1968, when there was a large drop off due to the Johnson administration programs. However, the percentage of total population at poverty level has declined slightly since 1968, from 12.5 to 11.6 since poverty is not increasing as fast as the population. In 1977, the median family income was $16,000, or more than double the poverty level.[22] Even after governmental assistance programs are taken into account, 14.1 million people remain at or below poverty levels.

If the calculations of the Social Security Administration are correct, and $6,191 is an essential minimum, as adjusted for inflation, then the conclusions become obvious; these families, including large numbers on welfare, do not feed, clothe, or house themselves or their children adequately. Since rent tends to be a fixed expense, it is often met first; then the problem becomes that of feeding the family until the next check arrives. This means that many people have periods of going without a meal. In 1970, a California legislative survey found that the 44 percent of the children of AFDC (Aid to Families with Dependent Children) in Sacramento County had involuntarily gone without food one or more days during the year, because the family had run out of money to buy food.[23]

Hunger is by no means a new phenomenon in the United States or elsewhere, although much of the public concern over malnutrition is of fairly recent origin. In the winter of 1965–1966, 35 blacks invaded an abandoned air force base in Greenville, Mississippi, because they said they were hungry, cold, and unemployed. Federal troops were sent in to evict the demonstrators, but a federal interdepartmental committee was set up to investigate the claims of the 35 that they and other residents of the area were starving.[24] Eventually, a delegation of United States Senators visited Mississippi in April 1967 to investigate poverty and hunger. The committee was shocked by what they saw. One member of the delegation, Senator George Murphy of California, regarded as one of the more conservative members, indicated that he was unprepared for what he saw. "I didn't know that we were going to be dealing with the situation of starving people and starving youngsters."[25]

The chairman of the investigating committee, Joseph S. Clark of Pennsylvania, briefly summarized the findings:

> We saw families who, without income with which to buy food or food stamps, were suffering from the effects of acute malnutrition and hunger. It is an exercise in semantics to argue whether

these and other families about whom we have heard and of whom we will hear today are "starving." Senator [Robert] Kennedy of New York observed that the conditions he saw in the delta were as bad as any he had seen in his extensive tour of South America. One of the doctors who will testify today, and who has had extensive experience in Africa has said that conditions he observed in this country are as bad or worse than those in Kenya and Aden.[26]

Testifying before the committee was a panel of six physicians who, with financial support from the Field Foundation, had made a personal inspection of the conditions in Mississippi with respect to malnutrition and medical care. These men reported that school children were unable to learn because of hunger and that signs of malnutrition were widespread. In an examination of a sample of 501 preschool children, one physician found that 81 percent of them were anemic, with hemocrit readings below 35. The diet of many Mississippi children was found to be practically devoid of animal protein. To complicate matters, the group reported that there was widespread evidence of discrimination in health care. One member went on to state a widespread belief that there was an unwritten but generally accepted policy of state officials to try to drive blacks out of the state or starve them to death.[27]

As might be expected, the report of these physicians to the Senate and to the world caused an uproar. The two Senators from Mississippi objected to the findings of both the Field Foundation project and the Senate subcommittee. They produced witnesses who argued that the reports were biased and unfair, and that Mississippi had wrongfully been singled out because hunger existed elsewhere.[28] On this last point, the Senators had the facts on their side. The Office of Economic Opportunity reported that hunger was a problem not only in Mississippi but also among Alaskan natives, the urban poor, rural Appalachia, and elsewhere.[29] The focus of the investigation of the hunger problem widened from what had seemed to be a Mississippi tragedy to a national problem, and the Senate committee went on to hold hearings and hear witnesses from throughout the country.

In the summer of 1967, a Citizens Crusade Against Poverty was set up, with Benjamin E. Mays, President Emeritus of Morehouse College in Atlanta, and Leslie Dunbar, Executive Director of the Field Foundation, as co-chairmen. This group also held hearings and collected data about the problems of hunger. Their findings were in substantial agreement with the findings of the official Senate subcommittee and other investigations carried out by journalists. It was suddenly agreed that hunger was a widespread phenomenon in this country, and the consequences of chronic malnutrition were found to be serious and widespread.

The incidence of anemia among poor infants was found to be particularly high. In a Washington, D.C., study of 460 children from low-income families, 29 percent were found to be anemic, with the highest rate recorded between the ages of 12 and 17 months, when 65 percent were so classified.[30] Similar statistics were found to be true for Chicago, New York, Pittsburgh, and Baltimore.[31] In the Senate hearings, physicians testified that the anemia they saw in small children tended to complicate other illnesses. One Kentucky pediatrician reported that the children from poor families spent twice as long in the hospital as those from more well-to-do families, because the handicaps of parasites and malnutrition tended to slow their recovery rate.[32]

Though there were few large-scale or carefully controlled research projects reported in these hearings on hunger, the cumulative evidence of reports by physicians who had examined the poverty population or who had compared patients across income levels was overwhelming. Not only did large numbers of poor children not have adequate diets, but many were actually hungry. One way in which this poor diet showed up clinically was in the development of nutritional anemia, a result of either iron or protein deficiencies. This anemia was most often manifest in infants below the age of two, in part because they were unable to eat the regular family diet, but also because their nutritional needs were so great during this most rapid growth period.

Investigators found even more serious protein deficiencies among some of the American Indians,[33] so serious that they were diagnosed as having kwashiorkor and marasmus, conditions usually associated with the most economically deprived areas of the world. Earlier research had also reported kwashiorkor among the children of migrant farm workers in Florida.[34] *Marasmus* is the term applied to a generalized undernutrition in which the intake of protein, calories, vitamins, and iron are all inadequate. *Kwashiorkor* is an old African tribal name for the syndrome that was frequently observed when infants were displaced from the breast by the birth of a younger sibling. The outstanding clinical symptom of kwashiorkor that differentiates it from marasmus is the development of a generalized edema. The edema is a result of a very low level of intake of the essential amino acids, which causes the protein level in the serum to fall to half or less than half of the normal

values. From 1966 to 1967, the authors of this book studied marasmus and kwashiorkor among a sample of 32 Egyptian infants and
concluded that no amount of nutritional health teaching could prevent kwashiorkor without an income level that would enable a
family to afford an adequate diet.[35] It is possible that health teaching would have more effect in this country where kwashiorkor and
marasmus are more sporadic events, but they still seem to be in
part the result of poverty. Two brief case histories illustrate the
problem:

> . . . . a one and one-half-year old Navajo girl, brought to the
> hospital because of swelling, irritability, and loss of appetite of
> one week's duration. Parents considered her well until the onset
> of swelling. She had received "no milk for a long time" and had
> rarely been given meat. Diet consisted primarily of tea, soda
> water and beans.
> . . . . a two-year-old Navajo girl admitted because of sudden
> swelling. One month before a mild diarrhea began. [It] ceased
> two days prior to admission at which point the swelling oc-
> curred. Child had been increasingly listless. For the month dur-
> ing which there was diarrhea the child was fed nothing except
> soup and soda water and occasionally whole milk.[36]

If these case histories are typical examples, it would seem that
malnutrition in the United States is not only directly attributable to
poverty but is also complicated by inadequate nutritional knowledge. Both of these children received soda pop. Many people fail to
realize the low level of food value in such readily available and
well-advertised foods such as soda pop, candy, potato chips, and
sweetened breakfast cereals. And the persuasive powers of nutrition-
ists are almost negligible compared to the influence exerted by ad-
vertising in the mass media.

Of course, it is very difficult to argue with hungry people, if you
are trying to dissuade them from eating. For generations, as indicated earlier, hungry black children have eaten clay to fill their
empty bellies and to stop the abdominal cramps that accompany
hunger. A whole folklore has grown up about clay eating, until now
there are people habituated to eating clay, even when they are not
hungry.

Malnutrition seems to be a particularly serious problem among
young children. Research reported in 1968 found that poor children lagged behing their peers in physical development, in part
because they were anemic and suffered from a lack of Vitamin A
and Vitamin C, as well as from other nutritional deficiencies.[37]

Migrant workers tend to be particularly disadvantaged, because social agencies find it more difficult to deal with migrants than they do with non migrants.[38] Even if food is available, however, it has to be available in sufficient quantities, since there is no guarantee that any particular diet would be nutritious. Still, the most significant variable in getting adequate nutrition is family income and ability to have a variety of food. For example, a California survey found that more than half of the 750,000 children in the state who were part of families receiving AFDC were required to live on incomes too low for their parents to purchase adequate diets.[39]

One of the most controversial yet serious consequences of malnutrition that has been reported is the possibility of brain damage. Although this sort of problem cannot be investigated in the political atmosphere of a Senate hearing, there is a substantial body of research knowledge related to this question. The negative consequences of inadequate nutrition start at least as early as the prenatal period, as undernutrition during pregnancy clearly affects reproductive outcomes. Recent research goes even further and suggests that the nutritional status of the mother before pregnancy occurs is also important. The correlation of malnutrition and intellectual development is easiest to demonstrate by using prematurity as a factor linking the two. This is because prematurity is most likely to occur among groups whose socioeconomic status is low, and there is growing evidence that children with birth weights below 2500 grams (5 ½ lb.) tend to score lower on intelligence tests than those with higher birth weights.[40] A controlled study of 500 prematures born in Baltimore in 1952, matched with term infants on such factors as race, age, parity of mother, hospital, season of birth, and socioeconomic status, showed that the premature infants were more intellectually retarded and more likely to have a physical or neurological problem when tested at ages three to five, six to seven, and eight to ten.[41]

One of the more innovative of the solutions adopted in the late 1960s was that found by H. Jack Geiger, a community health physician from Tufts Medical School who established a clinic in Mound Bayou, Mississippi, in 1967, through funds from the Office of Economic Opportunity. Geiger soon realized that the most pressing medical problem faced by his patients was hunger and that "pills without food" would be useless. He stocked food in his pharmacy on the theory that the "specific treatment for malnutrition is food." Though health professionals traditionally had given dietary advice, dispensed protein, vitamins, and mineral supplements, or pre-

scribed "formulas" for infants, they considered bags of food as belonging to the province of the welfare workers. Geiger simply added
food to the items that could be prescribed, and, since the project
was federally funded, the hungry were given food as part of their
medical treatment. The results in increased health were impressive,
although as a long-range solution to the problem the plan was not
without problems. One of Geiger's difficulties was in finding storage
space in the pharmacy.[42] Obviously, a long-term solution had to turn
to more traditional ways of distributing food.

Hunger was an issue in the 1968 elections. After his election,
President Nixon, in May 1969, pledged to "put an end to hunger in
America itself for all time." His recommendations for a change in
the food stamp program were passed by Congress in 1971. The
Nixon amendments represented an extension of food assistance that
had begun in 1935, been modified in 1939, become a part of our
agricultural policy in 1949, and been further extended in 1961. The
1971 amendments provided free stamps for the most needy, a ceil-
ing of 30 percent of income for the purchase price of food stamp
allotments, and uniform national eligibility standards, dependent
only on income and family size. In 1973, further amendments man-
dated that all counties switch from food distribution (some of which
the poor did not want) to distributing food stamps and allowing
people to have a choice. The result was a guaranteed minimum
income in food available to all low-income Americans, although,
like so many other programs, not everyone took advantage of it. In
fact, as of 1976, less than half the eligible population availed themselves of food stamps. Geography, social attitudes toward public
assistance, and historical influence of the farm lobby (in favor of
commodity distribution rather than food stamps) are some of the
reasons why, but it seems that administrative attitudes are also
important. Some county administrative areas make it more difficult
to apply for food stamps than others. Still, probably the most significant factor is the stigma that many people associate with letting
others know they are on welfare. For example, people over 65 are far
less likely to use food stamps than other eligible age groups. Eligible
working poor are less likely to get food stamps than those who are
long-time recipients of welfare.[43]

One of the traditional justifications for food stamps is that, if
given cash, the poor would spend the money on other things; society
also wants to insure the quantity and quality of food the poor consume. However, food stamps do not necessarily do this. Research
shows that less than 10 cents per bonus dollar seems to go for food
that would not otherwise be purchased. For this reason, President

Jimmy Carter in his proposed welfare overhaul, the Better Jobs and Income Programs, proposed limiting food stamps and supplementing this by a cash minimum for all. As of this writing, the proposal has not been enacted, instead, President Ronald Reagan has proposed stricter criteria. The problem remains that most Americans still fear that the poor are poor because they throw money around. Though most people do not want anyone to starve, they have not yet come to terms with the poor as people in more unfortunate circumstances than themselves.

Still, the existing programs, biased and inadequate as they are, have dealt with some of the problems of the poor. In 1978, about 16 million people participated in the food stamp program. The school lunch program reached 27 million students, 60 percent of all students enrolled.[44] Special programs such as meals on wheels have been established to help the poverty stricken oldsters. Though hunger still remains a problem in our affluent society,[45] the problem is not so much government unwillingness to deal with hunger or the public's lack of interest, but finding the needy poor and developing more effective programs. Whether the Reagan cuts in the food stamp program, in the school lunch program, and in other such programs will destroy what was accomplished by 1980 is unclear as of this writing. It appears however, that malnutrition will increase.

Hunger is not the only health problem of the poor. Others still remain. A 1979 report on California to the National Health Law Program reported that the poor are being priced out of the medical care market.

> Private physicians and hospitals treat the poor in need of medical care as pariahs. Physicians do not practice in rural poverty areas and the ghettos and barrios of our State. They continue to specialize in unneeded services at the expense of primary care, and they have all but foresaken the Medi-Cal [Medicaid] program. Throughout California, pregnant Medi-Cal patients have increasing difficulty finding a physician willing to treat them. Uninsured pregnant women find it impossible.
>
> Private hospitals, like physicians, shun the poor and continue to "dump" indigents onto County hospitals, despite their Hill-Burton "free care" and community service obligations. In Los Angeles County, nearly 2,000 patients per month are transferred from private to County facilities.
>
> California's emergency rooms have become a primary care provider for the poor. One ER physician has estimated that half of all visits to the emergency room are for Medi-Cal patients who have nowhere else to go. Care provided in this manner is very

costly and of very poor quality. There is a quality of inhumanity in the refusal of private physicians to care for the poor and "patient dumping" which is often ignored. In one Northern California city, a three-year-old boy was forced to wait for several hours with a "severely" broken arm in an ER room because the three Orthopedists on call refused to treat him as his parents were without insurance or money. Many private hospitals in Southern California are said to perform a "wallet biopsy" on all emergency room patients before they decide whether transfer to a County facility is "in order."

California's County hospital system remains the primary provider of health services for the poor. This system has long been under siege. Old and deteriorated physical plants, rapid inflation in health care costs and Proposition 13 threatened the life blood of County Hospitals and clinics throughout the state and the health of tens of thousands of poor Californians.[46]

What is described as the California situation is a national problem. It is also not just a problem of the medical establishment but of the government programs themselves. This problem can only worsen until there is a rethinking of the health care delivery system.

United Press International carried the story of the death of thirty-two-year-old Violet Guthrie on August 13, 1980. From Nashville, Georgia, Mrs. Guthrie became newsworthy because of her conflict with Medicaid. She had been diagnosed as having cancer in 1973, and the debilitating effects of the illness caused her to leave her job soon after. In 1978, her husband quit his job because his wife needed round-the-clock care and the family was too poor to hire anyone else to do it. The couple lived on the Social Security check of $239 a month that Mrs. Guthrie received. Unfortunately, this Social Security payment was $10.80 more than the maximum amount she could receive and still receive Medicaid. Medicare covered a portion of her bills for cancer, but the total costs soared to $50,000, which would have been covered if she had been eligible for Medicaid.[47] In her fight to get one part of the government bureaucracy to communicate with the other, she received national attention. Her efforts were unsuccessful.

Mrs. Guthrie symbolizes the fundamental difficulty with government programs as they now exist. They remain essentially patchwork efforts that do not deal with the basic problems of the poor. Much of the success of Medicare is due to the fact that everyone over a specified age is eligible. Age, not need, is the requirement. Once special requirements, such as income, family size, or others, are established for eligibility as they are in Medicaid, not only does the cost of administering the program rise, but so do the number of people who fall between the cracks. So does the stigma of utilizing such services. Wealthy as well as moderate income and poverty people utilize Medicare. Only poverty people are eligible for Medicaid. Obviously, the most effective ways to deal with the medical and nursing needs of all Americans is to have a national health insurance, something advocated by President Carter in his 1976 election, but which he failed to carry through. The Reagan administration has made no such promises.

Even guaranteeing health care for all still leaves open the problem of health care delivery. Many rural and urban poor lack qualified professionals to attend to them. Even in the cities, health care facilities are not always located where the poor can reach them. At present, there has been significant improvement in health services for the poor, but we still have a significant way to go, both in delivering effective health care and in getting the poor to effectively utilize what is available.

REFERENCES

1. Lewis, O. The Children of Sanchez. New York: Random House, 1961.
2. See: Haveman, R. H. A Decade of Federal Antipoverty Programs: Achievements, Failures, and Lessons. New York: Academic Press, 1977, passim.
3. Seeman, M. On the Meaning of Alienation. *American Sociological Review*, 1959, *24*, 783–791.
4. Moynihan, D. P. Maximum Feasible Misunderstanding: Community Action in the War on Poverty. New York: Free Press, 1969.
5. Moynihan. op. cit., p. 130.
6. Ibid., pp. 136–137.
7. Eisinger, P. The Community Action Program and the Development of Black Political Leadership. Research on Poverty Discussion Paper, No. 473–8. Madison, Wisconsin: Institute for Research on Poverty, 1979.
8. For example, see: Newman, P. with Wegner, J. Pass the Poverty Please. Whittier, California: Constructive Action, 1966.
9. U. S. Bureau of Census. Statistical Abstract of the United States, 1979. Washington, D.C.: U. S. Government Printing Office, 1979, Table 763, p. 464.
10. Orshansky, M. The Poverty Roster. In R. M. Ralson (Ed.), Sources: A Blue Cross Report on the Health Problems of the Poor. Chicago, 1968, p. 10. Statistical Abstract, 1979. p. 464, Table 761.
11. Ibid., Table No. 759, p. 462. For an earlier account, see: The People Left Behind: The Rural Poor, A Report by the President's Commission on Rural Poverty. In L. A. Ferman, J. L. Kornblugh, & A. Haber (Eds.),

Poverty in America. Ann Arbor: University of Michigan Press, revised edition, 1968, pp. 152–153.

12. Statistical Abstract, 1979. No. 686, p. 416.
13. Poverty in America. p. 155.
14. Statistical Abstract, 1979. Table 1175, p. 683.
15. For background, see; Vance, R. B. The Region: A New Survey. In T. R. Ford (Ed.), The Southern Appalachian Region: A Survey. Lexington: University of Kentucky Press, 1962, pp. 4–5. The 1979 figures are for an enlarged Appalachian area, because, in 1965, the definition of Appalachia was changed to include 397 counties in 13 states and data is easily available on these but not on the original counties. Statistical Abstract, 1979. No. 770, p. 468.
16. Ibid., p. 7. It also is the only region listed separately in the Statistical Abstract, 1979. Tables No. 770–771, p. 468.
17. Weller, J. E. Yesterday's People: Life in Contemporary Appalachia. Lexington: University of Kentucky Press, 1965. Caudill, H. M. Night Comes to the Cumberlands: A Biography of a Depressed Area. Boston: Little, Brown, 1963. Also see Robert Coles' study under the general title of The South Goes North. Volume two of this study deals with Migrants, Sharecroppers, Mountaineers. Boston: Little, Brown, 1971. Also see Chapter VI in The South Goes North. Boston: Little, Brown, 1971.
18. Brown, J. S. & Hillery, Jr., G. A. The Great Migration, 1940–60. In Ford, op. cit., p. 54. As of this writing, getting an update on the same area is difficult, for reasons listed above. The hard core of Appalachia continued to lose population, but the general area now called *Appalachia* showed a slight gain.
19. *New York Times*. August 2, 1980.
20. Randolph, V. Ozark Magic and Folklore. Reprint, New York: Dover Publications, 1964, chapter 6, pp. 92–93, and chapter 7, pp. 121–161.
21. Statistical Abstract, 1979. Table 1219, p. 703.
22. Ibid., No. 758, p. 462.
23. California Legislative Assembly Committee on Health and Welfare. Malnutrition: One Key to the Poverty Cycle. January 1970, p. 13.
24. Hunger, U.S.A.: A Report by the Citizen's Board of Inquiry into Hunger and Malnutrition in the United States. Boston: Beacon Press, 1968, p. 11.
25. Ibid., p. 3.
26. Hearings Before the Subcommittee on Employment, Manpower and Poverty of the Committee on Labor and Public Welfare. United States Senate, Ninetieth Congress, July 11 and 12, 1967. Washington, D.C.: U.S. Government Printing Office, pp. 1–2.
27. Ibid., pp. 4–62, ad passim.
28. Ibid., pp. 63–106.
29. Ibid., p. 188. Hunger, U.S.A., p. 194.
30. Hunger, U.S.A., p. 19.
31. Filer, J. L. The United States Today—Is It Free of Public Health Nutrition Problems Today—Anemia. Presented to the American Public

Health Association, Miami Beach, Florida, October 24, 1967. Cited in Hunger, U.S.A.

32. Ibid., p. 19.
33. Wolf, C. B. Kwashiorkor on the Navaho Indian Reservation. U. S. Public Health Service. In Hunger, U.S.A., pp. 20–21.
24. Delgado, G., Brumback, C. L. & Deaver, M. B. Eating Patterns Among Migrant Families. *Public Health Reports*, 1961, *76*, 349–355.
35. Bullough, B. Malnutrition among Egyptian Infants. *Nursing Research*, 1969, *18*, 172–173.
36. Wolf. op. cit. In Hunger, U.S.A., pp. 20–21.
37. Kotz, N. Let Them Eat Promises: The Politics of Hunger in America. New York: Anchor Books, 1971, pp. 186–187.
38. Hearings Before the Select Committee on Nutrition and Human Needs of the United States Senate. Ninetieth Congress, Second Session, and Ninety-first Congress, Part 5B, Florida, Appendix. Washington, D.C.: U. S. Government Printing Office, 1969, p. 1835.
39. California Assembly Committee. op. cit., pp. 1–26.
40. Birch, H. & Gussow, J. D. Disadvantaged Children: Health, Nutrition and School Failure. New York: Harcourt, 1970, pp. 123–153.
41. Knoch, H., Pasamanick, R., Harper, P. A. & Rider, R. The Effect of Prematurity on Health and Growth. *American Journal of Public Health*, 1959, *49*, 1164–1173. Weiner, G., Rider, R. V., Oppel, W. C., Fischer, L. & Harper, P. A. Correlates of Low Birth Weight: Psychological Status at Six to Seven Years of Age. *Pediatrics*, 1965, *35*, 434–444. Weiner, G., Rider, R. V., Oppel, W. C. & Harper, P. A. Correlates of Low Birth Weight: Psychological Status at Eight to Ten Years of Age. *Pediatric Research*, 1968, *2*, 110–118.
42. Kelly, C. Health Care in the Mississippi Delta. *American Journal of Nursing*, 1969, *69*, 759–763.
43. MacDonald, M. Food, Stamps, and Income Maintenance. New York: Academic Press, 1977.
44. Statistical Abstract, 1979. Table 208, p. 120.
45. White House Conference on Food, Nutrition and Health, Final Report. Chairman: Jean Mayer. Washington, D.C.: U. S. Government Printing Office, 1970.
46. See: Dallek, G. Health Care for California's Poor/Separate and Unequal. Mimeographed, Santa Monica, National Health Law Program, 1979, pp. 3–4.
47. United Press International. August 13, 1980.

8

Mental Health and Mental Illness

A dominant theme of this book has been that both poverty and ethnic identity need to be considered in any explanation of minority health problems. This is as true of mental health as it is of physical health. Nevertheless, some words of caution have to be given. There has always been a tendency to blame the ills of society on the poor—to indicate that the poor are poor because they are feeble, less able, or mentally ill. This was the implication of an 1856 report that stated that the "pauper class" in Massachusetts "furnished proportionately sixty four times as many cases of insanity as the independent class."[1] While there is a correlation between mental illness and socioeconomic status, the relationship is a complex one that has only begun to become evident through the research of the last 30 to 40 years.

A pioneering study in the field, done in Chicago by Robert E. L. Faris and H. Warren Dunham, was published in 1939. The two investigators found that patients who were diagnosed as schizophrenic were most likely to have home addresses near the central part of the city, in the slum and rooming-house neighborhoods, while patients who were diagnosed as manic depressive were scattered throughout the whole city. Since schizophrenia was the most common type of functional psychosis, the high rate of this disease found in poverty neighborhoods helped account for the correlation

157

between hospitalization and low socioeconomic status. In trying to explain their findings, Faris and Dunham hypothesized that schizophrenia might be more common in poverty neighborhoods because people in such areas felt a greater sense of isolation, owing to the social disorganization of their neighborhood.[2] This interpretation touched off a lively debate that is still going on. On the one hand, researchers have found that slums are not particularly disorganized, only that their social structure is different from that of the more affluent neighborhoods.[3] On the other hand, and much more basically, the interpretation has been challenged, because it implies a causal chain between poverty and schizophrenia. Later researchers, including Dunham himself, have argued that poverty might be a consequence of schizophrenia rather than its cause. The schizophrenic individual may drift down to live in a poor neighborhood because of the socially debilitating symptoms of his illness.[4]

Since the possible explanations have such great social consequences, the research has become voluminous. In a 1969 review of the major empirical studies investigating the relationship of socioeconomic status and psychological disorders, Bruce and Barbara Dohrenwend found that, in spite of differences in design, the vast majority of studies reported that psychological disorders were more common among poor people than among middle- or upper-class individuals. Usually, no matter how defined, it was the lowest class or stratum that had the largest population of the mentally ill. Although the interpretations of the data might be subject to debate, they concluded that there could be little quarrel with the basic correlation between poverty and psychological disorders.[5]

THE COMPLEXITY OF THE PROBLEM

The causes of this correlation are still being investigated. A methodological problem inherent in the research is how to define *mental illness*. A New Haven study, started in 1950 by a team of sociologists and psychiatrists headed by August Hollingshead and Fredrick Redlich, used "diagnosed illness" to define operationally what they meant by a psychiatric disorder. To find their sample of patients diagnosed as having mental illness, they contacted all of the mental hospitals, private psychiatrists, and clinics in the area. Then they classified the residents of New Haven into five social classes—a not particularly difficult thing to do, since New Haven, the home of Yale University, had already been the subject of several studies dealing with class structure. Again, they found that the poor were more likely to be diagnosed as having some type of psychiatric disorder than those who were richer probably due to the stress of living in a lower-class environment. They found that, depending upon a person's social class, there were significant differences in the type of diagnosis given. For example, psychoses were more commonly diagnosed among the two lowest of the five classes, while neuroses were more often found among the top three classes. The finding is not so clear-cut as it might seem. It could suggest either that the stress of poverty produces more serious types of mental illness, or that psychotherapists are more likely to diagnose an illness as a neurosis if the patient is from the middle or upper class, but will call it a psychosis, if the patient comes from a lower social class.[6]

The New Haven study was also criticized because it included only diagnosed illness. In 1954, a broad-scale study of the residents of midtown Manhattan was carried out under the direction of Leo Srole. The research team included both psychiatrists and sociologists. They attempted to broaden the definition of mental illness to include persons not under treatment. They gathered data by means of a lengthy interview, in which a random sample of people in different strata of society indicated their own feelings and problems. Their mental health status was determined by their answers to the questions. The procedure made the incidence of mental illness seem much higher, because it included all of the untreated cases, but the proportion of disorders was still highest among the lowest stratum.[7] This basic correlation between economic status and mental illness has held up over time. In 1974, a follow-up of the midtown Manhattan study was done, with as many people in the original sample as possible being relocated for interviews. This restudy seems to support the original findings.[8] Other research suggests that the strongest link between socioeconomic status and mental illness is in the area of depression.[9] In an epidemiological study of sixteen randomly selected adults from one southern county, researchers found a clear relationship between depressive symptomatology and low incomes, and low educational and occupational levels.[10]

In an attempt to determine whether poverty is the cause or consequence of these symptoms, investigators have also looked at the social class of the parents of the people they interviewed. Although persons whose parents are of low social class are more likely to report symptoms or be diagnosed as ill, the individual's own social class is more strongly related to the probability of having a mental disorder than that of the parents. In fact, mental illness occurs more often among the people who were downwardly mobile than those who moved up the social scale during their lifetime.[11]

The main reason for replication of studies and cautious concern about the link between socioeconomic status and psychiatric disorders is that researchers are still unsure about the cause of many mental illnesses. The studies linking poverty and mental illness suggest there is a sociogenic relationship. Following the lead of Sigmund Freud, psychiatrists have customarily attributed most symptoms of mental illness to stress of early childhood experiences and problems in family interactions. In turn, they have tended to discount most of the later stresses that sociologists feel are so important. A more recent trend, particularly in the research about schizophrenia, has been to reemphasize the role of biological determinants, particularly possible genetic causes. Several studies in which twins were utilized as research subjects have raised questions about the nature of schizophrenia. It has been found that a schizophrenic monozygotic twin is more likely to have a twin who is afflicted than a schizophrenic whose twin is not identical. These findings are also supported by other family surveys that reinforce the concept of the hereditary tendency to develop the disease.[12] Nevertheless, most authorities still believe that there are also environmental influences in the development of schizophrenia. A comparison with tuberculosis is often made, because tuberculosis is both an organic disease and an environmental disease. Similarly, schizophrenia now seems to be caused by a combination of biological, social, and psychological elements, with poverty implicated as one of the social elements in this causal chain.[13]

The unwillingness to discard the factor of environment is, in part, due to the fact that it enters into the mental health picture in so many other ways. The New Haven survey mentioned above had a ten-year follow-up study of the patients identified as mentally ill in the initial study. In this research, it was found that people received a different type of treatment, depending upon their social-class position. Middle- and upper-class patients were more likely to have received psychotherapy or somatotherapy and were able to be cared for on an out-patient basis or in a physician's office. Their families were not only better able to pay for the therapy, but they were also more willing to tolerate the ill person at home, either because they had more ample housing or could hire outside help if needed. On the other hand, lower-class patients had seldom received any effective therapy. They were more likely to have been committed to a long-term public facility, where they received little more than custodial care mingled with some drug therapy. They drifted into chronic mental illness, disappearing into the back wards of the state mental hospitals.[14] These differences in treatment patterns are important in explaining the higher overall percentage of mental illness among people with low incomes, regardless of the position one takes on the causes of mental illness. Most experts agree that the present state of psychotherapy leaves much to be desired but that it is still the most effective mode of treatment to date. At the crowded mental hospitals, where most of the poor end up, there are so few psychotherapists that the care offered must be classed as primarily custodial.

Related to this finding is the nature of long-term hospitalization itself. Erving Goffman believes that long-term hospitalization, in a total institution such as a mental hospital, actually causes people to behave in peculiar ways. The stress begins with the admission procedures themselves, which strip the patient of individual identity. In order to cope with inmate status, the patient then develops either an apathetic posture or takes on some special, peculiar coping mechanism that makes the individual seem not quite sane. What is diagnosed as psychopathology can well be a realistic response to the hospitalization experience. This means that the individual who is admitted to a mental hospital, particularly one of the larger public institutions, is at a marked disadvantage in comparison to the person who can be treated in accustomed surroundings.[15]

Finances are not the only barrier between lower-class patients and psychotherapists. Psychiatrists, clinical psychologists, and psychiatric social workers tend to be recruited almost exclusively from middle- and upper-class backgrounds, and, until recently, the only ethnic minority well-represented in the group were Jews. Since this is the case, it is possible that therapists are afflicted with a certain amount of class and racial ethnocentrism. This prejudice is clearly evident in the types of patients whom psychotherapists chose for therapy. For example, it has been shown that they tend to avoid patients whose education has been meager or whose occupations are unskilled. Such exclusion is justified on the grounds that the lower-class patient cannot verbalize adequately or does not have the necessary cognitive skills to participate in the therapeutic process. Undoubtedly, this is true, but the same type of statement can be made about children, and psychotherapists have found ways to deal with youngsters. Rather, it seems that the psychotherapists do not feel the same empathy for the problems of the lower-class patients that they do for those patients whose problems are similar to their own. Unfortunately, this generalization tends to be true even for those few therapists whose origins were lower-middle class or lower-class, because they tend to lose touch with their humble origins during the long training process. This means that, psychotherapy, in or out of the hospital, simply is not available to most poor or minority patients.[16]

FAMILY

A key variable in mental health is the family setting. In our society, the family nurtures and socializes the young, as well as gives psychological support to all of its members. It is the basic primary group, serving as a mediator or link between the individual and society, protecting its members yet also preparing them for the world.

The nuclear family consisting of the biological parents and their offspring exists in every known society, although there are some variants in which the biological father is replaced by an uncle or some other family member. Almost as common is the extended family, including grandparents, uncles, aunts, and cousins. Often, married siblings stay at home, adding their spouses and children. In some societies, such an intergenerational grouping becomes a tribe.

No one structure is best, although each has advantages and disadvantages. The nuclear family tends to maximize freedom for its members, while the extended family takes on more support functions, even including economic support and health care. For some, the extended family carries the support functions better than the nuclear, because the larger group allows for less intense feelings. Most of the immigrant groups discussed in this work came from societies in which extended families were the norm. However, this was more true for people from rural than those from urban areas, except for blacks, whose family life was much more restricted by slavery.

The immigration experience also tended to cut the immigrant off from the extended family, as parents and grandparents were left behind. This meant that the immigrant had to face the strain of a new environment without some of the traditional support groups. Inevitably, the immigrant tried to re-establish the traditional family patterns as soon as possible, and the first and second generations were often very closely knit. However, before the new family structure could be established, the immigrant was more vulnerable to the stresses of living than he or she might have been, and there was a high incidence of mental illness.

Families of any social class or background are subject to forces that often undermine them: death, illness, divorce, unemployment. However, those with the least economic resources are particularly vulnerable, since these forces often further weaken the stability of an already precarious existence. It is people from disorganized families who demonstrate the most social pathology: alcoholism, disease, mental illness, addiction, crime and delinquency.

Pavenstedt studied child rearing environments of preschool to first-year grammar school children of upper-lower class and very lower-class families. She found vast differences between them, but the stable family groups differed from what she called the *disorganized group*. In describing the disorganized familes, she stated:

> The outstanding characteristic in these homes was that activities were impulse-determined; consistency was totally absent. A mother might stay in bed until noon while the children also were kept in bed or ran around unsupervised. Although families sometimes ate breakfast or dinner together, there was no pattern for anything. The parents often failed to discriminate between the children. A parent, incensed by the behavior of one child, was seen dealing a blow to another child who was closer. Communication by means of words hardly existed. Directions were indefinite or hung unfinished in mid-air. Reprimands were often high-pitched and angry.... As the children outgrew babyhood the parents differentiated very little between the parent and child role. The parents' needs were as pressing and as often indulged as were those of the children. There was strong competition for the attention of helpful adults.[17]

Other studies of children from disorganized poverty families indicate that many aspects of their behavior predispose them to later chronic acting out and impulse disorders that society often classifies as mental illness. As children, they showed low frustration tolerance, impulsivity, and unreliable controls; dominant use of motor action for discharge; language retardation; tendency to concrete thinking; need-satisfying object relations; little evidence of constructive play or use of fantasy in play; poor sense of identity; and marked use of imitation.[18]

On the other hand, more stable families, even in the slum, had worked out a kind of community life that led to sharing problems, a regular routine, and leaning on one another, a sharp contrast to the disorganized families. Obviously, children from poor homes, just as those from minority or other stigmatized groups, grow up with many strikes against them, and not all of them become stable well-adjusted adults. Neither for that matter do those who come from more well-to-do homes. Still, a stable family life seems to be an important variable in predicting later probabilities of mental illness. Disorganization does not necessarily correspond to single-parent families, although the more handicaps a family labors under, such as poverty, discrimination, or single parenting, the more difficult it is to retain any kind of stability. The more apathetic and alienated the family members are, the more difficult it is to recruit them into programs aimed at bettering themselves. Thus, they continue to remain the most vulnerable.

ETHNIC IDENTITY AND MENTAL ILLNESS

Poverty clearly seems to be a factor in mental illness. Variables such as family are also important, but more debatable is the relationship of ethnic identity to the incidence of psychoses and neuroses. Much of the difficulty comes from the fact that, until recently, there was considerably more polemics than hard research in the field. Writers from the "right" try to prove that one group is inferior to another, while writers from the "left" argue that the present social structure needs reform. Although we fall into the second category, it seems apparent that the most effective reforms should be based upon objective findings. Unfortunately, the evidence is not at all clear since, as Benjamin Pasamanick pointed out, most of the investigators have demonstrated bias either in collecting data or in interpreting it. The controversy in the United States goes back at least to the census of 1840, which found that the rate of institutionalization for blacks was higher in the North than in the South. Advocates of slavery immediately interpreted this as meaning that the "innately inferior" blacks fared better under slavery than they did living as free men in the North. Ignored in the first burst of polemics was the fact that the South had fewer institutions than the North, and that the institution of slavery itself could afford to be somewhat tolerant of certain kinds of mental disorder that induce greater submission. Moreover, the South was much more rural than the North, and it is in the urban centers that the mentally ill were most likely to be institutionalized. However, the same kind of conclusion appeared in some of the studies in 1880, when there was growing hostility toward immigrants, particularly the Irish Catholics. The official census report of that year stated that there was an "extraordinary ratio of insanity among the foreign born."[19] Even as late as 1944, Malzberg published a well-accepted scholarly paper claiming a higher rate of mental disease for blacks.[20]

However, it is true, that nonwhites still represent a disproportionate share of those institutionalized (17 percent) in mental hospitals.[21] Whether or not this is due to race is debatable. One explanation is diagnositic errors that institutionalize patients who need not be institutionalized. In a study done by Simon in nine New York area state psychiatric hospitals, 192 patients who had been diagnosed by staff psychiatrists were re-interviewed by project psychiatrists, using a structured mental status examination. When the routine diagnostic procedures were used, more blacks were diagnosed as schizophrenic. Under the careful scrutiny of the project psychiatrists this was not true; race and diagnosis simply were not correlated. Giving further support to these findings of Simon was a four-year retrospective study of black patients admitted to Howard University Hospital by black psychiatrists. They reported that 32.5 percent of the patients were schizophrenic, while at a comparable time (1975), 46.5 percent of all nonwhites in nonfederal hospitals were diagnosed as schizophrenic. Even more striking was the comparison of the Howard figures with the rate of schizophrenia from the Walter Reed Army Medical Center, where 58 percent of the black patients were given that diagnosis.[22] The explanation for the differences lies in the fact that the black physicians at Howard University diagnosed a larger proportion of their patient population as suffering from other mental illnesses, including some less serious and more treatable conditions than schizophrenia.

The problem is a two-pronged one, with the professionals at times overestimating the seriousness of the black patient's illness from the cues presented, and the patient presenting a more restricted (i.e., sicker) personal picture to the therapist who comes from outside the ethnic group. To document this second process, Carkuff and Pierce examined the initial clinical interviews of hospitalized black and white female schizophrenics and found that patients are more self-exploratory with therapists whose race and social class are more similar to their own.[23]

In a study reported in 1959, Jaco found a lower incidence of diagnosed psychoses among the Spanish surname population than among either Anglos or nonwhites.[24] However, current epidemiological surveys suggest that the incidence of mental illness among Mexican Americans is probably comparable to that in the general population.[25]

Probably, the best synthesis of the literature related to mental illness and life stress has been done by Bruce and Barbara Dohrenwend. In a series of publications, they have analyzed the relationship of social class, race, and life stress to both psychological and physiological illnesses. One problem they point out is that *mental illness* is really a global term. Many disparate diagnoses have been clumped together so that contrary trends may well be cancelling each other out. However, in spite of this problem, they seem willing to conclude from available evidence that the major debilitating psychoses probably are not related to culture or ethnicity in any consistent fashion.

Socioeconomic status may be linked with mental illness, but it is not at all clear whether this is a cause or a consequence. Carefully controlled research is still needed.[26]

PERSONALITY DAMAGE

These findings do not mean that there are not much more subtle correlations between race and poverty and mental illness. In fact, the most serious health consequence of minority status might well be the damage that poverty and discrimination inflict on the attitudes and intellectual development of the growing child. Generations of researchers have found that both race and socioeconomic status correlate significantly with all of the common measurements of intelligence.[27] Moreover, the effects of both race and socioeconomic status tend to be additive, at least at times. This is evidenced by the fact that, in many studies of intelligence, poor white children score higher than poor black children, but neither group scores as well as families with adequate incomes.

Complicating the nature of the findings is another argument between nature versus nurture. A few years ago, Arthur Jensen was able to shake the scholarly world of educational psychology when he made a strong case for the genetic determinants of I.Q. Jensen believed that compensatory education was a failure, because educators had neglected to consider the importance of the genetic factor in predicting intelligence levels. He suggested that there might be inherited racial and social-class differences in ability that doomed all such educational efforts to failure.[28] Jensen became the focus of a sharp controversy, because many people felt that he was trying to revive racist ideologies about superior and inferior races. Certainly, Jensen tended to lend support to some of the racist arguments, although he has somewhat modified his original assertions.[29] The controversy still continues, but what is needed either to prove or disprove his assertions is more serious biological research.[30] Until such evidence is forthcoming, the debate is more or less meaningless. Our own research tends to indicate that I.Q. is not the most important variable in either intellectual or creative achievement, but that a whole host of other factors are significant.[31] This is not to say that biological factors are not important—they are—but the differences found by Jensen still might be influenced by environmental factors that we find are all important in fostering or hindering intellectual and creative achievement. It is also important to emphasize that environmental stresses can have biological consequences. As has been reported in earlier chapters, such factors as severe malnutrition, prematurity, and accidents at delivery—all of which are most commonly associated with low socioeconomic status—can have lasting negative consequences for mental development.

Unfortunately, as the child grows, disadvantages associated with poverty, ethnicity, and inadequate family support tend to be cumulative, so that he or she falls farther and farther behind in relationship to the peer group. This process can be observed in almost any school where there are children from poverty backgrounds. The child from such a background tends to come to school with cognitive deficits, because of less favorable preschool experiences; the child probably has seen fewer books, traveled less, had fewer verbal interchanges, and so on. The Head Start program was aimed at trying to supply some of these experiences by broadening the child's horizons, but even two years of Head Start cannot make up for the neglect and lack of opportunity before and after nursery school. In school itself, the comparative lack of experience and supportive action at home contributes to the child's failure in the early grades. This is most likely to happen if the child also has intestinal parasites or is malnourished. With these early failures, self-confidence is impaired. School becomes an unpleasant experience, so that there is little motivation for achievement. These factors reinforce each other, as low achievement leads to low grades and lack of positive reinforcement from the teacher leads to a further loss of self-esteem.[32]

Teacher expectations also enter this picture and further the process, since it is true that people tend to act as they are expected to act. Often on what seems to be quite reasonable grounds, a teacher may be convinced that children from minority and poverty backgrounds do not learn as fast or behave as well as children from more advantaged backgrounds. In a famous experiment in a northern California elementary school, the results of such attitudes were demonstrated effectively, where both teachers and pupils were unknowing guinea pigs. Students in all eighteen classes of the school were given a standard battery of intelligence tests, which the teachers were led to believe had predictive value for identifying future "academic blooming." Unknown to the teachers, the researchers then chose a random sample of about 20 percent of the children from each classroom and told the teachers that these children could be expected to show a burst of achievement. The teachers were also told to keep this information to themselves and not tell the students. All the children were tested again at four- and eight-month intervals, and a teacher rated each student at the end of the year. The results were just as the teachers thought the tests had predicted: the randomly selected academic bloomers had "bloomed." They were rated by their teachers as more interesting, curious, happy, and more likely to become successful in the future. These students also showed a more rapid gain on intelligence-test scores, particularly in their ability to reason, than did their class-mates.[33] The experiment demonstrated how crucial the teachers' attitudes were in determining success.

In addition to the cognitive and verbal deficits that accompany low socioeconomic status, the minority child also starts school with other disadvantages. By the age of five or six, the child often has developed feelings of racial prejudice against himself or herself. The black power movement proclaimed in a strident voice that "black is beautiful." This was an essential first step in developing a confident self-identity. But it can only be effective when this statement becomes accepted, and it is not at all clear that all blacks believe it. Hopefully, in the not too distant future, all black children will know that they are beautiful, just as white children know, for the most part, that they are beautiful. That day has not yet come. In spite of widespread popular beliefs that children do not know prejudice, a series of studies done by Kenneth and Mamie Clark found that pre-school children were not only aware of their own racial identity but had already acquired positive and negative feelings about that identity. The Clarks tested these feelings by presenting children with dolls of differing skin shades or having them color pictures with crayons. Quite consistently, black children chose light skins as more desirable and attractive. Their comments indicated that they had not only learned that they were black, but they were well aware of and believed in the negative stereotypes that accompanied such an identity.[34] The findings of other researchers have supported those of the Clarks. In sociometric tests in which children were asked to select the child in their class they would most like to play with or sit next to, both white and black chidren tended to select white children.[35] The denial of self as psychologically or physically beautiful was dramatically demonstrated one year in the early 1950s, when the black newspaper *The Chicago Defender* unwittingly selected a white girl who was passing as a black as their beauty queen. The reasons for the choice were obvious: she had the fewest black features of any of the candidates. Fortunately, the "black is beautiful" movement helped change some of these stereotypes.

The custom of human beings to search for their self-identity in the reflected image of others[36] places any despised minority group at a disadvantage when it comes to raising mentally healthy children. This is why racial prejudice has such serious consequences for mental health. Though there is little research about the evaluation of self that is made by Puerto Rican or Mexican-American children, it would seem that there would be similar forces at work as among the blacks.

Segregated schools also reinforce feelings of inferiority. In his comprehensive study of educational opportunities undertaken for the United States Office of Education, James Coleman concluded that segregated schools were very damaging to minority children. His team measured three types of attitudes related to academic motivation: (1) interest in school work, (2) self-concept regarding ability, and (3) sense of control over one's own rewards. He found that all three factors were related to academic achievement, but the most crucial was the third factor, control over one's own fate. Black children who felt the most powerless were the least likely to do well in school. As the proportion of white students in the school enrollment increased, the black student felt better able to cope with the dominant white world and both his feelings of control and his educational achievement increased.[37] Unfortunately, the feelings of powerlessness that develop out of segregated experiences have long-range consequences. In the Los Angeles study of housing segregation carried out by one of the authors of this book, it was found that feelings of alienation, including powerlessness and anomie, kept even successful middle-class blacks from making the effort to move to an integrated neighborhood, even though they placed value on this kind of residence. In effect, the ghetto builds its own walls, because the feelings of alienation of the adults were more strongly related to childhood experiences with segregated schools and neighborhoods than to childhood economic deprivation.[38]

The apathy, alienation, and negative self-image created by poverty, prejudice, and discrimination carry over to health in both direct and indirect ways. If mental health is defined positively as a sense of psychic well-being, rather than just the absence of certain debilitating behavioral symptoms, the person who has low self-esteem or feels he or she lacks power over his or her own fate rates low on a continuum of mental health. More importantly, feelings of hopelessness and powerlessness act as barriers to people seeking preventive health care because planning seems useless. Thus, they are more likely to develop preventable physical illness and to wait until their illness has progressed so far that they require long-term hospitalization. These negative feelings also fit into other causal sequences that have consequences for health. The child whose achievement in school is blocked by social-class background or minority status is likely to drop out of school before learning a useful occupational skill; this means that later employment is marginal. The cycle then continues, as the child is unable to furnish a good environment for his or her children or to buy good health care in a society in which health care is a commodity to be bought, and the complex Gordian knot becomes even more impossible to unravel.

ANGER

Apathy and withdrawal are the consequences of economic and racial discrimination; anger is still another. The psychiatrists William Grier and Price Cobbs have described an ever-present, gut-level rage as the outstanding race-related phenomenon they see in their black patients.[39] In the past, fear of violent reprisals and the conditioning for apathy and powerlessness had forced most blacks to suppress an overt expression of rage. However, as these barriers have begun to be dismantled, open violence has erupted. The race riots of the nineteenth and early twentieth centuries differed significantly from the more recent ones in that the earlier ones were instigated by white gangs who invaded black neighborhoods and attacked the residents, while those of the 1960s, 1970s, and 1980s were instigated by blacks.[40] The 1935 Harlem riots and the 1943 Detroit riots originated in the black ghettoes and were aimed at white-owned property. However, it was not until the decade of the 1960s that black rioting reached almost epidemic proportion and focused public attention on the problem of ghetto living.

To study the riots, President Lyndon B. Johnson appointed the National Advisory Commission on Civil Disorders. Somewhat to the surprise of most of its liberal critics, the commission reported that the basic cause of the riots was white racism. Translated into discrimination, this racism caused large numbers of blacks to feel angry, frustrated, and cut off from any legitimate outlet. To solve these problems, the commission advised basic reforms in the administration of justice, the opening-up of employment, housing, and educational opportunities, and a full-scale effort to lessen the level of frustration in the ghetto.[41] In 1970 and 1971, there were similar outbreaks of violence in the Mexican-American barrios of Los Angeles, with similar root causes. As the 1980 Miami riots indicate, problems still remain.

However, from a mental health standpoint, it could be argued that the open expression of this rage is a healthier response than the continued forced repression, although from the standpoint of public policy the riots are no solution. It is interesting to note that, while most ghetto residents understood and sympathized with the riots, usually only from 10 to 20 percent actively participated in them.[42] In effect, most people continued to control or repress their anger with the system. However, repression of anger shows up in other ways, one consequence is thought to be high blood pressure.

Hypertension is much more common among American blacks than Caucasians. When the criterion of a blood pressure reading of 160/95 is used as a definition of hypertension, 9 percent of the adult white population are hypertensive, compared to 22 percent of the black population. This results in a higher hypertensive death rate, particularly between the ages of 45 and 64, when black mortality rates for causes related to blood pressure are 6 to 7 times as high as that among whites. Since sex is also a variable, with males having the higher blood pressures, the young black male is greatly at risk for hypertension.[43] Dietary factors are probably involved in these statistics; the ghetto diet is high in carbohydrates, fats, and salt. Genetic factors may also be implicated. However, the hypothesis that repressed rage and blocked opportunities are involved may be fruitful. To date, the data are clearly suggestive, but more research is needed to pinpoint causes and suggest remedies.[44]

SUICIDE, ALCOHOLISM, AND DRUG ADDICTION

Also unclear is the correlation of race and suicide. Even the statistics that relate socioeconomic status to suicide are not always consistent. Using data from England, Louis Dublin found more suicides among the highest and the lowest social classes.[45] In most U.S. studies, a more simple correlation between low socioeconomic status and suicide has been found.[46] Nevertheless, most authorities hold that sex and race are more significant than income, when it comes to predicting suicide, although the psychodynamics and the precipitating cause of suicide tend to vary from one group to another. For example, more men kill themselves than women, and the stress that triggers their suicide tends to be work-related, while those women who destory themselves are more often disturbed by marital or family problems.[47]

The epidemic proportion of suicide and suicide-related behavior among Indians was pointed out in an earlier chapter. In order to explain this high rate, researchers turned to the concept of anomie, originated by Durkheim.[48] In effect, rapid social and cultural change has left the Indians without the societal underpinnings that usually constrain people from committing suicide. The same explanation seems to account for the high rates among foreign-born Americans, since immigrants are similarly cut off from the environment in which social norms were more stable and family relationships more available. Foreign-born males have a suicide rate that is almost double that of the population as a whole, while foreign-born females have a rate that is 74 percent higher than the female average.[49]

Contrary to expectations, however, suicide rates are not high among the major American ethnic minority populations. Blacks and Mexican Americans have low suicide rates. For example, Mexican-born residents of the United States have the lowest rate of any group of immigrants: 7.9 per hundred thousand in 1960, compared to the national average of 10.6 for that year. Even lower is the general nonwhite ratio (including blacks) of 4.5 per hundred thousand. Since most of the groups classed as nonwhite, including Orientals and Indians, have higher-than-average suicide rates, the black rate must be judged as very low.[50]

However, suicide statistics are misleading, because what constitutes suicide is dependent upon what various officials define as suicide. In general, suicide is more likely to be reported in the North than in the South and in urban areas than in rural areas. What constitutes suicide can also be debated; this causes difficulty, not only for theorists, but also for individuals who must decide as a part of their official duties whether an individual did or did not kill himself. To many people, suicide represents an escape from intolerable loneliness or the overwhelming problems of life.[51] It might be a major unreported cause of death among the elderly. Escape is also possible through drugs or alcohol, so that it has been argued that alcoholism and drug addiction can also be forms of suicidal behavior.[52] Obviously, such a conceptualization of suicide would change the statistical picture for minority group members. For example, there is a fairly high rate of problem drinking among blacks;[53] such drinking patterns can be a factor in accidental deaths and cirrhosis of the liver, or they can complicate other types of illnesses. The narcotizing effect of alcoholism is one way of dealing with frustration and escaping from painful realities. Drinking is not confined to lower socioeconomic groups but also seems to be common among middle-status blacks.[54] Alcoholism is the second leading cause of outpatient visits in the Indian Health Service.[55]

Most studies of drug addiction report that chronic users are likely to originate in the poorest neighborhoods and be members of minority groups. Addiction is rare in rural areas; it tends to be concentrated in the urban slums. Within these rural areas, users tend to come from the most disorganized families and from people in the most miserable circumstances. In fact, addiction correlates highly with almost any form of human misery, including poverty, unemployment, broken homes, low education levels, and substandard housing. Even with these common background factors, researchers are finding that no single explanatory principle can completely account for the high incidence of narcotic use in the urban slums. People start using drugs for a variety of reasons, including feelings of failure, alienation, or emptiness.[56] Then they continue with drug use to avoid withdrawal symptoms[57] or because the drug subculture gives them a way of life. Narcotics, which are readily available in the poverty neighborhoods, become an answer to feelings of hopelessness and frustration that otherwise seem to have no answer.

However, there are changes in the patterns of drug usage, particularly with hallucinogenic drugs, barbiturates, marijuana, and cocaine, which have been adopted by a broader youth culture. At the present time, marijuana and cocaine users are likely to come from higher-income families with better educated parents. Probably, in the period before 1960, the average marijuana user would have been black, lived in an urban slum, and suffered socioeconomic discrimination.[58] On the other hand, the hallucinogenic drugs and barbiturates had their beginnings with the youth culture, rather than with the poverty population. Although deaths are common among barbiturate users, the opiates are more debilitating, and they remain the most serious drug problem among minority group members.

From this brief survey, it seems evident that the association of poverty and ethnic identity with mental illness is a complex one. The relationship between local socioeconomic status and the psychoses is clear, but diagnostic and treatment differences may be the reason for this correlation. Poverty, family disorganization, and discrimination are obviously implicated as factors causing school failures and creating a ghetto attitude marked on the one hand by apathetic withdrawal and on the other by a bubbling anger that can break through in violent revolt. The Indian minority has a high suicide rate, but blacks, Puerto Ricans, and Mexican Americans are less likely to be victims of suicide, unless the anesthetizing destruction of alcoholism and drug addiction are defined as suicide.

REFERENCES

1. Sandifer, Jr., M. G. Social Psychiatry A Hundred Years Ago. *American Journal of Psychiatry*, 1962, *188*, 749–750.

2. Faris, R. E. L. & Dunham, H. W. Mental Disorders in Urban Areas: An Ecological Study of Schizophrenia and Other Psychoses. Chicago: University of Chicago Press, 1939, reprinted 1965.
3. Suttles, G. D. The Social Order of the Slum: Ethnicity and Territory in the Inner City. Chicago: University of Chicago Press, 1968.
4. Dunham, H. W. Community and Schizophrenia: An Epidemiological Analysis. Detroit: Wayne State University Press, 1965.
5. Dohrenwend, B. P. & Dohrenwend, B. S. Social Status and Psychological Disorder: A Causal Inquiry. New York: Wiley-Interscience, 1969, pp. 10–19.
6. Hollingshead, A. B. & Redlich, F. C. Social Stratification and Psychiatric Disorders. *American Sociological Review*, 1953, *18*, 163–169. Hollingshead, A. B. & Redlich, F. C. Social Class and Mental Illness. New York: Wiley, 1958.
7. Srole, L., Langner, T. S., Michael, S. T., Opler, M. K. & Rennie, T. C. Mental Health in the Metropolis: The Midtown Manhattan Study, Vol. 1. New York: McGraw-Hill, 1962.
8. Srole, L. Measurement and Classification in Socio-Psychiatric Epidemiology: Midtown Manhattan Study (1954) and Midtown Manhattan Restudy (1974). *Journal of Health and Social Behavior*, 1975, *16*, 347–363.
9. Warheit, G. J., Holzer, III, C. & Arey, S. Race and Mental Illness: An Epidemiological Update. *Journal of Health and Social Behavior*, 1975, *16*, 243–256.
10. Warheit, G. J., Holzer, III, C. E. & Schwab, J. An Analysis of Social Class and Racial Differences in Depressive Symptomology: A Community Study. *Journal of Health and Social Behavior*, 1973, *14*, 291–299.
11. Srole. op. cit., 1962.
12. Heston, L. L. The Genetics of Schizophrenia and Schizoid Disease. *Science*, 1970, *1967*, 249–256. Dohrenwend & Dohrenwend. op. cit., pp. 32–38.
13. LaPouse, R., Monk, M. A. & Terris, M. The Drift Hypothesis and Socio-Economic Differentials in Schizophrenia. *American Journal of Public Health*, 1956, *46*, 978–986.
14. Myers, J. K. & Bean, L. L. in collaboration with Pepper, M. P. A Decade Later: A Follow-Up of Social Class and Mental Illness. New York: Wiley, 1968.
15. Goffman, E. Asylums: Essays on the Social Situation of Mental Patients and Other Inmates. New York: Anchor Books, 1961.
16. Rowden, D. W., Michel, J. B., Dillehay, R. C. & Martin, H. W. Judgments About Candidates for Psychotherapy: The Influence of Social Class and Insight-Verbal Ability. *Journal of Health and Social Behavior*, 1970, *11*, 51–58.
17. Pavenstedt, E. A Comparison of the Child-Rearing Environment of Upper-Lower and Very Low-Lower Class Families. *American Journal of Orthopsychiatry*, 1965, *35*, 89–98, quotation is from pp. 94–95.

18. For a discussion of this, see: Minuchin, S. et al. Families of the Slums. New York: Basic Books, 1967, pp. 26–27, and passim.
19. Pasamanick, B. A Survey of Mental Disease in an Urban Population. In M. M. Grossack (Ed.), Mental Health and Segregation. New York: Springer, 1963, pp. 150–157.
20. Malzberg, B. Mental Disease Among American Negroes: A Statistical Analysis. In O. Klineberg (Ed.), *Characteristics of the American Negro.* New York: Harper, 1944.
21. Data on institutionalization can be found in Kramer, M. Psychiatric Services and the Changing Institutional Scene 1950–1955. U.S. Department H.E.W., National Institute of Mental Health Series B, No. 12. Washington, D.C.: U.S. Government Printing Office, 1977, pp. 24–25, 32–33, 38–39.
22. Simon, R. J., Fleiss, J. L. & Gurland, B. J. Depression and Schizophrenia in Hospitalized Black and White Mental Patients. *Archives Gen Psychiatry,* 1973, *28,* 509–512. Collins, J. L., Rickman, L. E. & Mathura, C. B. Frequency of Schizophrenia and Depression in a Black Inpatient Population. *Journal of the National Medical Association,* 1980, *9,* 851–856.
23. Carkuff, R. R. & Pierce, R. Differential Effects of Therapists' Race and Social Class upon Patient Depth of Self Exploration in the Initial Interview. *Journal of Counseling Psychology,* 1970, *31,* 632–634.
24. Jaco, E. G. Mental Health of the Spanish-American in Texas. In M. Opler (Ed.), Culture and Mental Health: Cross Cultural Studies. New York: Macmillan, 1959, pp. 467–485.
25. Roberts, R. E. Prevalence of Psychological Distress Among Mexican Americans. *Journal of Health and Social Behavior,* 1980, *21,* 135–145. Quesada, G. M., Spears, M. W. & Ramos, P. Interracial Depressive Epidemiology in the Southwest. *Journal of Health and Social Behavior,* 1978, *19,* 77–85.
26 Dohrenwend & Dohrenwend. op. cit., pp. 13–16. Dohrenwend, B. S. & Dohrenwend, B. P. Stressful Life Events: Their Nature and Effects. New York: Wiley, 1974. Dohrenwend, B. P. Sociocultural and Social-Psychological Factors in the Genesis of Mental Disorders. *Journal of Health and Social Behavior,* 1975, *16,* 365–392.
27. Pettigrew, T. F. A Profile of the Negro American. Princeton, N.J.: D. Van Nostrand, 1964, pp. 100–135. Whiteman, M. & Deutsch, M. Social Disadvantage as Related to Intellective and Language Development. In M. Deutsch, I. Katz, & A. R. Jensen (Eds.), Social Class, Race, and Psychological Development. New York: Holt, 1968, pp. 86–114.
28. Jensen, A. R. How Much Can We Boost I.Q. and Scholastic Achievement? *Harvard Educational Review,* 1969, *39,* 1–123. The controversy between Jensen and other scholars is well presented in the issues of the *Harvard Educational Review* that followed this presentation.
29. Jensen, A. R. Bias in Mental Testing. New York: Free Press, 1980.
30. Gottesman, I. I. Biogenetics of Race and Class. In Social Class, Race and Psychological Development. op. cit., pp. 11–51.

31. For a convenient summary of our own research, see: Bullough, V. L. Dissenting Thoughts on Intellectual and Creative Achievement. *Humanist*, January-February 1980, pp. 43–46, 56.
32. Whiteman, M. & Deutsch, M. op. cit.
33. Rosenthal, R. & Jacobson, L. Self-Fulfilling Prophesies in the Classroom: Teacher's Expectations as Unintended Determinants of Pupils' Intellectual Competence. In Social Class, Race and Psychological Development. op. cit., pp. 219–253. Rosenthal, R. & Jacobson, L. Pygmalion in the Classroom: Teacher Expectation and Pupils' Intellectual Development. New York: Holt, 1969.
34. Clark, K. B. Prejudice and Your Child. Boston: The Beacon Press, 1955. Clark, K. & Clark. M. Emotional Factors in Racial Identification and Preference in Negro Children. In Mental Health and Segregation. op. cit., pp. 53–63.
35. Proshansky, H. & Newton, P. The Nature and Meaning of Negro Self-Identity. In Social Class, Race and Psychological Development op. cit., pp. 178–218. This article includes a comprehensive review of such studies.
36. The Social Psychology of George Herbert Mead. Edited by Anselm Strauss. Chicago: University of Chicago Press, 1956.
37. Coleman, J. S., Campbell, E. Q. et al. Equality of Educational Opportunity. Washington, D.C.: U. S. Office of Education, 1966.
38. Bullough, B. Social Psychological Barriers to Housing Desegregation. Los Angeles: University of California, Housing, Real Estate, and Urban Land Studies Program, 1969.
    Bullough, B. Alienation and School Segregation. In Integrated Education, 1972, 2, pp. 29–35.
39. Grier, W. G. & Cobbs, P. M. Black Rage. New York: Basic Books, 1968.
40. Tuttle, Jr., W. M. Race Riot. New York: Atheneum, 1970.
41. Kerner, O. Chairman. Report on the National Advisory Commission on Civil Disorders. Washington, D.C.: U. S. Government Printing Office, 1968.
42. Kerner. op. cit., pp. 73–77. Fogelson, R. M. & Hill, R. B. Who Riots? A Study of Participation in the 1967 Riots. In O. Kerner, Chairman, Supplemental Studies for the National Advisory Commission on Civil Disorders. Washington, D.C.: U. S. Government Printing Office, 1968, p. 223.
43. Holm, D. Understanding Hypertension. In B. Bullough (Ed.), The Management of Common Human Miseries: A Text for Primary Health Care Practitioners. New York: Springer, 1979, pp. 250–251.
44. J. Stamler (Ed.), et al. Hypertension in the Inner City. Minneapolis: Proforum, 1974. Hosten, A. O. Hypertension in Black and other Populations: Environmental Factors and Approaches to Management. *Journal of the National Medical Association*, 1980, 72, 111–117. Benson, H., Kotch, J.B. & Crassweller, K. D. Stress and Hypertension: Interrelations and Management. *Cardiovascular Clinic*, 1978, 9, 113–124.

45. Dublin, L. I. Suicide: A Sociological and Statistical Study. New York: Ronald Press, 1963, pp. 61–65.
46. Maris, R. W. Social Forces in Urban Suicide. Homewood, Ill.: The Dorsey Press, 1969, p. 160.
47. Breed, W. Suicide, Migration and Race: A Study of Cases in New Orleans. *The Journal of Social Issues*, 1966, *22*, 30–43.
48. Durkheim, E. Suicide: A Study in Sociology. Translated by J. A. Spaulding & G. Simpson. Glencoe, Ill.: The Free Press, 1957, pp. 241–276.
49. Dublin. op. cit., p. 31.
50. Ibid., Tables II, X, XI, pp. 211, 216, 21–19. Breed. op. cit. Labovits, S. Variation in Suicide Rates. In J. P. Gibbs (Ed.), Suicide. New York: Harper, 1968, pp. 57–73.
51. For a discussion of the various meanings of suicide, see: Douglas, J. The Social Meaning of Suicide. Princeton: Princeton University Press, 1967.
52. Menninger, K. A. Man Against Himself. New York: Harcourt, 1938.
53. Maddox, G. L. Drinking Among Negroes: Inferences from the Drinking Patterns of Selected Negro Male Collegians. *Journal of Health and Social Behavior*, 1967, *8*, 114–120.
54. Frazier, E. F. Black Bourgeoisie. New York: Collier Books, 1962, p. 190.
55. Rhoades, E. R. et al. Mental Health Problems of American Indians Seen in Outpatient Facilities of the Indian Health Service, 1975. *Public Health Reports*, 1980, *95*, 329–335.
56. Chein, I. Psychological, Social and Epidemiological Factors in Drug Addiction. In Rehabilitating the Narcotic Addict. Report of the Institute of New Developments in the Rehabilitation of the Narcotic Addict. Washington, D.C.: U. S. Government Printing Office, 1966, pp. 53–66.
57. Lindesmith, A. R. Basic Problems in the Social Psychology of Addiction and a Theory. In J. A. O'Donnell & J. C. Ball (Eds.), Narcotic Addiction. New York: Harper & Row, 1966, pp. 91–109.
58. Goode, E. The Marijuana Smokers. New York: Basic Books, 1970, pp. 35–39.

9

Discrimination and Segregation

In the twentieth century, U.S. medicine has been regarded as an occupation for the upper-middle classes. Costly and time-consuming education has made it difficult if not impossible for a poor person to become a high-status health professional. In fact, with only slight exaggeration, it can be argued that, until the advent of the GI Bill in the aftermath of World War II, college education itself was primarily a middle-class phenomenon. Since those students who continued their studies beyond the bachelor's degree had to have even greater economic resources, the fact that physicians came from the more affluent sections of society seems self-explanatory. As late as 1961, about 40 percent of all medical students came from families whose income was in the top 8 percent of the population.[1]

In a sense, medicine was not particularly different from other professional occupations in its educational demands; but, in another sense, it was much more elitist in orientation because, unlike law or college teaching, medicine demanded that the training be taken in a concentrated dose. Long hours of duty and study made it difficult for the would-be physician to have a part-time job on the side. There were occasional scholarships, and, in spite of all obstacles, some students from a poverty background made it through medical school. However, to do so required greater intelligence and dedication than that demonstrated by the average medical student; the less affluent student also needed better luck and a devoted family, since the student and the whole family had to sacrifice. The very structure of medical training was designed to exclude almost all but the more well-to-do.

Medical schools were also geographically concentrated. Until after World War II, many states and regions were without medical schools, making it necessary for the would-be student to relocate in an area far from home and to maintain a second household, a task that added to economic burdens. If only because the course of studies was shorter and the entrance requirements less rigorous, dentistry offered slightly greater opportunities to students from the lower economic levels.

Even those professional groups that had started out with a more "lower-class origin"—nursing and pharmacy—attempted to adopt the same procedures as medicine to raise their status. Undoubtedly, becoming middle-class is part of the professionalization process, at least in the Western world, but it also has positive and negative implications for medical care. Since the establishment of formal nursing educational programs more than a century ago, nursing has been struggling to raise its standards and its status. The hospital schools, the dominant nursing educational institution for the past century, gave students room and board and helped them keep the financial barriers to a minimum. As collegiate nursing education has grown and educational standards have been raised, even hospital schools have turned to charging tuition or fees, making nursing less accessible to students from lower socioeconomic backgrounds. Pharmacy, which originally had an apprenticeship system, has also become much more middle-class oriented, as it transferred into the colleges and the universities.

However, regardless of their social-class background, once health professionals entered practices, their patients, at least until World War II, were most likely to come from the middle class, and their professional success was dependent upon their ability to attract such patients. This was because medicine, nursing, and dentistry were practiced on a fee-for-service basis, in which the relationship between the patient and practitioner was one-to-one. Pharmacists differed from these groups in that they were not usually paid directly for services but for a commodity, drugs. Nonetheless, the implications of such relationships for all health professionals was clear. Even though an individual from a poverty background might have become a professional, the individual's success in monetary terms was dependent upon the ability to escape from social-class origins.

Outside the system, although not entirely overlooked, were the poor—those unable to pay for the services of an individual practitioner. To deal with these people, society established institutions, hospitals, or clinics staffed by medical students, student nurses, interns, or residents who were supervised by a few paid practitioners and several volunteers. At the same time, these institutions served as training grounds for the future professionals. In effect, as we have stated earlier, the poor were guinea pigs so that the would-be health professionals could acquire enough expertise to deal effectively with the paying patient.

One reason why there is a crisis in medicine today is that the institutions originally designed to serve the poor are now also serving the rich. As indicated earlier, the great revolution in medicine of the past 50 years has been the removal of the patient from the home to the hospital and the change from a one-to-one relationship to the health care team. The change was dictated by several facts, not the least of which was economics. Technical advances in medicine required the purchase of more and more costly equipment and greater and greater specialization. This meant that services and equipment had to be concentrated, and the hospital was the logical place for such concentration. Giving further impetus to this trend was the development of medical insurance, which required hospitalization before reimbursement could be made. This encouraged transferring to the hospital many services previously carried out in a physician's office or in a patient's home.

The first group to experience the change was nursing; as hospitals grew, nurses changed from being private-duty practitioners to institutional employees. Forced into the hospital, middle-class patients demanded better care than was available in the student-run charitable institutions. They proved extremely reluctant to be experimented upon by unsupervised nursing and medical students. Hospitals were forced to upgrade their training programs, and in doing so they found it much less costly to hire an all-professional nursing staff than to maintain their nursing schools. The change in the nature of the hospitals also coincided with nurses demands for higher educational standards. As educational requirements were increased, nursing became much more middle class. In the process of upgrading itself, nursing delegated many of its functions to new auxiliary nursing personnel: the licensed practical or vocational nurse and the nursing aide, who generally came from a lower economic background than the nurse.[2]

The transfer of the medical practitioner into the hospital led to further schooling for the physician and the surgeon, since the hospital setting required greater and greater specialization. This meant that medical education became even more expensive. Unfortunately, the physician was less able to adjust to the real changes in the nature of medical practice than the nurse. As expressed by the official statements of the American Medical Association, the physician continued to think of medicine as a one-to-one relationship, although in reality he (and the overwhelming majority of physicians were male) was little more than a member of the medical team. Even though he might still be captain of the team, many of his "subordinates" acquired greater expertise in their specialty than he did, and this caused a crisis in the physician's view of himself, as well as his subordinates. Dentistry is only now beginning to face up to the same kind of pressures, since it has lengthened its period of training and increased its specialization, but the profession is still struggling to avoid team care and is maintaining a one-to-one relationship with the patient. Dentistry still serves the most middle-class clientele of the four groups, since only the middle class can afford this type of health care. The one group that has been downgraded in this process is the pharmacist, who in many ways is overtrained for the tasks of the profession. The pharmacist is no longer called upon to personally compound prescriptions, but rather to dispense prepared prescription drugs; in most settings, the pharmacist counts pills and measures liquids. As an employee of a chain store, the pharmacist has also lost the place of the individual entrepreneur in the corner drug store. To deal with this crisis, pharmacy has followed nursing into the hospital, with the rapidly expanding field of clinical pharmacy.

The middle-class bias so evident in the selection and training of health professionals might well be unconscious; at least it does not appear to be deliberate. The same cannot be said of the professions' handling of either the minority-group patient or the would-be professional from an ethnic minority. Here in the past, the exclusion has been conscious and deliberate, and this has had tragic consequences for the health care of Americans.

DISCRIMINATION IN MEDICAL EDUCATION

Until recently, the vast majority of medical schools operated on either a discriminatory or a segregated basis. Members of certain minority groups were either trained in segregated institutions or admitted only on quota to a few others. The result of such practices was to keep medicine a much more exclusive profession than it otherwise would have been. Not all segments of the health care community were as segregated or discriminatory as others. For example, nursing was somewhat less prone to discriminatory practices than medicine, and within medicine, osteopathic schools were more willing to tolerate minority group members than others. Inevitably, a significant percentage of osteopaths were Jewish, a group that, in spite of middle-class origins and aspirations, was discriminated against in most medical schools until the era following World War II. The breakdown of discrimination against Jews in medicine was partly due to a reaction against the ideology of Hitler and a consciousness of what discriminatory attitudes might lead to. Also important was Jews' willingness to organize and support medical schools of their own—such as Einstein College of Medicine or Mount Sinai College of Medicine (now part of the City University of New York)—or to give large-scale financial support to existing schools such as the Chicago College of Medicine. Today, it seems that most of the barriers based upon religious identity are in the process of disappearing.

However, much more serious barriers were erected against blacks. As late as 1947, only 20 of the "white" medical schools had black students, and then they had only 93 black students in total. There were two segregated medical schools: Howard University Medical School in Washington, D.C., largely funded by the United States Government; and Meharry Medical College, located in Nashville, Tennessee, near Fisk University. The black student who wanted to study medicine had to travel to either of these two centers for medical education or wait until a black quota slot was available nearer to home. The effective result was to deny most blacks the opportunity to become physicians. In 1958, only 2.2 percent of all physicians were black.[3] The percentage has moved up somewhat since then, as blacks and other minorities have been allowed into medical schools in greater numbers, and as financial assistance has been provided through federal support programs that came out of the civil rights struggle. For example, in 1974 to 1975, 6.3 percent of all medical students and 7.2 percent of the entering class were black.[4]

The same discriminatory practices existed in dentistry. Howard University had a dental school, and so did Meharry for a time, but no other dental schools admitted blacks in any significant number until after World War II. For example, in 1940, there was only one black dentist for every 8,745 blacks, compared to the overall ratio of one dentist to 1,865 people.[5] The ratio inched up slightly in the 1960s and 1970s. By 1975, ten percent of the students in dental colleges were classified as minority, with blacks making up the most significant proportion of this group.[6] Pharmacy likewise discriminated, and most black pharmacists until fairly recently were graduates of Howard or Meharry.

Nursing was equally discriminatory. In 1950, nonwhite nurses (including Orientals and Indians, as well as blacks) amounted to only 3.5 percent of the total nurse population.[7] Most of these who did graduate came from segregated nursing schools.[8] As the discriminatory barriers dropped, nursing schools appeared willing to admit black students but did little about this until after 1960. In a 1962 survey of 1,128 schools of nursing, 22 were predominantly black— that is, they had originally been segregated black schools—but only 9 of these were accredited. Of the remaining schools, 912 said they would accept blacks as students if and when they applied, 162 stated they would not, and 29 were in the process of closing down. This was about eight years after the 1954 Supreme Court school desegregation decision. One of the most disappointing findings was that the number of blacks entering into nursing education at all levels had declined to about 3 percent of the total number,[9] due in large part to the decline of the segregated nursing schools. Rather than helping blacks, integration seemed on the surface to have harmed them. For the most part, nursing school officials responded that they were willing to admit blacks, but a willingness to admit blacks and actually admitting them proved to be two different things. A century of segregation could not be wiped out overnight.

Beginning in 1966, there was a concentrated effort to recruit minorities, but the results have not always been successful, as interest has waxed and waned. In 1975, the number of blacks admitted to basic RN programs (associate, diploma, and baccalaureate) amounted to 9.1 percent, but this declined to 7.2 percent in 1978. Some 5.7 percent of the 1975 graduating class were black, but this fell to 4.7 in 1978. There had been a slight increase in Spanish-speaking minorities, from 2.3 percent of the admission in 1975 and 1.8 percent of those graduating, to 2.5 percent in 1978 and 3.1 percent of those graduating. American Indians and Orientals had also increased slightly, from 1.2 percent in 1975 to 1.4 percent in 1978, and from 1 percent of the graduates in 1975 to 1.3 percent in 1978. Minorities were represented in greater numbers proportionately at the practical or vocational level, better at the associate degree than at the baccalaureate degree and most underrepresented in the diploma programs.[10]

During their efforts to recruit minorities, health professionals became conscious of the fact that many of their admission requirements were designed to exclude minorities. Particularly in medical schools, admission committees were faced with the fact that only a small proportion of their applicants could be admitted and tried to find rational and quantifiable criteria for selection. In an earlier age, money had been more important, and the cost of medical education has proven beyond the dreams and aspirations of most students. However, as the money barrier decreased and the number of applicants increased, there was an attempt to objectify grades and tests. Believing that some of the high achievers were better qualified to become research scientists than medical practitioners, admission committees occasionally went farther down the grade point ladder to admit students, but these efforts were half-hearted and sporadic. Certain groups, such as children of physicians, also were often favored, but increasingly medical students became a highly selective intellectual elite; dental schools made an effective effort to imitate medicine in this regard.

As has been indicated earlier, intellectual achievement at this level is not merely a product of individual genius; it is also a product of social background and schooling. Only a few middle-class minority families could afford to give their children similar advantages, and their numbers were not sufficient to satisfy the sudden demand for more identifiable minority students. The ghetto students from segregated schools who made it through the basic baccalaureate training were at a disadvantage when they were thrown in with the student body of a medical school at the graduate level, because there were so many gaps in their own backgrounds. Thus, in effect, those schools that admitted minority students without regard to their educational background and preparation programmed them for failure.[11]

The failure of some of these specially admitted minority students forced a further re-examination of recruitment efforts. It was found that solid compensatory education could give some students the background they needed to compete. Some programs of this type started with financing through private foundations, such as the Josiah Macy, Jr. Foundation, or through federal grants. Another alternative, and one which received little support, was lowering the level of medical and dental education for the primary practitioner, or at least allowing such students to go part-time as they can in many other graduate schools. On the contrary, as medical specialties have developed and become more complex, each of them has competed for a place in the basic medical program, until now medical students are required to cover each of the various fields far beyond the level needed by the ordinary general practitioner, or even beyond the needs of the specialist who does not practice in that area. In a 1970 study, the Carnegie Foundation suggested that, if medical and dental education was re-evaluated, the number of years spent in training could be lessened to three years for the basic medical and dental degrees.[12]

Theoretically, nursing was in a somewhat better position to recruit minority students than the more prestigious professions. The entrance requirements for the baccalaureate-level nurse training programs are not so high as those for medicine and dentistry, and the associate degree and hospital training program are somewhat lower. In spite of this, it was not until deliberate efforts were made that the number of minority students began to increase in any appreciable way. One of the earliest and most successful recruitment programs was started by Boston University Alumni in 1965. Called *ODWIN*, an acronym for Opening the Doors Wider in Nursing, volunteers visited high schools in minority neighborhoods to counsel students and start "future nurse" clubs. With financial assistance from the Rockefeller and Seatlantic funds, they set up tutoring services and programs to provide compensatory education. ODWIN members not only increased the number of successful minority students at Boston University, but in the following years they spread their programs to include other schools in the New England area.[13] Other programs such as the East Los Angeles Health Task Force relied upon federal funds to recruit.

Overall, however, most recruitment programs have not been successful in retaining the students they recruited. In trying to determine why some programs were more successful in retaining minorities than others, John Buckley examined programs in 16 geographically dispersed states. Though all of the least successful schools enrolled a sizeable black student body (at least 10 percent), retention rates were 50 percent or less. The key to success was flexibility in scheduling and administering the program, integration of faculty and staff, and the commitment of the teaching faculty to minority education.[14] However, recruitment is also a two-way street, and the minorities themselves have to bear some of the blame. In the developmental phases of recruitment, some of the minority groups visualized the new emphasis on minority status as a power tool. In their desire to build a power base, they ignored many a willing Anglo worker. The key to success, however, is cooperation of both majority and minority groups. Without this, even the most successful recruitment project is doomed to fail.

Volunteer cooperation has become more crucial, as the courts have ruled out some of the procedures used to choose students from a variety of applicants. One of the first challenges to the use of special admission was that of Marco De Funis, who was one of 1,600 applicants to the University of Washington School of Law. The school's enrollment was limited to 150 in the first-year class, so most applicants were denied admission. However, the law school did admit some minority students who had grade point averages below that of De Funis and whose Law School Admission Tests were also lower. De Funis sued and, though he gained admittance to the law school through a lower court decision, the Washington State Supreme Court held that a racial classification was constitutionally permissible if it could be shown as necessary to serve a "compelling interest." Law school admissions should not be arbitrary and capricious but should remain sensitive and flexible to meet the great public need. The United States Supreme Court refused to intervene, because by the time the case could be decided, De Funis would have graduated.[15]

Though schools might undertake special admission policies, they could not set quotas. This was the ruling in *Bakke v. Regents* of the University of California in November 1974. Conditions in the medical school at Davis were similar to those of the law school in Seattle, except that the medical school had clearly established a quota. The decision of the superior court was appealed to the California Supreme Court, which held similar to the Washington court that the university is not required to make admissions strictly on the basis of academic grade but could take the background of the candidate into consideration, so long as admission standards were applied in a racially neutral fashion.[16] The U.S. Supreme Court upheld the decision of the California Supreme Court. Although some liberals were disappointed by the Bakke decision, it is not a serious barrier to recruitment. The quota system is a two-edged sword, and it has been used most often to exclude minorities rather than encourage them. Since the Bakke decision, programs have focused on the disadvantaged student, regardless of race, and this seems to be a mechanism that can withstand court tests. Through such recruitment efforts, the number of blacks in the health professions is slowly rising to match their percentage in the population, while Spanish-speaking Americans, Indians, Puerto Ricans, are beginning to grow. Some minorities, such as the Japanese or Chinese, have entered the higher status health occupations disproportionately to their numbers.

In view of past discriminatory practices against ethnic minorities in this country, an anomolous situation is the broad-scale admission of foreign medical graduates. The United States has drained neighboring countries of their physicians, because once an individual has graduated from medical school, even a foreign one, the individual has comparatively little difficulty in getting a job in the United States. State licensure usually requires special internship, but the obstacles are not so great as to prevent large numbers of physicians from emigrating to the United States. In 1970, for example, it was estimated that one doctor in every 20 trained in Latin America eventually left for the United States.[17] Though few of the Latin American medical schools would meet the U.S. standards of medical education, they nonetheless supply a large number of U.S. physicians. Thus, while U.S. medical schools might be the world's best, a significant number of American physicians come from schools throughout the world that do not match the better U.S. schools in education. A significant number of foreign-educated physicians attended schools where students enter as freshmen rather than as graduate students, and many attended medical schools where there is little clinical training. The issue is further complicated by the fact that many Americans, unable to get into U.S. medical schools, turn to third-world medical schools or to schools where there are no limits on enrollment or registration, such as the University of Bologna. In such schools, there are so many students that it is impossible for students even to attend classes. Though a dedicated student can get an adequate education at even the most inadequate of medical schools, providing he or she has the determination to do so, the student does so in spite of the school rather than because of it. This alternative recruitment of physicians to the medical community serves as a safety valve for U.S. medical colleges, allowing them to claim they are keeping standards very high when, in reality, a significant minority of new practicing physicians do not meet these standards. We then compensate by requiring foreign physicians to serve years of additional internships and residencies in order to overcome their dubious preparation. Only now that medicine is worrying about an oversupply of physicians is there an attempt to deal with the foreign medical student.

In the United States, medicine traditionally discriminated against women. Even as late as 1970, a study conducted by Harold I. Kaplan for the National Institute of Mental Health found that many medical schools were reluctant to accept women as students. Kaplan found that women who were admitted to medical schools were academically more exceptional than their male counterparts.[18] Since this study was completed, increasing numbers of women have entered medical school. Current enrollment figures include 22.4 percent women, but practicing physicians who are women[19] remain a minority. Countries like Great Britain, where 24 percent of the physicians are women, or the Soviet Union, where 65 percent are, have far better records than the United States. Once the barriers for women are lowered, the major obstacle to admission of women turned out to have been, as it has in the case of other minorities, the prejudices of the admission committees in medical schools. These prejudices undoubtedly were a reflection of most American medical practitioners and have only been lessened by the threat of government intervention. Dentistry has been even more closed than medicine; in 1970, less than two percent of the practicing dentists were women.[20]

Although the causal sequence is different, the sex segregation in nursing is as severe as that in medicine and dentistry. As late as 1969, only 3.5 percent of the registered nurses and 4.4 percent of the practical nursing students were men.[21] By 1978, the rate had almost doubled, until 6.3 percent of the students admitted to nursing schools were men, and 5.5 percent of those graduating from various R.N. programs were men. On the other hand, the percentage of men in practical nursing programs remained the same, at about 4.5 percent.[22] Perhaps the major reason for sex discrimination in the past was that student nurses were required to live in dormitories on hospital grounds and dormitories for men were not available. This same reason was used by medical schools to refuse admission to large numbers of women, although women medical students were welcome in the nurses' dormitories. As it became more identified with women, men also avoided nursing because of the threat to their status. Generally, men have been more reluctant to enter a "woman's" profession than women have been to enter a so-called "man's" profession. Gradually, however, men have entered nursing in increasing numbers, and there are probably enough male nurses now that larger and larger numbers of men will feel comfortable enough to become nurses.

The recital of this background is important, because it emphasizes how discrimination against various minority health practitioners has affected patient care. Obviously, a health professional who is white and from the middle class will have trouble communicating with patients who are black and from the lower class. His or her task is made even more difficult if the patient's knowledge of English is less than adequate, as is the case with many Puerto Ricans or Mexican Americans. Until 1970, there were Mexican-American patients in Los Angeles County Hospital who were being treated without the benefit of a case history, since neither the nurse nor the physician spoke Spanish; until pressured to do so, the hospital did not always furnish an interpreter. Much of medical treatment was carried out through sign language. This in a city where Spanish has always been spoken and where Spanish surnames make up the majority of large selections of the county.

A patient from a different ethnic group than the professional often has difficulty in communicating, even when both speak the same language. Much of the information we transmit to each other is conveyed by facial expression, body movement, voice tone, and so forth. Professionals who regularly deal with ethnic minorities and who make the effort to understand the subculture can pick up this kind of communication, but most professionals, particularly those who only occasionally deal with the poor members of minority groups, are totally unaware of their lack of communication.[23] The sex barriers in the health care professions also have implications for patient care, because many patients have great difficulty communicating with a professional of the opposite sex. The horror of having to be examined by a male physician keeps many shy Mexican-American women from seeking prenatal care or contraceptive advice. As the level of sophistication of the patient increases, communication becomes easier, but this does not help the poverty-stricken minority patient.

DISCRIMINATION IN TREATMENT

Lack of ability to communicate is only one of the lesser effects of discrimination. A much more serious difficulty that too often has proven fatal to the patient has been the denial of actual health care to individuals on the basis of race. This aspect of medical discrimination must be counted as one of the most disgraceful chapters in all of U.S. history. In 1954, the year the Supreme Court ordered the desegregation of schools, medical care, both in the North and the South, was delivered on a highly discriminatory basis. A study conducted by the authors of this book in Chicago in that year found that, though 15 percent of the city's population (about 590,000 people) were black, 50 percent of the blacks were treated in one hospital, Cook County. This was true in spite of the fact that some of the patients who went there had paid-up hospitalization policies that nominally would have allowed them to be treated at private hospitals. Unfortunately, most of the 65 hospitals in the city, many of which were located in or near the ghetto, refused to admit black patients. The results of such discriminatory admission practices were evident in birth statistics. In 1951, 82 percent of the black births in Chicago took place in only four hospitals or under the supervision of the Chicago Maternity Center, which delivered babies at home. Of the remaining 18 percent of the black births, 80 percent were concentrated in eight nongovernmental hospitals. Cook County Hospital alone recorded 54 percent of all black births but only 2 percent of the white births.

When a black person attempted to get treatment at other hospitals, the results were often fatal. We found that a black employee of a manufacturing company that had a medical agreement with a hospital was denied admission to the hospital, even though he was seriously ill with a massive lobar pneumonia. The hospital admitted blacks only to "hall" beds, which were filled at the time, although there were vacant wards and rooms. Equally as tragic, a black journalist from Trinidad who was struck by an automobile and rushed to a nearby hospital with a skull fracture was denied admission because of his color. After considerable delay, he was transferred to Cook County Hospital, where he died shortly afterward. Whether he could have been saved with prompt treatment is perhaps debatable, but a 3-hour delay was certainly fatal.

A 15-year-old black boy with an intestinal obstruction was brought by his mother to a private hospital and was denied admission because of his color, despite the woman's ability to pay. He died shortly after arriving at Cook County Hospital. The list of cases compiled in Chicago and elsewhere by the Medical Committee Against Discrimination was full of such incidents.

The extent of discrimination was most effectively revealed when Altgeld Gardens, a public housing project on the far south side of Chicago, contracted with an ambulance service to carry emergency cases past 28 hospitals to Cook County Hospital, because of the inability to get treatment any closer. There was an average delay of 1 hour and 20 minutes between the time the ambulance was called and the time the ambulance arrived at Cook County Hospital. A few of the hospitals on the route did not discriminate, notably Provident Hospital, an all-black institution, but it was not equipped to deal with the emergencies from such a large population. In a sense, Illinois was a leader against racial discrimination among northern states, since it had a public accommodation law making it illegal to bar anyone because of race, creed, or color, but hospitals had been ruled as not being "public accommodations."[24] They remained exempt until the legislature amended the state statute in 1955. Still, in 1963, the United States Commission on Civil Rights found medical discrimination in Chicago to be as bad as in Memphis, Tennessee. Most of the black patients were still cared for at Cook County Hospital or at three predominantly black hospitals, one a proprietary hospital with only 15 beds. With 206 beds, Provident Hospital was the largest black institution, but the Commission found its facilities outmoded and its treatment for most cases inadequate, since its prime purpose was to care for maternity cases.[25]

Compounding the problem was the fact that large numbers of physicians in the United States refused to treat "colored" patients. Even when a physician consented to do so, he or she could not always gain admission for the patient to a hospital. If the physician did gain admission for the patient, the patient was usually put into a segregated wing, ward, or hallway, and occasionally in a broom closet. Most black physicians lacked hospital affiliations, since to have staff or courtesy privileges required membership in the county or state medical society and this in most states was a discriminatory body. To counter such discrimination, black physicians had organized the National Medical Association, which proved over the years to be an effective voice, but this still did not get them staff privileges.

When students of today hear of such practices, their first reaction is to demand that the government do something about it. Unfortunately, in the case of medical discrimination, the federal government in the past has tended to encourage rather than discourage such practices. Even after segregation in education had been ruled unconstitutional, the federal government continued to support segregated medical delivery systems and training programs. In fact, because so much of the past history of discrimination and segregation has been caused by government intervention, many people now feel it takes positive effort on the government's part to undo the damage that it has caused in the past.

One of the most notable examples of the government encouraging discriminatory practices was the Hill-Burton Act of 1946, often cited as the Hospital Construction Act. The purpose of this legislation was to provide a government subsidy for the construction of hospitals, since a medical census taken at that time found that the number of hospital beds in the United States would have to be doubled to meet the expected demand. Under the legislation, the government contributed roughly one-third of the costs incurred in building hospitals in those areas or neighborhoods that met its criteria. Hospital construction immediately zoomed until the three-year period, 1958 to 1961; hospital construction totaled $1,825,000,000, approximately a third of which came from federal funds.[26]

However, the Hill-Burton funds provided for hospital construction on a separate-but-equal basis, which meant that very few hospitals were ever constructed for blacks. By 1963, only 13 new hospitals had been specially constructed for blacks, while 76 had been specifically designed to exclude blacks. Inevitably, the disparity between white and black medical care increased rather than decreased. In Atlanta, it was found in 1963 that only 630 of the 4,500 hospital beds in the city were available to blacks—who comprised approximately 50 percent of the population. In Birmingham, Alabama, in that same year, 574 beds were allocated to blacks and 1,762 to whites— although 40 percent of Birmingham's population was black. In some of the smaller southern towns, where only one hospital had been built with Hill-Burton funds, the hospitals refused to admit blacks under any condition. This was the case in Augusta, Georgia. In fact, Georgia had about 83 hospitals built with grants from the Hill-Burton fund, almost all of which were for whites only.[27]

It was not until 1963, after an estimated 1,000,000 hospital beds had been constructed and over $1,600,000,000 of federal money spent, that the separate-but-equal doctrine in hospital construction finally received a court hearing. In that year, six black physicians and dentists plus two black patients in Greensboro, North Carolina, charged that they were discriminated against by two hospitals, Moses Cone Memorial Hospital and Wesley Long Community Hospital, both constructed with Hill-Burton aid. The physicians and dentists sought staff or clinic privileges and the two black patients sought admission to the hospitals and the right to treatment by their personal physicians. The suit brought by the National Association for the Advancement of Colored People also received support from the Department of Justice. After an adverse decision in the local court, the Fourth Circuit Court of Appeals in Richmond, Virginia, struck down the separate-but-equal clause as unconstitutional, and this decision was affirmed by the United States Supreme Court.[28]

Known in the law books as *Simkins vs. Moses H. Cone Memorial Hospital*, the decision forced the government to change its policy from that of promoting segregation to that of being an advocate of nondiscrimination. The Public Health Service then charged with administering the Hill-Burton funds, eventually passed regulations prohibiting discrimination by any hospital that in the future received construction funds. More positive action came in 1964, with the passage of the Civil Rights Act. Title VI of that act prohibited any program or activity receiving federal financial assistance from denying benefits on grounds of race, color, or national origin. Each federal department or agency extending financial assistance, other than by contract or insurance or guarantee, was directed to effectuate this prohibition by rules approved by the President, and was authorized to terminate assistance to those agencies that failed to comply. In spite of Title VI, most hospitals that had discriminated in the past (including those previously built with Hill-Burton funds) continued to do so, since reimbursements for patients usually came third-hand, from local welfare agencies, and since the state agencies that managed the federal funds were reluctant to enforce the prohibitions against discrimination. In a survey made by the United States Commission on Civil Rights one year after the passage of the act, health care discrimination was found to be widespread. Blacks were housed in segregated wings or floors, forced to use separate waiting rooms, nurseries, cafeterias, and clinics, and, in many cases, blacks were entirely excluded from the medical facilities. Black physicians were refused staff privileges at any but all-black or inner-city hospitals. Most nursing homes were restricted to whites, although a large percentage of the patients were supported by federally-assisted public welfare agencies. Those nursing homes admitting blacks were usually all-black institutions. Even state owned or operated health facilities, such as mental health institutions, tuberculosis sanitariums, and charity hospitals, were often segregated by state law.[29]

The most effective instrument in encouraging a change in past practices was the enactment of Medicare on July 3, 1965, since in line with Title VI all participating hospitals and nursing homes, public or private, had to drop their discriminatory practices in order to qualify for funds. This was emphasized in 1966 by a White House directive stating that no hospital that discriminated would be eligible for Medicare funds. To make certain the directive was enforced, the Office of Equal Health Opportunity (OEHO) was established in the Public Health Service in February 1966 to screen hospitals applying for Medicare funds to see that they did not discriminate. In July 1966, when Medicare became effective, OEHO reported that more than 35,000 hospitals, which in the past had used discriminatory assignments or had segregated facilities, had agreed to integrate. This was one-third of the 9,200 hospitals in the United States at that time. By 1968, it was estimated that over 98 percent of the hospitals applying for Medicare met the nondiscriminatory provisions of the Civil Rights Act.

Regarded as typical of the changes taking place was the example of St. Dominic Jackson Memorial Hospital in Jackson, Mississippi. Before 1963, no black physicians had been allowed staff privileges at the hospital, no black students had been accepted into the nursing training program, and all black patients had been confined to a first-floor ward. Black newborns had been kept in a segregated section of the nursery on the second floor. In 1965, the hospital

admitted blacks to its nursing school and granted staff privileges to
a few black physicians. Shortly afterward, black fathers were allowed to visit the second floor to see their babies in the nursery, a
privilege previously denied them. Still, by 1968, the hospital had
little biracial occupancy. In order to speed up integration, the
OEHO took legal action in cities such as Pittsburgh, Baltimore, and
Camden (New Jersey) to break down entrenched patterns of staff
privileges and patient referrals.[30]

In extreme cases, the government acted to cut off funds. An early
test case involved the Alabama Board of Mental Health, which administered Bryce, Searcy, and Partlow Hospitals. At Bryce, black and
white patients were housed in different buildings and no black professional staff members were employed, although black psychiatric
aides were assigned to black wards. The treatment center, an adjunct
to Bryce Hospital, admitted only black patients and provided inferior
services and facilities. Searcy Hospital was an all-black hospital with
inferior facilities. Partlow Hospital assigned patients to wards on a
racial basis, segregating psychiatric aides' dining rooms and assign-
ing them patients only of their own race. Because of such practices, a
hearing officer ordered termination of all federal funds on October 4,
1967. In spite of objections from the hospitals, the hearing officer's
decision was upheld.

Though this might be interpreted as a forward step, the difficulty in carrying integration much beyond tokenism is indicated by
the case of the Mobile Infirmary, the largest hospital in Alabama
but the one with the fewest blacks. In 1966, it was found that only
20 of the 1,767 patients admitted during a one-month period were
black. The Infirmary's application for Medicare funds was deferred
for three months while an investigation was carried out, but the
Infirmary successfully argued that it was in compliance with Title
VI, since few blacks chose to go there. Though it was assumed that
there was an active policy of discouraging blacks, and it was evident
that blacks feared the treatment they would receive if they did attend the clinic, the OEHO ruled that it could find no blacks who
claimed to have been denied admission.[31]

The original Hill-Burton legislation had also included a requirement that hospitals receiving construction monies would provide a
reasonable volume of services for the poor. This feature of the law
was never operationally defined, so it was essentially not enforced;
in effect, any service to the community could be considered "reasonable services." Starting in 1970, a group of public interest law
groups, including most notably the National Health Law Program,
started campaigning for enforcement of this provision. They wrote

papers urging enforcement and fought a series of law suits. Finally in 1972 (26 years after the writing of the law), the Department of Health, Education, and Welfare issued draft regulations suggesting that hospitals use 5 percent of their total costs or 25 percent of their net income, whichever was more, to provide services for those who could not pay.[32] This proposal was vigorously questioned by the American Hospital Association, which had by that date emerged as a powerful lobby and, as of this writing, possibly the most powerful lobby in the health care field, a position it took over from the AMA. The AHA eloquently argued that hospitals had a crucial responsibility to stay solvent in order to serve the community, that such a provision was unnecessary, that the poor could be cared for in some other way, and that many hospitals had had their new wing in place for almost twenty years, so their obligations to the poor were too old to be enforced.[33] After three years of delays, watered-down regulations were passed.[34] Hospitals now have an obligation to give some services to the poor, but it still remains difficult to actually admit a poor person who does not have proof of an outside third-party payer in hand.

Another problematic area related to government intervention is that of the elderly. In a comprehensive review of the laws and regulations related to Medicare and Medicaid, Patricia Butler concluded that the two programs had created almost insurmountable obstacles to out-patient services for the elderly. She pointed out that there were three dominant powers that shaped the 1965 legislation: the American Medical Association, the American Hospital Association, and the insurance industry. These lobbies favored a medical rather than a social definition of the problems of aging, and they supported expensive institutional care over home-support services.[35] Clinics, visiting nursing services, nurse practitioners, social work services, and health maintenance organizations have difficulty being reimbursed for care to the elderly, but institutional care is covered. In many cases, the 1972 reforms establishing utilization reviews have cut off payments to hospitalized patients but have not replaced those services with less expensive formats for care. Our society is now faced with an expensive system that is tied to beds rather than essential services. The system cannot be scrapped, because there are many needy elderly persons who do need beds. But most do not. Obviously, major reforms are needed, since the number of aged is growing as the population ages. Many aged also need assistance, as inflation destroys the incomes of even the most prudent among them. The problem is complicated by the fact that the declining birth rate of the last twenty years will cut the number of workers who can support the burgeoning elderly population in expensive depressing nursing homes.

CONCLUDING COMMENTS

The history of past discriminatory practices of medical institutions and medical practitioners is something that still handicaps effective medical care today. Though race or ethnic identity are becoming less important as grounds for being denied medical care, there is still a double standard for medical treatment. Many minority persons and most poor people still receive second-rate medical care from practitioners who have little understanding of their problems. The result is that our health care delivery system remains uneven, and, until there are changes, the United States will lag behind less rich and less educated countries in the health of its citizens.

REFERENCES

1. Somer, H. M. and Somer, A. R. Doctors, Patients and Health Insurance: The Organization and Financing of Medical Care. Washington, D.C.: The Brookings Institution, 1961.
2. Bullough, V. & Bullough, B. The Care of the Sick: The Emergence of Modern Nursing. New York: Prodist, 1978.
3. Reitzes, D. C. Negroes and Medicine. Commonwealth Fund Study. Cambridge, Mass: Harvard University Press, 1958, pp. xxi and xxii.
4. Standard Medical Almanac. Chicago: Marquis Academic Media, 1917, pp. 350, 358. Johnson, D. G. Smith, V. C. & Tarnoff, L. Recruitment and Progress of Medical School Entrants, 1970–1972. *Journal of Medical Education*, 1975, *50*, 713–755. Gray, L. C. The Geographic and Functional Distribution of Black Physicians: Some Research and Policy Considerations. *American Journal of Public Health, 1977, 67*, 519–526.
5. The Carnegie Commission on Higher Education. Higher Education and the Nation's Health: Policies for Medical and Dental Education. New York: McGraw-Hill, 1970, p. 28.
6. Dummett, C. O. The Growth and Development of the Negro in Dentistry. Chicago: The Stanek Press for the National Dental Association, 1952.
7. American Nurses' Association. Facts About Nursing. New York: ANA, 1958, p. 10.
8. *Nursing Outlook*, February 1965, p. 63, a boxed extract from *The Trained Nurse and Hospital Review*, 1925, *74*, 260.
9. Carnegie, M. E. Are Negro Schools of Nursing Needed Today? *Nursing Outlook*. 1964, *12*, 52–56. Reprinted in B. Bullough and V. Bullough (Eds.), New Directions for Nurses. New York: Springer, 1971, pp. 292–303.

10. Vaughn, J. C. & Johnson, W. L. Educational Preparation for Nursing, 1978. *Nursing Outlook*, 1979, *27*, 608–614.
11. Stanley, J. C. Predicting College Success of the Educationally Disadvantaged. *Science*, 1971, *171*, 640–644. de Tornyay, R. & Russell, M. L. Helping the High Risk Student Achieve. *Nursing Outlook, 1978, 26*, 576–580. Malhiot, G. & Ninan, M., A Seminar for Minority Students. *Nursing Outlook*, 1979, *27*, 473–475.
12. The Carnegie Commission on Higher Education. op. cit., pp. 35–59.
13. Scheinfeldt, J. Opening Doors Wider in Nursing. *American Journal of Nursing*, 1967, *67*, 1461–1464.
14. Buckley, J. Faculty Commitment to Retention and Recruitment of Black Students. *Nursing Outlook*, 1980, *28*, 46–50.
15. Odegaard, C. E. Minorities in Medicine. New York: Josiah Macy Jr. Foundation, 1977, pp. 46–50.
16. Ibid., pp. 50–54.
17. Kent, F. B. Latin America Losing Much Needed Doctors. *Los Angeles Times*, September 17, 1971.
18. A summary of this report was written by E. Shelton. Prejudices Hit Women in Medicine. *Los Angeles Times*, October 4, 1970.
19. Minorities and Women in the Health Fields. Health Manpower References DHEW Publication No. 79–22. Washington, D.C.: Public Health Service, Bureau of Manpower, October 1978, pp. 64–66.
20. The Carnegie Commission on Higher Education. op. cit., p. 26.
21. Educational Preparation for Nursing—1969. *Nursing Outlook*, 1970, *18*, 52–57.
22. Vaughn and Johnson. op. cit., p. 613. The Carnegie Commission on Higher Education. op. cit., p. 26. Educational Preparation for Nursing— 1969. op. cit.
23. Bigham, G. D. To Communicate with Negro Patients. *American Journal of Nursing*, 1964, *64* 113–115.
24. The information was collected together in a pamphlet by B. Bullough, V. Bullough, & L. Tannenbaum. *What Color Are Your Germs? Chicago Committee To End Medical Discrimination, 1954.*
25. U.S. Commission on Civil Rights. Civil Rights '63. Washington, D.C.: U.S. Government Printing Office, 1963, pp. 137–138.
26. Harris, S.E. The Economics of American Medicine. New York: Macmillan, 1964, p. 170.
27. U.S. Commission on Civil Rights. op. cit., p. 131.
28. Seham, M. Discrimination Against Negroes in Hospitals. *New England Journal of Medicine*, 1964, *271*, 940–943.
29. 323 F. 2d 939 (4th Cir)., cert. denied, 376 U.S. 938 (1964). See also: Seham. op. cit.
30. U.S. Commission on Civil Rights. Title VI Circuit One Year After: A Survey of Desegregation of Health and Welfare Services in the South. Washington, D.C.: U.S. Government Printing Office, 1966.
31. The Impact of Title VI on Health Facilities. *The George Washington Law Review*, 1968, *36*, 980–993.

32. Hill-Burton. *Health Law Newsletter,* 1972, *13,* 1.
33. Letter from Kenneth Williamson, Deputy Director of the American Hospital Association to Elliot Richardson, Secretary of Health, Education, and Welfare, April 20, 1972.
34. *Federal Register,* October 6, 1975, p. 46203. Hill-Burton. *Health Law Newsletter,* 1975, *55,* 3. Federal Regulation of Service to the Poor Under the Hill-Burton Act: Realities and Pitfalls. *Northwestern University Law Review,* June 1, 1975.
35. Butler, P. Assuring the Quality of Care and Life in Nursing Homes: the Dilemma of Enforcement. *North Carolina Law Review,* 1979, *57,* 1317–1382.

10

Improving Health Care Delivery

Today's world is radically changed from that of the past. Yet in spite of its tremendous technical advances, the American health care industry often seems to act as if the United States were still primarily a nation of small towns and rural farms. Over the past century, millions of people have moved from the country to the large urban complexes, until today less than 5 percent of the population is engaged in agriculture. In the rural environment, a person could be self-reliant within limits, making clothes, growing crops, and calling on neighbors or family to help when calamity threatened. Medically, a person could learn to know and love a physician who, in a time of crisis, would spend long hours with the patient. If it was necessary, a nurse came to the patient's home and cared for the individual on a one-to-one basis.

In the city, on the other hand, almost everything a person does is dependent upon the impersonal activities of large numbers of other people, as the city is preeminently the home of the specialist. Such a simple task as getting to work takes the coordinated efforts of dozens of people, whether one takes a subway, a bus, or drives a car. In health care, the individual has been replaced by a team of specialists, who often do not know what the others are doing. At best, the system is often confusing, and all too frequently it breaks down. An example of the difficulties was outlined by Milton Ro-

199

emer, a physician and Professor of Public Health at UCLA, in his testimony before the Senate Subcommittee on the Health of the Elderly:

> May I take the time of a distinguished committee of the U.S. Senate to tell of one aged patient who, like most old people, suffered from multiple diagnoses?
>
> He had a serious eye problem—actually two diseases: glaucoma and keratitis—for which he received care at a nearby medical center, in the department of ophthalmology.
>
> His personal doctor, a good internist, however, had diagnosed a mild diabetes and for this periodic visits were necessary to an office eight miles away.
>
> Painful corns and bunions, impairing the ability to walk, were not within the specialty of the personal doctor, so these required periodic visits to a podiatrist at an office six miles in another direction.
>
> Dental care, in an effort to save the few remaining teeth, so that dentures would fit more firmly and food could be more properly chewed, required numerous visits to a dentist at still another location.
>
> Then a bladder problem developed and prostatic disease was suspected. At about the same period, the patient showed lethargy and confusion, suggesting a mild cerebrovascular accident. The personal doctor made a home call and the decision was to hospitalize.
>
> A bed was not immediately available—except in a small proprietary hospital which the family refused—and it was not till ten days later that he could be admitted to a good voluntary general hospital fifteen miles away.
>
> After x-rays, cystoscopy, and other examinations there, his treatment was stabilized. In the workup, it was discovered that a drug the ophthalmologist had been prescribing for many months was causing serious side effects that had been missed by the internist since these two specialists had never communicated with each other.
>
> The patient was then admitted to a sanitarium selected for its closeness to the family home, so that daily visits from the patient's children would be possible.
>
> This was one of the "better" nursing homes—it was certainly expensive enough at $32 a day paid by Medicare—but this was evidently not costly enough to support a proper staff. After a few days, because of lack of proper surveillance, this aged patient was found roaming on the street. When this happened a second time, the commercial proprietor decided to discharge the patient as "too difficult to care for." It took five weeks of nursing

care at home, with daily problems of incontinence of urine and feces, before a bed in another nursing home became available.

The latter facility proved to be better managed and the patient improved. After only two weeks, however, he was getting up from a chair one day when he fell and fractured his left hip.

This required an orthopedic surgeon, readmission to the hospital, and preparation for a major operation. But then complications to the diabetes set in, because of the traumatic shock of the fracture. A delay in over twenty-four hours in reporting a critical laboratory test nearly cost the patient's life at this time. Had the hospital been adequately staffed, this delay would not have occurred.

A skillful operation, with a pinning of the broken bone was done. Special-duty nurses costing $111 a day—over and above the Medicare coverage of the hospital bill—had to be hired because of the shortage of regular hospital nurses.

I have not recounted the other details of multiple drug prescriptions, special services of an appliance shop to adjust the bed at home, the physical therapy required for a knee injury, and much more.[1]

Dr. Roemer added that the patient in question was his widowed father, who had retired after fifty-one years of medical practice. If Roemer, with his medical background and knowledge, found it difficult to wend his way through the maze of specialists in securing adequate medical care, it should be evident that those with much less ability to deal with the medical establishment would have even greater difficulties. With its great potential for specialization, urbanization has encouraged a jungle of specialists and an impossible medical care delivery system.

Tied in with urbanization has been the growth of technology, which has made labor less important as machines have taken over more of the functions once reserved for brains and muscles. Many types of work have been upgraded, so that the average worker now has to have more skills or be better educated than in the past. In the case of medicine, this trend has led to a proliferation of devices and techniques, higher educational standards, and greater gaps between the various levels of health practitioners. Not too long ago, most health care was in the hands of a physician, nurse, or pharmacist, but now there are dozens of major categories of jobs within the health care industry. In terms of total manpower, the health care industry is the third largest industry in the United States and one of the most rapidly growing segments of the economy.

Together, technology and urbanization have tended to widen

the gap between the "haves" and "have nots" in all societies. In the United States, many of the "have nots" are members of groups that traditionally have been discriminated against in American life, and their immediate situation is likely to worsen before it improves. In fact, the hardest hit by the changing employment standards have been the undereducated, particularly members of minority groups, who, in spite of the civil rights legislation of the last two decades, often find themselves still at a disadvantage because of past economic and educational discrimination.

This means that health care, more than ever before, is inevitably tied in with the economic conditions of mass numbers of people. Over the past century, Americans have taken steps to lessen the economic extremes, through graduated income tax, a system of social security, and various kinds of government-supported welfare programs. Medically, we have enacted Medicare and Medicaid as supplements to Social Security, as well as various smaller-scale programs aimed at certain groups of people or specific disease entities. However, most health care is still privately paid for on a fee-for-service or insurance basis. This means that people who do not have money to buy good health care are not likely to get it. Nearly 200 years ago, Thomas Malthus, an English clergyman, wrote *An Essay on the Principle of Population*, in which he said:

> I believe it has been generally remarked by those who have attended to bills of mortality that of the number of children who die annually, much too great a proportion belongs to those who may be supposed unable to give their offspring proper food and attention, exposed as they are occasionally to severe distress and confined, perhaps to unwholesome habitations and hard labor.

Alonzo Yerby has claimed that Malthus summarized contemporary conditions in the United States: a system of medical care for the poor that Yerby described as piecemeal, poorly organized, and without compassion or concern for the dignity of the individual.[2]

THE GORDIAN KNOT

There are no easy answers to our current health deficiencies. Problems are intertwined and interrelated until there is almost a Gordian knot, impossible to unravel except as Alexander the Great did—by cutting it with a sword and starting over. Although we are not advocating a revolution, it does seem obvious that a drastic revision of the health care delivery system is needed to replace the present complex patchwork nonsystem with a comprehensive and accessible plan for the delivery of health care to all people. However, even with a rational system of health care, there will still be inequities in health, until problems of discrimination and poverty are solved.

As was indicated in the previous chapter, continued effort is still needed to eliminate the barriers in health care institutions due to segregation and discrimination. The schools that prepare health professionals must make sure their doors remain open so that members of minority groups can be better represented in the ranks of their graduates. Health workers at all levels have to keep examining their own attitudes toward poor and minority patients. There are probably enough laws on the books to deal with discrimination; what is needed is better enforcement of these laws, both at the overt level and on the more subtle personal level.

This book is not the place to go into the whole strategy of ending poverty, since our primary emphasis is on health, but health itself, as it has been emphasized before, is dependent on ending poverty. The complexity of dealing with poverty makes us cautious in proposing any one solution. Investigators advocate several different solutions: a Guaranteed Annual Wage as a means of fighting poverty, the development of WPA-like projects to provide jobs, a cut in working hours, and a vast overhaul of the welfare system.

Robert Heilbroner has argued that a good measure of a country's greatness is the way in which it treats its sick, its poor, and its deviants. If such a measure is applied on a world basis, it becomes obvious that the United States, in spite of its great power and strength, is overshadowed by many nations in the world. Heilbroner believes that our relative failure in this regard is due to an American antiwelfare animus, a feeling that those who do not succeed have no one to blame but themselves. This attitude has led to an anesthetizing of America's social conscience that, coupled with a profound suspicion of government, has caused us to regard poverty with mixed feelings of indifference and impotence.[3] If Heilbroner is right that Americans are indifferent to social neglect and reluctant to use public authority to deal with it, then health care will continue to be in a crisis and poverty will grow. In an earlier and more rural day, personal charity could help ease the burdens, but in this day of urban problems, government action becomes imperative, and, fortunately or unfortunately, even local governments are no longer able to deal with poverty. In the past, when government has entered into the poverty area, it has mostly been through the city or county, less often through the state, and only rarely through agencies of the federal government itself. The result has been a patchwork of welfare programs that vary from state to state and even from locality to locality, with the greatest crisis in the largest urban areas—the political unit least able to deal with the problem because of the present tax structure and distribution of political power. In order to work effectively toward a solution, we have to recognize that poverty and health care are national problems.[4]

As indicated earlier, there are approximately 25 million people in the United States who fall below the poverty line. Though the percentages of those so classified have been declining over the past decade, the total number has remained about the same.[5] Generally, those so classified are among the least educated, least skilled and most alienated of society. Since the most severe contraction in the job market has been at the lowest levels, and since those workers who still can find jobs at this level traditionally have lacked the union organization or professional association of the more sophisticated workers, even when they do work, they have no organized advocates for bettering their position. Trying to solve this poverty problem has proven to be extremely difficult.

Since President Lyndon B. Johnson declared a "War on Poverty" in 1964, the U.S. government has continued to work for the alleviation of poverty under succeeding presidents, both Democratic and Republican, but only with partial success. The government programs have been most successful in dealing with some of the effects of poverty and least successful in eliminating poverty. The government has also not been particularly successful in getting the private sector to deal with poverty. One of the most successful early program of the Office of Economic Opportunity was the training and employment of home health aides and social work assistants whose origins were in the community being served. One reason for the success of the programs is that they did the obvious: they offered jobs to the unemployed. Agencies found that their new employees were valuable in their ability to understand and interpret the clients' and agency's point of view.[6] However, the number of health aides and social work assistants who could be employed, was limited, because there were a limited number of low-level jobs. When agencies attempted to expand the scope of these new employees, they were unable to do so, since they lacked the sophistication and knowledge (with some exceptions) to go beyond the lower levels. Many who were stuck in these jobs became disenchanted after a few years, because the barriers to advancement were formidable. Overcoming these barriers required considerable education and special efforts by the professionals involved to develop career ladders for alternative entry points into the profession. Even where a career ladder developed, as it has in nursing, upward mobility was difficult for those at the bottom.

Another success of the OEO funded projects was the demonstration health centers, such as the two clinics opened by the Tufts University School of Medicine in the Columbia Point housing project in Massachusetts and in Mound Bayou, Mississippi, or the multipurpose Health Center in Watts. Such centers effectively demonstrated that it was possible to give comprehensive health care and that members of the poverty community could be involved in planning and in giving health care.[7] However, moving from a demonstration unit to implementing the program on the national level proved difficult. Part of the difficulty was the fact that the centers often were never fully integrated into the health care system but remained grant-funded, and grant funding is not a particularly efficient way to run a health center. The most innovative centers were also likely to be the least efficient and most expensive.[8] Still, they served as an alternative to the hospital and, as of this writing, could still be regarded as a possible alternative, if they were widespread, had effective backup services, and more effectively utilized professionals such as nurse practitioners. Tokenism in this area, as in so many others, created more problems than it solved.

HEALTH CARE DELIVERY SYSTEM

This country desperately needs to replace its patchwork nonsystem for financing health care with a comprehensive, federally run system of national health insurance. For many years now, the United States has been the only industrialized country that does not have some kind of national health insurance or national health service.[9] Usually, the failure to develop such a system is blamed on the American Medical Association. Although this is a much too simplistic explanation, the AMA has certainly been a significant force in "saving us from socialized medicine." For a long time, the organization was in the hands of general practitioners who were fighting against the increasing specialization of medicine. In part, the physicians who were most active in organizational activities were also likely to come from smaller towns, so that in a sense, the twentieth-century struggle within the AMA represented an alliance of the small towns against the big cities, of rural versus urban, and of old American values against the new. Over the years, while the ultraconservative forces held sway, the organization fought against private health insurance, maternal health programs, various aspects of the social security legislation, medical care for military dependents, and even against Veterans Administration hospitals.[10]

While the AMA is no longer dominated by general practitioners, it is still a conservative organization—partly because the very nature of medical practice tends to leave the average physician with little time for organizational activities. This means that the work of the association is often carried out by the older retired physicians who are still thinking both politically and medically in terms of their own youth. Too often they assume that medical care is still given on a one-to-one basis, with a fee for service. While physicians have generally been noted for their compassion, the heavily science-oriented focus of medical education has given them little background with which to understand the problems of the modern world, and their too-heavy work schedule has left them little time for independent study.

Although the attitudes and actions of the AMA still affect the way in which the medical establishment works today, as will be indicated later, no lobby—and the AMA is a lobby—can be effective unless it expresses the views of a large segment of its members, as well as the general population. For a long time, the AMA attitudes were the dominant American ones, but this is no longer the case. If any group is most influential, it is the American Hospital Association and the Health Insurance industry as a group. Within the AMA, the balance of power has shifted to a more urban practitioner. The result has been a modification of some of the earlier political positions. There is also a growing number of physicians, usually young ones, who have refused to join the organizations. Some of these rebels have joined with other health workers to form dissident groups, such as the Medical Committee for Human Rights or Physicians for Social Responsibility, but many others remained unorganized. The AMA also lacks the kind of power it once had. For example, lawsuits have forced the association to be less hostile to chiropractors than it once was. Specialty groups also are of more interest to the average physician. Denial of hospital affiliation is not the negative sanction it once was in many parts of the country.

BACKGROUND: OTHER COUNTRIES

Under Prince Otto von Bismarck, Germany was the first country in the world to establish a compulsory national sickness insurance program. The original program, started in 1883, gave free care only to enrolled workers, but benefits were soon extended to the families of employed persons. Following the German example, several other European countries took steps to have their government enter into the medical field, including Austria in 1888, Sweden in 1891, Denmark in 1892, Belgium in 1894, and Switzerland in 1912. Great Britain acted much more slowly and in a more piecemeal fashion. Some compensation was given to a few workers in 1880, and a limited national health insurance program was enacted in 1911, but complete health coverage was not established until the inauguration of National Health Insurance in 1948. The Union of Soviet Socialist Republics nationalized all health care in 1917, as part of the Russian Revolution, and other countries that came under the Russian sphere of influence following World War II patterned their health care delivery system after that of the Russians. Numerous other countries have also adopted some form of government-sponsored or controlled health care.

In spite of the fact that the various government-sponsored programs are usually labeled "socialized medicine," each country administers its programs very differently: programs may be based on a fee for service, cash reimbursement, capitation, or straight salaries. Each system has its advantages and disadvantages. The difficulty with the negotiated or set fee-for-service system is that the better-paid procedures tend to be more frequently performed than those paid less, because the physician is likely to opt for the more expensive treatment than the lower-cost one. Moreover, failure to pay adequately for certain procedures can result in the underdevelopment of an entire speciality. Fee-for-service benefits the surgical specialties more than the medical or preventive specialties, since the surgical specialties can easily be itemized and priced. In those systems in which any physician can be paid for any procedure, general practitioners become more alike in skills and income and specialists become more versatile, since the narrower the specialization the more difficult it is to establish a set fee. Fee-for-service systems also enable the physician to bill the funds without the patient's knowledge, since there is little witness to the actual work as against the physician's claims. Under this system, it is possible to write fee schedules with variable payment formulas that discourage the unnecessary multiplication of work, but the problem is to prevent these formulas from discouraging justified long-term care.[11]

Germany is an example of a country where fee-for-service is practiced. Originally, the German system arranged for individuals to join a sickness fund; this fund then contracted for care from groups of physicians. At the present time, about 200 such funds operate in West Germany, covering about 87 percent of the population. Within the group, patients can choose their own general practitioner but are referred to specialists only as needed. Physicians are paid on the basis of a fee-for-service, with fee levels being negotiated by the sickness funds and the local association of physicians. Hospitals are run by local government and their staffs of physicians and nurses are salaried. In surveys, 90 percent of those enrolled in sickness funds recently indicated they would remain if the funds were voluntary instead of compulsory.

Although satisfaction with the fee-for-service system is high, it is not without problems. In order to get reimbursement, physicians with few patients tend to require more visits per patient than busy physicians. In a 1966 study, it was found that physicians who saw 2,500 to 3,000 patients per calendar quarter provided 5.06 services per person, while those seeing 1,000 to 1,500 provided 6.24 services, and those seeing fewer than 1,000 provided 8.90 services. From this it would seem that at least some of those extra visits to the practitioner with the small patient load may have been motivated by a desire to keep up income. From the physician members, the greatest complaint is the amount of paperwork required to obtain reimbursement. From the governmental point of view, the system is expensive to operate unless there is very rigid fee control.[12]

Closely allied to the negotiated fee-for-service system, but with more difficulties and complications in operation, is the cash benefit system. Instead of receiving a fee for service, the physician charges cash and then the patient is reimbursed. This system has the advantage of being the most politically feasible in those countries where there are well-established medical practitioners, such as the United States. The physicians are usually more willing to accept this reimbursement procedure; they believe that it will preserve their autonomy in full, because the patient, not the physician, communicates with the sick fund. When this system has been tried, these beliefs of the medical profession have been proven wrong, because physicians who charge higher rates for the same service soon find themselves being queried by the reimbursement agency, and those who persist find themselves under investigation. Inevitably, many physicians are placed under sanctions by the government, even to the point that patients going to them are not reimbursed. Most cash benefit systems also anticipate that the patient will pay part of the initial charge, but the effect of this is to discourage the poor from ever seeking needed medical care or to wait until an emergency arises. In order to get around this, it has become necessary to impose means tests—the very thing that national health insurance was supposed to eliminate. The cash payment system also has most of the other difficulties of fee-for-service. Nevertheless, both France and Sweden have established cash benefit systems, which, from the physician's point of view, have the advantage of giving high incomes to the physicians. Both countries have also achieved better results in medical care for the poor than the United States.[13]

As it is operated in Great Britain, capitation is much simpler to administer than fee-for-service or cash benefit systems, but it also has difficulties. Under the British system, a physician is responsible for a panel of patients, with the quality of service depending upon personal conscience or the informal sanctions of other members of the profession. At worst, the system gives little encouragement for the physician to do more than the minimum required for the patient, but it also discourages unnecessary or drastic medical procedures. If a physician has a time-consuming patient, he or she might want to transfer the individual to another panel or to an outpatient department or hospital unless there are effective administrative or ethical deterrents for the physician not to do so. The British system also reinforces a distinction between the general practitioner and the specialist by depriving the general practitioner of any financial motive to perform tasks assigned to the specialist. From the physician's point of view, the system has the merit of preserving the individual practitioner in the office. In Britain and Holland, where the capitation system is most firmly established, general practitioners were traditionally based in private offices, separate from the specialists who were attached to the hospitals.[14]

The British system has the advantage of offering almost universal coverage. Each patient is assigned to a panel, with similar panels for dental care and drugs. Specialists and hospital employees are on a salary, under the direction of the Ministry of Health. The chief dissatisfaction with the capitation system comes not from patients but from physicians. Many physicians feel their pay is low; to increase it, they take on rather large patient panels, an average of 2,300 patients. To handle so many patients, they then have to work long hours and cannot spend as much time with each patient as careful medical practice would indicate is desirable. Separation of the general practitioner from the hospital patient and lack of contact with specialists also reduces the intellectual stimulation of seeing the seriously ill patient or working with colleagues. This is not so much a difficulty with capitation per se, but with the way health care delivery is organized in Great Britain.[15]

Most countries that have national health schemes rely heavily upon salaried physicians, although even here there is great variance in medical care, because the delivery system seems to be dependent on past tradition within the country. In many ways, the salary system encourages desirable characteristics, such as nonmercenary attitudes, close colleague relationships, interest in personal professional growth, and it also has the virtue of simpler administration than the other systems. The salaried system also discourages unnecessary treatment or medically unjustified multiplication of procedures, although in the few systems in which physicians earn overtime or can select the amount of salaried work time, this is a problem. Also, under a salary system medical care can be more equitably distributed, through encouraging medical practitioners to go into areas of greatest need by giving them higher salaries. In salaried systems that also allow the physician to have a private practice, the more affluent patients are often referred to the individual physician during private practice hours, thus subverting the system somewhat. This is particularly true in countries like Egypt, where salaries for physicians are low.[16]

Russia and most of those countries that have followed the Russian lead have adopted the salary system. In Russia, all levels of health workers are salaried, and care is given through a system of polyclinics, health centers, and hospitals. In line with earlier Russian tradition, there is considerable opportunity for advancement within the system; theoretically, a hospital orderly or an ambulance driver can work his way up through a system of additional training programs to become a physician. In actuality, this sort of upward mobility is uncommon, although nurses and feldshers, the middle-level medical workers, occasionally move up the career ladder to become physicians. Soviet doctors give fewer diagnostic tests and treatments than do Western physicians, but this may be due less to salary than to a clinical tradition that for a long time suffered from a shortage of equipment, technicians, and laboratories. The Soviet system of medicine is one of the most popular governmental services in the USSR, and even the personnel shortages and time pressures of World War II did not lead to dissatisfaction. For example, the Harvard Russian Research Center interviewed Russian emigres shortly after the war and found a remarkably high level of satisfaction with the physician-patient relationship. Those refugees who eventually settled in the U.S. felt that one of the few advantages Russia had over the U.S. system was their medical care delivery system.[17]

There are other variations of payment for health care delivery;

in fact, many countries have combinations of several, as does the United States today. All of the systems, however, at least in the industrialized nations, tend to offer adequate medical care and have the advantage of reaching segments of the population not reached by the U.S. system. This does not mean that the United States should adopt any of the systems per se—partly because U.S. medicine has a different tradition—but there are many variations possible, even in "socialized" medicine.

THE STRUGGLE FOR HEALTH INSURANCE IN THE UNITED STATES

The attempt to gain a national health insurance in this country has been, and continues to be, a long and bitter struggle. In the process of the struggle, U.S. medicine has developed along certain lines that have to be considered in planning a better health care delivery system. In order to understand the importance of this early struggle in forming medical practice today, it is necessary to examine some of the past history of medical insurance, if only briefly. One of the early leaders in the campaign for government-sponsored health insurance was Dr. Alexander Lambert, an AMA leader, who was also personal physician to President Theodore Roosevelt. When Theodore Roosevelt attempted to regain the presidency in 1912, Lambert had enough influence to get compulsory health insurance included in the Progressive Party platform. However, it was several decades before the Democratic or Republican parties picked up this part of the Bull Moose or Progressive party platform. With the failure of the Roosevelt campaign, much of the early efforts to gain some sort of health service was directed by a private reform group called the American Association for Labor Legislation, which had originally been established to lobby for workmen's compensation laws in various states. As this movement succeeded (some 41 states had enacted laws by 1920), the association turned its attention to health problems. In its early attempt to establish health insurance, the AALL for a brief time had the support of the AMA. From 1915 to 1920, the AMA was at its progressive best, under the influence and leadership of Lambert, I. M. Rubinow, and others who were members of an AMA Social Insurance Committee established in 1915. By 1920, however, partly because of grass-roots opposition by physicians, the AMA had adopted a policy of official opposition to any kind of health insurance, private or public.

The model health insurance bill drawn up by AALL, providing

broad hospital and medical coverage for workers and their families on a state level, was introduced into 20 state legislatures between 1914 and 1920. None of the bills passed and the movement almost died during the 1920s. Employers were generally antagonistic toward the bill on the ground that their costs would be increased. Commercial life insurance companies became active opponents, even though at that time they wrote little health insurance. However, the AALL plan included a funeral benefit that the insurance companies opposed, because death benefits were included in the six billion dollars of industrial insurance then in effect. Even organized labor, particularly in the person of Samuel Gompers, president of the AFL, opposed the health scheme on the grounds that it would lead to government control of the union movement. However, many state federations were in favor, and it was the state labor organizations that gave the greatest support to the effort. Large pharmaceutical houses also opposed the various bills, as did an increasing number of local medical societies and individual physicians, whose opposition eventually led the AMA itself to oppose the plan. In California, where the state constitution permitted a referendum, an attempt to set up a state-sponsored health insurance plan was overwhelmingly defeated at the polls.[18]

The issue was not dead, only dormant. By 1925, continuing concern over the cost and organization of medical care had resulted in a Washington Conference on the Economic Factors Affecting the Organization of Medicine. A second conference was held in 1926 and, in 1927, this led to the formation of a Committee on the Costs of Medical Care, under the chairmanship of Ray Lyman Wilbur, Secretary of the Interior. For the next five years, the Committee, with the support of various private foundations, investigated the costs of medical care. Its findings and recommendations filled 28 volumes, in addition to a number of subsidiary reports. The final summary, entitled *Medical Care for the American People*, appeared in 1932, when the country was at the depth of the Depression.[19] It included both a majority and a minority report. The majority favored medical and hospital insurance on a voluntary basis, until adequate experience could be accumulated to serve as a sound basis for a comprehensive system based upon compulsory tax deductions. The majority also approved group medical practice organized around health centers, and grants-in-aid to provide hospitals, physicians, and nurses to poor and thinly populated areas. It also urged government support of the cost of medical care for the indigent, the tubercular and the mentally ill. On the other hand, the minority opposed any kind of prepaid medical care, even on a voluntary basis, and vehemently objected to the proposal for group practice. However, the minority was willing to accept hospital insurance plans, provided they were sponsored and controlled by organized medicine. In general, its view coincided with the emerging view of the AMA. The hostility with which the majority report was greeted by the medical profession is evident from the pages of the *Journal of the American Medical Association*, which labeled it as "inciting to revolution." The words of the then-editor of the *Journal*, Dr. Morris Fishbein, indicate better than any other statement we could make the racist and antigovernment attitude so characteristic of organized medicine at the time:

> One must review the expenditure of almost a million dollars by the committee and its final report with mingled amusement and regret. A colored boy spent a dollar taking twenty rides on the merry-go-round. When he got off, his mammy said, "Boy, you spent yo' money but where you been?"

Fishbein felt this was the same as the committee's efforts. He even went so far as to call the recommendation for group practice an attempt to establish medical "soviets."[20]

In spite of such vehement opposition, national health insurance became a major issue during the early years of President Franklin D. Roosevelt's administration. The Depression, with its resulting desperation, once again created a climate of opinion favorable to social legislation. Many physicians found themselves with rapidly declining incomes and were unable to collect from their out-of-work patients. This helped change their attitudes, at least temporarily. In 1933, Congress, with AMA approval, appropriated money to help pay physicians' fees. This temporary measure was soon found to be inadequate. To deal more effectively with this and other problems, President Roosevelt in 1934 appointed a cabinet-level Committee on Economic Security, under the chairmanship of Frances Perkins, Secretary of Labor. Mrs. Perkins immediately announced that she favored enacting into law substantially all of the social insurance measures that European countries earlier had set up. Harry Hopkins, who held various jobs under Roosevelt and acted as his close adviser, was also in favor of health insurance. The omens seemed favorable, but, by the time the committee completed its report, the AMA had once again announced its opposition to health insurance. Fearful that medical opposition would prevent passage of any social security legislation, Roosevelt requested the House Ways and Means Committee to strike most provisions dealing with medical care from the bill establishing Social Security. With these deletions, Social Security was enacted into law. Token concession to health insurance supporters was given in the form of increased grants-in-aid to states for maternal and infant preventive care and a strengthened public health program; both of these measures were passed over the opposition of the AMA.

The extent to which organized medicine was prepared to go was demonstrated by the case of the Milbank Fund, set up by Albert G. Milbank, chairman of the Borden Company. The Milbank Fund had granted money for local studies of preventive medicine, and its secretary, John A. Kingsbury, had criticized the AMA for its opposition to the then-pending Social Security bill. A number of medical journals began hinting through editorials that a boycott of Borden products would have a salutary effect on the fund. Not surprisingly, physicians' recommendations of Borden's irradiated evaporated milk for babies fell off and so did the company profits. Milbank was led to deny his fund had ever endorsed compulsory health insurance or "any other plan to distribute the costs of medical care." Shortly afterward, Kingsbury lost his post as secretary of the fund.

In spite of such actions, the leaders of the AMA realized there was a growing demand for some kind of health insurance. To head off any government-sponsored plan, they reversed their opposition to voluntary insurance plans. The first to gain support were the hospital plans, particularly the Blue Cross, which had its origin at Baylor University in Texas in 1929. By 1935, hospitals had enrolled about 23,000 people in more than 400 different employee groups. In 1933, the American Hospital Association's Board of Trustees approved the principle of hospital insurance as a practical solution to the more equitable distribution of the costs of hospital care. The American College of Surgeons, whose members were dependent upon hospitals, endorsed a similar scheme, in spite of AMA opposition. By 1937, the American Hospital Association had approved various hospital plans that met its criteria by allowing such plans to use its trademark of the blue cross. In the first list of Blue Cross subscribers published in 1938, some million and a half people were enrolled. By 1953, about 41.8 million persons were enrolled in Blue Cross plans.

Hospital insurance was one thing, while prepaid medical care was quite another. Here, the opposition of the AMA was much more vigorous. The matter came to a head in the case of the Group Health Association established in 1937 in Washington, D.C., by employees of the Federal Home Owners Loan Corporation. This nonprofit prepayment hospitalization and medical care program contracted with physicians to serve its members. The physicians employed by the group soon found themselves expelled from the District of Columbia Medical Society and barred from the seven district hospitals, because of their lack of AMA certification. The District Medical Society even went so far as to warn physicians of a rule barring medical consultation with nonsociety members. Hospitals were also warned that, if they accepted patients from the group, they would lose the AMA approval for their intern-training programs. The effect of such action was to deny hospitalization to members of the Group Health Association. Because of these and other "criminal actions" against the health group, the United States Government instituted a suit for criminal violation against the American Medical Association and the District of Columbia Medical Society. The resulting conviction was eventually affirmed by the United States Supreme Court in 1943. In the meantime, to prevent similar plans, the AMA set up a Council of Medical Service and Public Relations designed to encourage state medical societies to make some type of health insurance plans available to the public, something that several state medical societies had already initiated. To coordinate these plans, Associated Medical Care Plans was created in 1945 and adopted the Blue Shield as its copyrighted symbol.[21]

MEDICARE

It was not until 1939 that Robert F. Wagner of New York formally introduced a national health insurance proposal into the United States Senate. Though it failed to get out of committee, Wagner continued to introduce it in successive sessions. In 1943, he was joined by Senator James Murray and Representative John Dingell, and in this and subsequent years it was known as the Wagner-Murray-Dingell bill. In spite of public opinion polls indicating strong national support for governmentally sponsored health insurance, the AMA and its allies were able to prevent the bill from coming to a vote.[22] After repeated failures to secure a vote, health reformers decided to concentrate on a lesser goal: health benefits for social security beneficiaries. This concept had great appeal because the financial drain of serious illness was the most devastating for the elderly and for the welfare recipient, and it was these groups that were the least likely to be covered by voluntary insurance plans. Moreover, the growing numbers of the elderly in the population represented a politically potent interest group. In 1957, Congressman Aime J. Forand of Rhode Island introduced a bill to furnish hospital, surgical, and nursing benefits to all social security beneficiaries. Opposition sprang almost immediately from the AMA, the National Chamber of Commerce, the National Association of Manufacturers, the Health Insurance Association, the Pharmaceutical Association, and the American Farm Bureau Federation. Support came from organized labor, from the National Association of Social Workers, the National Farmers Union, and, most importantly, the American Nurses Association. The nurses' support was crucial, because it indicated that a significant number of health professionals were opposed to the AMA stand. The support of the nurses was also a factor in encouraging the American Hospital Association to re-evaluate its position on health insurance. Though the AHA did not at this time come out in support, it did not oppose the bill, and the association took the opportunity to point out that something had to be done to help elderly patients pay their bills, if only because so many hospitals were being left with uncollectable debts.

In 1960, Senator Robert Kerr of Oklahoma and Congressman Wilbur Mills of Arkansas introduced a substitute bill providing for federal subsidies to states, in order to help pay for the health care of welfare recipients, including aged indigents. Though this was a weak compromise for the Forand bill, it had the merit of being enacted. The new legislation soon proved to be ineffective, because many states never bothered to institute the programs necessary to utilize the grants. In 1962, the Medicare bill, a revision of the original Forand bill, was again introduced, but this time it had the full support of President John F. Kennedy. Although it failed to get out of committee in that session of Congress, it gathered support and was enacted into law in 1965 under President Lyndon B. Johnson.[23]

Financed through the social security system, Medicare provides two separate but coordinated coverages: hospital insurance for most persons aged 65 or over, and supplemental medical insurance for those persons in the same age group who voluntarily enroll and pay the required monthly premiums. Although the patients are required to pay a portion of their hospital bill, the coverage is substantial. A companion bill, upgrading the provisions of the Kerr-Mills bill, was also passed in that year and is generally known under the term *Medicaid*, although various states have given it a different name. This bill gave funds to states to set up health care programs for welfare recipients covered under the federal programs for families with needy children, the totally or partially blind, and the totally disabled. In order to cut down the opposition of the insurance lobby, Medicare was administered through voluntary insurance carriers, usually Blue Cross. This has added an extra administrative cost to

Medicare and hampered governmental cost-control mechanisms. More troublesome was the fact that little control was put over fees, and one of the immediate results of the passage of Medicare and Medicaid was the escalation of physicians' fees, which had been predicted by almost everyone who had ever studied medical care delivery systems. Hospital costs also skyrocketed, although the connection of these increases to the legislation was due more to past practices than to any new ones. The health industry has never been a particularly efficient one, and the lack of government controls did little to encourage economy.

THE CURRENT SITUATION

In spite of these improvements in the medical care delivery system, health care remains in a crisis, simply because it still is not organized to meet the needs of today. In fact, the very opposition of the organized medical profession to past health schemes has so changed U.S. medicine that programs such as Medicare, which fail to take these changes into account, are bound to be in difficulty. The reluctance of physicians to accept medical insurance caused more and more medical plans to concentrate upon hospital insurance. Most such hospital plans were set up on a cost-plus basis, which means that hospitals were free to expand or buy new equipment to meet needs, both anticipated and hoped-for. Hospitals were able to do this because the costs, almost any costs in fact, would be automatically covered by insurance. Moreover, physicians' opposition to health insurance put more and more medical activities into the hospital, in order to gain reimbursement for the patient; in the process, physicians became more and more dependent upon the hospital. Hospitals became a place not only for the sick or injured but for patients undergoing diagnostic work, since the physician knew that the only way the patient could have the insurance company pay was to put the patient into the hospital.

At the same time, the nature of medical education in the United States changed, mainly because the federal government poured billions of dollars into biomedical research. In fact, so much money was available that the central activity of the country's major medical schools changed from teaching medical students to carrying out medical research. This not only tremendously increased the cost of medical education, both to the student and the taxpayer, but in the process it also erected an ever-escalating ladder of medical costs. For example, during the 10-year period from 1959 to 1969, the budget for the Stanford University School of Medicine rose from $5.7 million to $25.5 million, without any basic increase in the number of students being graduated. During the same period, federal grants rose from $2.3 million to $15 million, or from 41 to 60 percent of the budget; yet the total cost to Stanford, to its students, and to its patients also rose. The bulk of this increase did not go to patient care, but to research—until, in 1970, Stanford had 375 full-time faculty members and only 357 medical students.[24] It also had several hundred part-time faculty members who came in occasionally for consultation or who maintained a university connection for prestige reasons. The availability of federal funds for medical research had created new glamour positions in medicine for the university medical professors.

In the process, university affiliation has also become a matter of great importance to hospitals who want to attract interns and residents for their ongoing medical care. Almost all hospitals and health centers in major metropolitan areas have affiliated with medical schools. In Baltimore, John Hopkins Medical College, and in Boston, Harvard, are the medical centers from which affiliations radiate out to nearby hospitals. In cities like New York, there are several influential medical schools. The resulting medical empires, networks of affiliated institutions, are replacing the individual hospital as the basic unit of practice, just as hospitals earlier replaced the private physician's office.

Increasingly, major medical institutions also have begun to display an internal dynamic of their own, expanding to larger and larger proportions through more and more affiliations in order to maintain their status and their prestige. However, in building these medical empires, the whole nature of patient care has been downgraded, because the rewards come from other directions. The result has been what some have called a *medical industrial complex*. In 1978, Americans spent more than 192 million dollars on medical care, which represented a 45 percent increase over the amount spent in 1975 and more than six times the amount spent in 1960. The 1978 expenditure amounted to 9.1 percent of the gross national product and was almost double the percentage spent in other industrialized countries.[25] The health industry is big business: despite the fact that much of it claims to be nonprofit, it has billions in after-tax profits. The implications for health care become clear. For instance, community hospitals spent 13 percent more money in 1979 than in 1978 but provided only 1.6 percent more days of inpatient care and had 3.2 percent *fewer* outpatient visits. In turn, the year 1978 had expenditures of 13 percent over 1977, with only a 1.1 percent increase in patient care, while the amount spent in 1977 was 17.1 percent higher than that spent in 1976.[26] Average medical expenditures per family rose from $101.18 in 1950, to $195.55 in 1960, to $903.50 in 1975.[27] Little of the increase in cost went for higher salaries or wages for low-level hospital employees. Actually, the proportion of wages to other costs has consistently declined year after year. Instead, most of it paid for the escalating costs of drugs, supplies, equipment, and in many cases for profits to the physicians and the hospitals. Much of the equipment purchased each year had a planned obsolescence; in many of the smaller hospitals, such equipment, particularly of the more specialized nature, largely went unused.

Bringing these escalating costs under control has proved difficult to do. Almost all plans have required greater and greater government intervention. The most comprehensive effort so far has been the National Health Planning and Resources Development Act of 1974 (Public Law 93–641), signed into law on January 4, 1975. This act replaced three former federal programs: the Hill-Burton Hospital Construction Act, the Comprehensive Health Planning Program, and the Regional Medical Program. The goal of the legislation is to monitor federal spending but, at the same time, to see that better and more effective health care is given to more people. To do this, the act set up a series of state, regional, and local boards, Health Service Agencies, which have the power to determine whether new facilities are needed or whether old ones should go on getting federal funds. In order to insure consumer participation in decision making, the law stipulates that 51 percent of the members of the Board be consumers. However, consumers are essentially disorganized, so this has meant that the organized groups, not engaged in health care delivery, control a simple majority of the votes. These groups, labor unions, special community interest groups, and so forth, have their own special interests. Inevitably, decision making is a result of horse trading between various groups. The agencies are more effective in making negative decisions than in doing anything positive to improve health care, and, instead of eliminating the usual decision makers in the community, they gain more power. In spite of these and other criticisms, the HSAs are the only thing in existence and they do represent an historic step forward. Part of their difficulty is the historical setting in which they find themselves. Historically, health care has been an unorganized and entirely entrepreneurial system. Trying to bring organization into this system without at the same time stifling innovation is a difficult if not impossible task. Traditionally, the health care industry has been very unbusinesslike in terms of cost accounting, equipment, supplies and so forth, and often each medical section chief in a hospital has acted as if he or she commanded a separate fiefdom. Trying to bring control where there has been almost no control is extremely difficult.[28]

Many of the developments in medical care are beyond the ability of the HSA to control. For example, a high proportion of the new building and investment in health care went for research facilities rather than specifically to patient care. If the cost of research is applied to patient care, then inevitably the cost of medical care rises astronomically, and this is just what has happened. In 1950, the nation spent 3.8 billion dollars on hospital care; by 1965, the figure rose to 13.8 billion; in 1978, twelve years after Medicare and Medicaid, expenditures for hospital care alone were running at 76 billion dollars a year.[29] Without materially serving a large number of patients, county hospitals have also found their costs mounting. For example, the city of Chicago saw public expenditures for health care go up fourfold between 1960 and 1970, from $100 million to $400 million. As statistics are gathered on a statewide basis rather than on a citywide basis, the same escalation of costs appears. For example, the state of Illinois spent five times as much in 1978 on health care as it spent in 1968, with costs going from $200 million to over $1 billion. In 1970, it was estimated that it cost $104 a day to keep a patient in Cook County Hospital; in 1978, it cost $217.79.[30] By 1979, costs on a national basis had risen to $229.59 per day, up 11.4 percent over the same time in 1978.[31]

EXTENSION OF GOVERNMENT-SUPPORTED MEDICAL CARE

The escalating crisis in medical care has led an increasing number of people publicly to advocate some form of national health insurance. So great is the need, in fact, that experts for the past decade have been predicting the enactment of some sort of comprehensive medical program.[32] As of this writing, this still has not happened. Although a single well-thought-out health care package might be the ideal way of solving the growing problems, political realities would indicate that reform is more likely to come about in a piecemeal fashion. From this perspective, in 1965 Medicare and Medicaid legislation can be viewed as opening wedges in the gradual reform process. The 1967 and 1972 amendments to the social security act, which added provisions for early and periodic screening of preschool Medicaid eligible children, was a step forward in the reform process. Similarly, the complete coverage of kidney dialysis services in 1972 added another piece to the package. However, the trouble with this piecemeal approach is that long-range goals are neglected, and, for any system to be effective, no matter how it is enacted, it is essential that long-range goals be established.

In our minds, one of the most important long-range objectives should be the establishment of a comprehensive health care system, something that is now almost totally lacking. This was not true so much in the past, but in recent decades the patchwork financing system and the growing trend toward specialization in medicine have created a fragmentation of care. Though poor people and minorities can now receive a certain amount of health care, the value of the care is not so great as it could be because of fragmentation. For example, the federal government furnishes care through various agencies to many people, including the aged, the blind, the totally disabled, families with dependent children, veterans, and members of the armed forces. As we have indicated, research hospitals sometimes give outstanding care to a patient with a rare disease or someone who fits into a given study sample, but other seriously ill patients are ignored. Private funds sometimes finance the care of a specific disease, but often the funding specialized agencies or hospitals are located far from the point of need. Health departments give preventive care to mothers and infants but usually do not give acute care. This maze of eligibility categories is difficult enough for the expert to comprehend, but it is truly formidable for the poor, the uneducated, and those with a language barrier. Moreover, even when services are available in scattered specialty facilities, someone with multiple health problems often must travel around to various specialists, because there is no one worker who looks at the total health problem of the patient or evaluates the total regimen. This is true in private-patient care as well as in charitable or governmental medical care.

Any effective plan to deal with health care must do away with the complex eligibility rules and simply give health care to all people, employed or unemployed, rich or poor, citizen or alien, young or old. In effect, health care must be thought of as a right for all, instead of a privilege for those who have money or accidentally qualify under some special program. Some means must also be established by which one worker can take the primary responsibility for coordinating the patient's care. In the past, this was the role of the general practitioner, but, because of the trend in medical education away from producing family physicians and toward gathering ever-more-specialized knowledge, it is possible that the primary-care role will fall to less expensive workers, such as the nurse practitioners or the physicians' assistants. Whether they are general practitioners, nurse practitioners, or physicians' assistants, these workers should be allowed to treat the less complex illnesses and refer the problems to the various specialists. They should also coordinate the care so that the welfare of the total patient is not overlooked, as the specialists narrow their focus on diseases or organs.

A second important goal in establishment of a health care plan is an economically feasible system. The already existing Medicare-Medicaid legislation needs revision to cut out its inflationary characteristics that have increased costs but not necessarily improved medical care. Fee controls and cost-accounting procedures are badly needed, and the unnecessary administrative cost of using intermediate carriers, such as Blue Cross, to do work that the government can do cheaper should be eliminated. Planning for economy is always a difficult aspect of reform, because each of the various lobbies works to see that its group gains economic advantages, but it is a crucial step in order to make a health plan workable in the long run.

Both of these major objectives, making health care comprehensive and economically efficient can best be furthered by the encouragement of government-sponsored health maintenance organizations. Basically, these organizations are a form of group practice, something pioneered by Americans. The first group practice was the famed Mayo Clinic in Rochester, Minnesota, in which the various professional and paraprofessional groups worked together to treat the patient. Dating from the nineteenth century, the Mayo Clinic was originally developed not for preventive reasons but to deal with the seriously ill patient. Its example has been followed by various other specialized clinics, such as Cleveland Clinic, the Ochsner Clinic in New Orleans, and the Lahey Clinic in Boston. The consultation of the experts assembled in these clinics probably furnishes the best medical care in the world. These "clinics" had little opposition from organized medicine, but when the concept of the clinic was combined with the prepaid factor and preventive care, and was opened up to a wider public, organized medicine went into opposition. In fact, on the urging of their medical associations, many states passed laws prohibiting group practice of any kind, and such laws still exist in some states.

The two best-known of the prepaid group practice insurance plans are the Health Insurance Plan (HIP) in New York and Kaiser-Permanente on the West Coast. Both have the advantage of adjusting to the realities of how the best medicine is increasingly practiced in this country, and they also have the additional advantage of costing less than other insurance plans. Kaiser-Permanente was started by Henry J. Kaiser, the California contractor, as a plan for his employees when he was building Grand Coulee Dam. It was expanded during World War II, as Kaiser turned to building ships, and then further expanded as the industrialist turned to manufacturing steel, aluminum, and automobiles. Shortly after the end of the war, the system went public and, through contracts with various unions and other organizations, Kaiser-Permanente began offering total prepaid medical care to all subscribers.[33] For those who belong to the complete Kaiser plans, everything is paid except drugs used in outpatient care, and these are sold at less than wholesale prices. From the first, Kaiser-Permanente has insisted that all companies and organizations offering their plan also offer competing ones. This has tended to keep subscribers from feeling trapped within the Kaiser system, and it has also served as an effective cost-accounting procedure. The great virtue of the Kaiser system and similar ones is that they emphasize preventive medicine. The difference that effective preventive care makes was demonstrated by a study of federal employees on the West Cost, some of whom were insured by Kaiser-Permanente and others by Blue Cross–Blue Shield. The study found that, although Kaiser subscribers had greater contact with physicians and other health practitioners, they spent far less time in the hospital. Each unit of 1,000 federal employees spent a total of 433 days in the hospital per year under the Kaiser plan, while those under Blue Cross–Blue Shield spent an average of 865 days per 1,000 employees. This enabled Kaiser to keep its costs about 20 percent lower than the cost of California's voluntary hospitals and to keep the rate of increase to less than half of the national rate.

Prepaid group plans achieve these lower costs by practicing effective preventive medicine and by cutting out unnecessary operations or other medical procedures. For example, Kaiser surgery rates are little more than one half of the Blue Cross figures. As one Kaiser official stated, Kaiser has a vested interest in keeping the patient well—a few pennies spent on prevention saves dollars spent on cure. Kaiser physicians and employees are salaried, but those at the higher levels are also eligible to become partners and share in the profits from the plan. In a 1966 study of various prepaid group practice plans, it was found that, for each 1,000 enrollees, physicians in the group practice performed fewer than one-quarter the number of tonsillectomies, half the number of appendectomies, and only slightly more than half the hysterectomies done by fee-for-service physicians. This same trend appeared with those welfare patients enrolled in group practice plans. In 1962, for example, New York City's HIP undertook to treat welfare recipients, and it was found that its physicians made but one-quarter the number of premium-priced home calls and ordered but one-half the highly profitable (and highly expensive) laboratory tests that fee-for-service, solo practitioners were accustomed to doing.[34]

Under a national health insurance plan, such health maintenance organizations would contract to care for a given number of patients for an annual fee, rather than be paid for each service rendered.[35] Recognizing the value of the HMO and their cost effectiveness, the federal government supported legislation to help establish them. The result was Public Law 93-222, the Health Maintenance Organization Act of 1973, which was signed into law in December 1973. Without actually defining HMOs, the law established minimum requirements that HMOs had to meet in order to qualify for grants, contracts, loans, and loan guarantees that would be given to offset the costs of planning, development, and initial operation. Minimum benefits included physicians' services, in-patient and out-patient hospital services, medically necessary emergency services, short-term ambulatory evaluative and crisis-intervention mental health services, medical treatment and referral services for alcohol and drug abuse and addiction, laboratory and diagnostic and therapeutic radiological services, home health services, and preventive services, including voluntary family planning services, infertility services, preventive dental care for children, and children's eye examinations. Gradually, HMOs have spread out of the New York City and West Coast areas into other areas of the country, in spite of the fact that some government stipulations about minimum benefits have put HMOs at a competitive disadvantage with other insurance plans. HMOs' big advantage is not only in the ability to practice more effective preventive health care but also to more effectively mix primary health-care givers, including nurse practitioners and physicians' assistants, with specialists, without losing sight of the patient.

This book is not the place to decide how any national health plan is financed. Such a topic deserves a study in its own right. However, it still is possible to speculate, if only briefly. An insurance principle in which each worker contributes a portion of his or her salary, as is done under Social Security, seems a likely possibility. Although payment out of general revenues would be easier for the marginal worker to afford because general revenues receive a greater share from higher-income levels in society, it would be more difficult to get this method through Congress. Probably some combination of these two sources of financing is the most pragmatic suggestion we have to offer.

However, government-supported health care also raises problems. What should tax money be used for? Public awareness of this problem has focused on such issues as abortion and life-support systems. In terms of public health, funding for abortion lowers maternal mortality,[36] increases the likelihood of a child being wanted, and, in terms of tax money, decreases the long-term medical costs of unwanted and often abandoned children. However, a significant portion of the American population regards abortion as murder. What once might have been a matter of individual conscience has now become an issue of public policy.

Life-support systems allow patients to remain technically alive for long periods of time without any hope of recovery or, in many cases, without the possibility of regaining consciousness. In the past, such decisions were largely made upon economic grounds; those who could afford the necessary special services, which then included round-the-clock nursing, received them, while those who could not usually did not. With tax money involved, the problem remains an economic one, but it also is an ethical one, because a decision must be made as to when life-support systems should be discontinued.

Any long-range planning for health reform also requires considering how to better use health workers. One of the most obvious consequences of any extension of health care will be the need for more health workers. One of the easiest ways to solve the problem is to make more effective use of present workers. Laws that bar workers from performing tasks they can safely and effectively perform need to be reconsidered. Although current trends suggest that there may soon be an oversupply of physicians,[37] this still does not solve the problem of staffing a well-planned health care system, because the present organization of medical schools makes this oversupply of physicians too expensive and too specialized. Perhaps financial incentives now being used to encourage research and specialization should be reconsidered. Some of the funds might be better spent to educate more nurse practitioners and family practitioners. The suggestion of the Carnegie Foundation that medical education be shortened also has merit.[38] As the health care industry expands, care must be taken to see that many people will not be trapped at the bottom of the economic ladder in no-advancement jobs, such as nurses' aides and orderlies. Many such workers are at near-poverty levels of income, which in itself is not a healthy phenomenon. More important, however, is the fact that workers who have no chance for advancement tend to lose interest in their jobs over the years. Unless some means can be found to interest them in helping to deliver better health care, all the best-laid plans of scholarly investigators and government planners will fail. Not only should these workers be paid more, but they should also be given in-service training and encouraged to work to the full level of their capacity. The health care team must be democratized.

In this book, we have tried to present the health care problems of the major ethnic minority groups in perspective. We believe that poverty is the most crucial variable in the genesis of these problems. Poverty breeds disease, and, until the environmental, social, and economic circumstances of the poor are changed, they will continue to suffer from unnecessarily high morbidity and mortality rates. Yet, the conditions of poverty can be alleviated, and it is a demonstrable fact that quality health care mitigates the effect of poverty on health. Effective health care cannot prevent the deformities visited upon a child whose mother contracted rubella during the first trimester of pregnancy, but it can protect women from contracting the disease; it cannot keep a child from developing a strep throat or an ear infection, but it can prevent these illnesses from progressing to rheumatic fever and hearing loss; it cannot prevent strabismus, but it can protect a child from losing sight in one eye because of the eye muscle disorder. Health care has no effect on crowded unsanitary housing, but it can treat the communicable diseases easily spread under these conditions. Health care can do nothing about racism in the society and the stresses of being black in the United States, but it can control the level of high blood pressure and the associated risks of heart disease and stroke brought on by that stress. Health care can do nothing about environmental pollution and the high exposure to that pollution among inner city minorities, but it may be able to prevent death from environmentally caused cancer.[39]

Evidence for these assertions is not hard to find. Denver, Colorado, has perhaps the most integrated and comprehensive system of city-run neighborhood health centers and Children and Youth projects in the entire country. The city also has the lowest differential between white and black infant mortality rates in the nation. Nurse midwivery programs in Mississippi, Kentucky, and New York City have shown similar results in their success in reaching previously unserved populations.

Effective preventive care in poverty areas means lower cost for health care in the long run. A Medicaid study compared Medicaid-eligible children who had been screened under the EPSDT program (Early and Periodic Screening, Diagnosis, and Treatment) with eligible children who had not been screened. The study found that the screened children needed significantly less hospital care, and 55 percent fewer patient days, and 26 percent fewer physician visits outside of physicians' offices. Similarly, the need to hospitalize children was reduced by 36 percent in two years, following the introduction of a comprehensive child-care program at Boston Pediatric Center.[40]

The list could go on, and, in fact, many similar cases have been recorded earlier in this book. Poverty is also associated with many subtle and not so subtle forms of discrimination based on color or ethnic identity. In other aspects of American life, discrimination has also had consequences for health and, in turn, poor health helps perpetuate the cycle of alienation and poverty that so many minorities live in. We have tried to emphasize that there are no simple solutions but that problems come together into a kind of Gordian knot. However, there are rational and possible steps to take to cut that knot, including (1) eliminating poverty, or at least the effects of poverty; (2) effectively enforcing the laws against discrimination; and (3) revising our health care delivery system to provide total coverage for all people. To some, these might seem utopian steps, but, until we take effective action against these barriers, the United States will not fully live up to its potential in the health field. No matter how we look at it, health care in the future will be costly;[41] the question is whether all segments of the population will benefit from our costly system.

REFERENCES

1. Costs and Delivery of Health Services to Older Americans. Hearings Before the Subcommittee on Health of the Elderly of the Special Committee on Aging, United States Senate, Ninetieth Congress, 1st Session, Part I. Washington, D.C.: U.S. Government Printing Office, 1967, pp. 84–85.
2. Yerby, A. S. Health Departments, Hospitals, and Health Services. Mimeographed copy of an address given at the Fiftieth Anniversary Celebration, October 6, 1966, at The Johns Hopkins School of Hygiene and Public Health.
3. Heilbroner, R. L. Benign Neglect in the United States. *Transaction*, 1970, 7, No. 12, 15–22.
4. For example, see: Schorr, A. L. The Case for Federal Welfare. *The Nation*, May 3, 1971, pp. 555–557. Mr. Schorr was a former Deputy Secretary of the Department of Health, Education, and Welfare.
5. See: U.S. Bureau of Census. Statistical Abstract of the United States. Washington, D.C.: U.S. Government Printing Office, 1979, Table 143, 145, pp. 100–101. For earlier information, see: U.S. Bureau of Census. Current Population Reports, Series P-60, No. 76. 24 Million Americans— Poverty in the United States, 1969. Washington, D.C.: U.S. Government Printing Office, 1970.
6. See: Riessman, F. Strategies Against Poverty. New York: Random House, 1969, pp. 21–40. Also see: R. E. Haveman (Ed.), A Decade of Federal Antipoverty Programs. New York: Academic Press, 1977.

7. Kelly, C. H. Fighting Poverty in Urban Areas, & Fighting Poverty in Rural Areas. In B. Bullough & V. Bullough (Eds.), New Directions for Nurses. New York: Springer, 1971, pp. 248–259, 259–266.

8. Breye, P. R. Neighborhood Health Centers: An Assessment. *American Journal of Public Health*, 1977, *67*, 179–181.

9. U.S. Social Security Administration. Social Security Programs Throughout the World. Washington, D.C.: U.S. Government Printing Office, 1967.

10. For a popular account of the opposition of AMA, see Cray, E. In Failing Health: The Medical Crises and the AMA. Indianapolis: The Bobbs-Merrill Company, 1970, pp. 40–59.

11. Glasser, W. A. Paying the Doctor: Systems of Remuneration and Their Effects. Baltimore: The Johns Hopkins University Press, 1970, p. 178. Also see: Roemer, M. I. & Axelrod, S. J. A National Health System and Social Security. *American Journal of Public Health*, 1977, *67*, 462–465.

12. Roemer, M. I. The Organization of Medical Care Under Social Security. Geneva: International Labour Office, 1969, pp. 31, 46–47.

13. Glasser. op. cit., pp. 202–203.

14. Ibid., pp. 286–287.

15. Roemer. The Organization of Medical Care. pp. 52–55. Also see: Jagdish, Community Medicine in the British National Health Service. *American Journal of Public Health*, 1978, *68*, 54–57.

16. Glaser. op. cit., pp. 52–53.

17. Ibid., pp. 206–207. Roemer, M. I. Highlights of Soviet Health Services. *Milbank Memorial Fund Quarterly*, 1962, *15*, No. 4, 381–385.

18. Corning, P. A. The Evolution of Medicare: From Idea to Law. Research Report, No. 29. Washington, D.C.: U.S. Government Printing Office, 1969, pp. 5–16.

19. Committee on the Costs of Medical Care. Medical Care for the American People. Chicago: University of Chicago Press, 1932. Reprinted by U.S. Government Printing Office, 1970.

20. Cray. op. cit., p. 65.

21. Rosen, G. A History of Public Health. New York: M. D. Publications, 1958, pp. 456–562. Bullough, V. & Bullough, B. Care of the Sick: The Emergence of Modern Nursing. New York: Prodist, 1978, pp. 170–271.

22. Social Security Administration. The Evolution of Medicare. pp. 53–57.

23. Ibid., pp. 74–115. Cray. op. cit., pp. 90–109.

24. Walsh, J. Stanford School of Medicine (1) Problems over More than Money. *Science*, February 12, 1971, 551–553. Also see: Bullough, V. L. Financial Crisis on the Campus. *Progressive*, October 1971, 37–40.

25. Statistical Abstract, 1979. Tables 143, 145, pp. 100–101.

26. The American Health Empire: Power, Profits and Politics. A Health PAC Book prepared by B. Ehrenreich & J. Ehrenreich. New York: Random House, 1970, pp. 96–103.

27. Leffler, K. National Health Insurance: A Social Placebo. *Current History*, 1977, *73*, 17–21.

28. There has been much written about HSAs. For discussion of Act, see:

The Nation's Health, June 1975, pp. 1, 4, 5. For discussion of later problems, see: Vladeck, B. C. Interest Group Representation and the HSAs: Health Planning and Political Theory. *American Journal of Public Health,* 1977, *67,* 23–29. Berry, D. E. & Candia, G. R. Voluntary Coordination as a Strategy of Plan Implementation for Health System Agencies. *American Journal of Public Health,* 1979, *69,* 1035–1039.

29. *Hospitals,* 1979, *53,* 47–50, 54.

30. Starr, J. Cook County Hospital: The Terrible Place. *Look,* May 18, 1971, pp. 24–33. *Chicago Tribune,* December 17, 1979, Sec. 1, p. 1; December 18, 1979, p. 12, col. 1.

31. *Hospitals.* op. cit.

32. For example, see: Cohen, W. J. National Health Insurance—problems and prospects. The Michael M. Davis Lecture for 1970 at the Center for Health Administration Studies, Graduate School of Business, University of Chicago, 1970.

33. For a discussion of this and other plans, see: Somers, H. M. & Somers, A. R. Doctors, Patients and Health Insurance: The Organization and Financing of Medical Care. Washington, D.C.: The Brookings Institution, 1961.

34. Cray. op. cit., pp. 190–191. Also see: Tunley, R. The American Health Scandal. New York: Harper, 1966, pp. 112–125.

35. Ellwood, Jr., P. M. Health Maintenance Organizations: Concept and Strategy. *Hospitals,* 1971, *45,* 53–56.

36. Petiti, D. B. & Cates, Jr., W. Restricting Medicaid Funds for Abortion: Projects of Excess Mortality for Women of Childbearing Age. *American Journal of Public Health,* 1977, *6,* 860–862. Quick, J. B. Liberalized Abortion in Oregon: Effects of Fertility, Prematurity, Fetal Death and Infant Death. *American Journal of Public Health,* 1978, *68,* 1003–1008.

37. Report of Graduate Medical Education, National Advisory Committee to the Secretary of the Department of Health and Human Services, Vol. 6, Nonphysicians Health Care Procedures Technical Panel. U.S. Department of Health and Human Services, Public Health Service Health Resources Administration, Office of Graduate Medical Care. September 1980.

38. Carnegie Commission on Higher Education. Higher Education and the Nation's Health: Policies for Dental and Medical Education. New York: McGraw-Hill, 1970.

39. See: Dallek, C. Health Care for California's Poor/Separate and Unequal. Mimeographed report by the National Health Law Program, Inc., 2401 Main Street, Santa Monica, California 90405.

40. Children's Defense Fund. Doctors and Dollars Are Not Enough. Washington D.C., 1976, pp. 12–13. Children's Defense Fund. EPSDT: Does It Spell Health Care for Poor Children? Washington, D.C., 1978. Johnson, R. W. Foundation Annual Report, 1976, p. 16. Dallek. op. cit., pp. 87–92.

41. Gori, G. B. & Richter, B. J. Macroeconomics of Disease Prevention in the United States. *Science,* 1978, *200,* 1124–1130.

BIBLIOGRAPHY

Acosta, F. X. & Sheehan, J. G. Self-Disclosure in Relation to Psychotherapist Expertise and Ethnicity. *American Journal of Community Psychology*, 1978, *6*, 545–553.

Acosta, F. X. Barriers Between Mental Health Services and Mexican Americans: An Examination of a Paradox. *American Journal of Community Psychology*, 1979, 7, 503–520.

Adair, J. & Deuschle, K. W. The People's Health: Medicine and Anthropology in a Navaho Community. New York: Appleton, 1970.

Aday, L. A. Anderson, R. & Fleming, G.V. Health Care in the U.S.: Equitable for Whom? Beverly Hills, California: Sage Publications, 1980.

Addams, J. Twenty Years at Hull House. New York: Macmillan, 1912.

Alford, R. R. Health Care Politics: Ideological and Interest Group Barriers to Reform. Chicago: University of Chicago Press, 1975.

Alford, R. R. The Political Economy of Health Care: Dynamics Without Change. *Politics and Society*, 1972, *2*, 256–259.

Alpert, J., Kosa, J., & Haggerty, R.J. A Month of Illness and Health Care Among Low Income Families. *Public Health Reports*, 1967, *82*, 705–713

American Indian Nurses Association. Survey of Schools of Professional Nursing: American Indian Involvement in Professional Schools of Nursing 1974–1975. Norman, Oklahoma: American Indian Nurses Association.

American Nurses' Association, Affirmative Action Task Force. Affirmative Action: Toward Quality Nursing Care for a Multiracial Society. Kansas City, Missouri: American Nurses' Association, 1976, Publication No. M–24 2500 5/76.

American Nurses' Assocation, Commission on Human Rights. A Strategy for Change. Kansas City, Missouri: American Nurses' Association, 1979.

American Public Health Association. Evaluatory Study on Operation of the Migrant Health Program Under the Migrant Health Act. New York: mimeographed, December 30, 1964, pp. 1–49.

Anderson, E. H., & Lesser, A. J. Maternity Care in the United States: Gains and Gaps. *American Journal of Nursing*, 1966, *66*, 1539–1544.

Anderson, G. & Tighe, B. Gypsy Culture and Health Care. *American Journal of Nursing*, 1973, 73, 282–285.

Anderson, R. Lewis, S. Z., Giachello, A.L., Aday, L.A. & Chiu, G. Access to Medical Care among the Hispanic Population of Southwestern United States. *Journal of Health and Social Behavior*, 1981, *22*, 78–89

Atunes, G. C., Gaitz, C. M., & Scott, J. Ethnicity, Socioeconomic Status and the Etiology of Psychological Distress. *Sociology and Social Research*, 1974, *58*, 361–368.

Armstrong, R. L. & Holmes, B. Counseling for Socially Withdrawn Indian Girls. *Journal of American Indian Education*, January 1971, 4–7.

Baca, J. Some Health Beliefs of the Spanish Speaking. *American Journal of Nursing*, 1969, *69*, 2172–2176.

Badgley, R. F. & Wolfe, S. Doctors' Strike: Medical Care and Conflict in Saskatchenwan. New York: Atherton, 1967.

Baird, K. & Twining, M. Sea Island Culture. Editors of a special issue of *Journal of Black Studies*, 1980, *10*.

Ball, R. M. National Health Insurance: Comments on Selected Issues. *Science*, 1978, *200*, 864–870.

Barnett, S. E., Gillespie, J., & Call, R. L. Migrant Health Revisited: A Model for Statewide Health Planning and Services. *American Journal of Public Health*, 1980, *70*, 1092–1094.

Barrett-Conner, E. Latent and Chronic Infections Imported from Southeast Asia. *Journal of American Medical Association*, 1978, *239*, 1901–1906.

Barron, M. L. *Minorities in a Changing World. New York: Alfred A. Knopf, 1967.*

Bazell, R. J. Health Insurance: Battle Focuses on Nixon and Kennedy Schemes. *Science*, 1971, *171*, 783–785.

Bell, C. C. & Mehta, H. The Misdiagnosis of Black Patients with Manic Depressive Illness. *Journal of the National Medical Association*, 1980, *72*, 141–145.

Bell, C. C. & Mehta, H. Misdiagnosis of Black Patients with Manic Depressive Illness: Second in a Series, *Journal of the National Medical Association*, 1981, *73*, 101–107.

Bell, D., Longfellow, C., Makosky, V., et al. Income, Mothers' Mental Health, and Family Functioning in a Low-Income Population. In The Impact of Changing Resources on Health Policy. American Academy of Nursing, 1981, 28–37.

Bennett, F. The Condition of Farm Workers. In L. A. Ferman, J. L. Kornblush, & A. Haber (Eds.), Poverty in America. Ann Arbor: University of Michigan Press, revised edition 1968, pp. 303–314.

Benson, H., Kotch, J. B., & Crassweller, K. D. Stress and Hypertension: Interrelations and Management. *Cardiovascular Clinic*, 1978, *9*, 113–124.

Bergner, L. & Yerby, A. S. Low Income and Barriers to Use of Health Service. *New England Journal of Medicine*, 1968, *278*, 541–546.

Berkanovic, E. & Reeder, L. G. Can Money Buy the Appropriate Use of Services? Some Notes on the Meaning of Utilization Data. *Journal of Health and Human Behavior*, 1974, *15*, 93–99.

Berle, B. B. Eighty Puerto Rican Families in New York City: Health and Disease Studied in Context. New York: Columbia University Press, 1958.

Berry, D. E. & Candia, G. R. Voluntary Coordination as a Strategy of Plan Implementation for Health Systems Agencies. *American Journal of Public Health*, 1979, *69*, 1035–1039.

Berthol, C. Prayer as a Coping Mechanism Among Mastectomy Patients. Unpublished master's thesis. Long Beach: California State University, 1979.

Bigham, G. D. To Communicate with Negro Patients. *American Journal of Nursing*, 1964, *64*, 113–115.

Birch, H. G. & Gussow, J. D. Disadvantaged Children: Health, Nutrition and School Failure. New York: Harcourt, 1970.

Blau, P. M. & Duncan, O. D. The American Occupational Structure. New York: Wiley, 1967.

Blum, R. et al. Society and Drugs; Social and Cultural Observations, Vol. 1. San Francisco: Jossey-Bass, 1969.

Bogardus, E. S. The Mexican in the United States. New York: Arno Press, 1934. Republished 1970.

Boles, D. & Boles, J. The Gypsies' Doctor in Georgia. *Journal of the Gypsy Lore Society*, 1959, *38*, 55–63.

Bongarts, R. Who Am I? The Indian Sickness. *The Nation*, April 27, 1970, 496–498.

Branch, M. F. & Paxton, P. P. Providing Safe Nursing Care for Ethnic People of Color. New York: Appleton, 1976.

Breed, W. Suicide, Migration and Race: A Study of Cases in New Orleans. *The Journal of Social Issues*, 1966, *22*, 30–43.

Breslow, L. Risk Factor Intervention for Health Maintenance. *Science*, 1978, *200*, 908–912.

Breyer, P. R. Neighborhood Health Centers: An Assessment. *American Journal of Public Health*, 1977, *67*, 179–181.

Brisbane, R. H. The Black Vanguard: Origins of the Negro Social Revolution 1900–1960. Valley Forge: Judson Press, 1970.

Brooks, C. H. Social, Economic, and Biologic Correlates of Infant Mortality in City Neighborhoods. *Journal of Health and Social Behavior*, 1980, *21*, 2–11.

Brosseau, J. D., Eelkema, R. C., Crawford, A. C., & Abe, T. A. Diabetes Among Three Affiliated Tribes: Correlation with Degree of Indian Inheritance. *American Journal of Public Health*, 1979, *69* 1277–1278.

Brown, C. Manchild in the Promised Land. New York: Macmillan, 1965.

Brown, L. Hunger USA: The Public Pushes Congress. *Journal of Health and Social Behavior*, 1970, *11*, 115–126.

Bruhn, J. G., Philips, B. U. & Wolf, S. Social Readjustments and Illness Patterns: Comparisons Between First, Second, and Third Generation Italian-Americans Living in the Same Community. *Journal of Psychosomatic Research*, 1972, *16*, 387–394.

Bucher, K. A., Patterson, A. M. Jr., Elson, R. C., Jones, C. A., & Kirkman, H. Racial Difference in Incidence of ABO Hemolytic Disease. *American Journal of Public Health*, 1976, *66*, 854–858.

Buckley, J. Faculty Commitment to Retention and Recruitment of Black Students. *Nursing Outlook*, 1980, *28*, 46–50.

Bullock, P. Watts: The Aftermath. New York: Grove Press, 1969.

Bullough, B. Alienation in the Ghetto. *American Journal of Sociology*, 1967, *72*, 469–478.

Bullough, B. Malnutrition Among Egyptian Infants. *Nursing Research*, 1969, *18*, 172.

Bullough, B. (Ed.) Management of Common Human Miseries New York: Springer, 1979.

Bullough, B. Social-Psychological Barriers to Housing Desegregation. Los Angeles: University of California, Graduate School of Business Administration, 1969.

Bullough, B. Alienation and School Segregation. *Integrated Education*, 1972, 29–35.

Bullough, B. Poverty, Ethnic Identity and Preventive Health Care. *Journal of Health and Social Behavior*, 1972, *13*, 347–359.

Bullough, B. The Measurement of Alienation as it Relates to Family Planning Behavior. *Communicating Nursing Research 8:* In Nursing Research Priorities Choice or Chance, M.V. Batey. (Ed.) Boulder Colorado: Western Interstate Commission for Higher Education, 1977, pp. 41–52.

Bullough, B. The Expanding Role of the Registered Nurse. In J. R. Folt & E. S. Deck (Eds.), A Sociological Framework for Patient Care (2nd ed.) New York: Wiley, pp. 142–152.

Bullough, B. The Law and the Expanding Nursing Role (2nd ed.). New York: Appleton, 1980.

Bullough, B. & Bullough, V. Issues in Nursing. New York: Springer, 1966.

Bullough, B. & Bullough, V. New Directions for Nurses. New York: Springer, 1971.

Bullough, B. & Bullough, V. A Career Ladder in Nursing. *American Journal of Nursing*, 1971, *71*, 1938–1943.

Bullough, V. Financial Crisis on the Campus. *Progressive*, October 1971, 37–41.

Bullough, V. L. Dissenting Thoughts on Intellectual and Creative Achievement. *Humanist*, January-February 1980, 43–46, 56.

Bullough, V. & Bullough, B. What Color Are Your Germs? Chicago: The Committee to End Discrimination in Chicago Medical Institutions, 1955.

Bullough, V. & Bullough, B. The Untouchables. Chicago: Committee Against Discrimination and the Southern Conference on Education, 1955.

Bullough, V. & Bullough, B. Care of the Sick: Emergence of Modern Nursing (3rd ed.). New York: Prodist, 1978.

Bunker, J. P., Hinkley, D., & McDermott, W. V. Surgical Innovation and Its Evaluation. *Science*, 1978, *200*, 937–941.

Bureau of Maternal and Child Health, California State Department of Public Health. Health for the Harvesters: A Ten Year Report by the Farm Workers Health Service. State of California, 1970.

Burgess, E. W. Urban Areas. In T. V. Smith & L. White (Eds.), Chicago: An Experiment in Social Science Research. Chicago: University of Chicago Press, 1929, pp. 113–138.

Burrell, L. & Rayder, N. F. Black and White Students Attitudes Toward White Counselors. *Journal of Negro Education*, 1971, *40*, 48–52.

Cabot, R. C. Social Service and the Art of Healing. New York: Dodd, Mead, 1931.

Cahalan, D., Cisin, I., & Crossley, H. M. American Drinking Practices: A National Survey of Behavior and Attitudes Related to Alcoholic Beverages. Washington, D.C.: Social Research Group, George Washington University, Report No. 3, 1967.

California Legislative Assembly Committee on Health and Welfare. Malnutrition: One Key to the Poverty Cycle. January 1970.

Campbell, A. A. Fertility and Family Planning Among Non-White Married Couples in the United States. *Eugenics Quarterly*, 1961, *12*, 124–131.

Cannon, M. S. & Locke, B. Z. Being Black is Detrimental to One's Mental Health: Myth or Reality? *Phylon*, 1977, *38*, 408–428.

Cappannori, S. C. et al. Voodoo in the General Hospital, A Case of Hexing and Regional Enteritis. *Journal of the American Medical Association*, 1975, *232*, 939–940.

Carkuff, R. R. & Pierce, R. Differential Effects of Therapists' Race and Social Class Upon Patient Depth of Self Exploration in the Initial Interview. *Journal of Consulting Psychology*, 1967, *31*, 632–634.

Carnegie Commission on Higher Education. Higher Education and the Nation's Health: Policies for Dental and Medical Education. New York: McGraw-Hill, 1970.

Carnegie, M. E. Are Negro Schools of Nursing Needed Today? *Nursing Outlook*, 1964, *12*, 52–56. Reprinted in Bullough, B. & Bullough, V. (Eds.), New Directions for Nurses, New York: Springer, 1971, pp. 292–303.

Carp, F. M. & Kataoka, E. Health Care Problems of the Elderly of San Francisco's Chinatown. *Gerontologist*, 1976, *16*, 30–38.

Carr-Saunders, A. M. World Population. Oxford: Clarendon Press, 1936.

Carter, J. H. Mental Health Service in a Black Community. *Urban Health,* 1977, *6,* 36–37.

Caudill, H. M. Night Comes to the Cumberlands: A Biography of a Depressed Area. Boston: Little, Brown, 1963.

Chadek, M. Nursing Service for Migrant Workers. *American Journal of Nursing,* June 1965, 62–65.

Chapman, C. B. Doctors and Their Autonomy: Past Events and Future Prospects. *Science,* 1978, *200,* 851–856.

Chapman, C. B. & Talmadge, J. M. The Evolution of the Right to Health Concept in the United States. The Pharos of Alpha Omega Alpha, 1971, *34,* 30–51.

Chase, H. C. Perinatal and Infant Mortality in the United States and Six West European Countries. *American Journal of Public Health,* 1967, *57,* 1735–1748.

Chein, I. Psychological, Social and Epidemiological Factors in Drug Addiction. In Rehabilitating the Narcotic Addict. A report of the Institute on New Developments in the Rehabilitation of the Narcotic Addict. Washington, D.C.: U.S. Government Printing Office, 1966, pp. 53–66.

Chenault, L. R. The Puerto Rican Migrant in New York City. New York: Columbia University Press, 1938.

Chinatown, U.S.A., 1970. *California's Health,* 1970, *27–28,* 1–3.

Chisholm, N. Letter: Restriction of Medical Aid in Abortion. *British Medical Journal,* 1975, *1,* 629.

Christian, J. R., Celevycz, B. S., & Andelman, S. L. A Three Year Study of Lead Poisoning in Chicago, Epidemiology. *American Journal of Public Health,* 1964, *54,* 1241–1245.

Civil Rights '63. Report of the United States Commission on Civil Rights. Washington, D.C.: U.S. Government Printing Office, 1963.

Clark, K. B. Dark Ghetto: Dilemmas of Social Power. New York: Harper, 1965.

Clark, K. B. Prejudice and Your Child. Boston: Beacon Press, 1955.

Clark, K. & Hopkins, J. A Relevant War Against Poverty, A Study of Community Action Programs and Observable Social Change. New York and Evanston: Harper, 1970.

Clark, M. Health in the Mexican-American Culture: A Community Study. Berkeley: University of California Press, 1959, Reprinted 1970.

Clark, Sr., M. F. Adequate Health Care: One Step Toward Social Justice. *Hospital Progress,* 1978, *59,* 6, 8, 10.

Clebert, J. The Gypsies. Baltimore: Penguin Books, 1963.

Coakley, T. A., Ehrlich, P. R., & Hurd, E. Health Screening in a Family Clinic. *American Journal of Nursing,* 1980, *80,* 2032–2035.

Coburn, D. & Pope, C. R. Socioeconomic Status and Preventive Health Behavior. *Journal of Health and Social Behavior,* 1974, *15,* 67–78.

Cogan, L. Negroes for Medicine: Report of a Macy Conference. Baltimore: Johns Hopkins Press, 1968.

Cohen, R. E. Principles of Preventive Mental Health Programs for Ethnic Minority Populations: The Acculturation of Puerto Ricans to the United States. *American Journal of Psychiatry*, 1972, *128*, 1529–1533.

Coleman, E. Financial Feasibility Under Hill-Burton Act: An Accountant's Perspective. *Clearing House Review*, June 1975.

Coleman, J. S., Campbell, E. Q. et al. Equality of Educational Opportunity. Washington, D.C.: U.S. Office of Education, 1966.

Coleman, J. S. Resources for Social Change: Race in the United States. New York: Wiley Interscience, 1971.

Coles, R. Migrants, Sharecroppers, Mountaineers. Vol. II of Children in Crisis. Boston: Little, Brown, 1971.

Coles, R. The South Goes North. Boston: Little, Brown, 1971.

Collins, J. L., Rickman, L. E., & Mathura, C. B. Frequency of Schizophrenia and Depression in a Black Inpatient Population. *Journal of the National Medical Association*, 1980, *9*, 851–856.

Committee on Labor and Public Welfare, United States Senate, Special Subcommittee on Indian Education: A National Tragedy—A National Challenge. Washington, D.C.: U.S. Government Printing Office, 1969.

Committee on the Costs of Medical Care. Medical Care for the American People. Chicago: University of Chicago Press, 1932. Reprinted by U.S. Government Printing Office, 1970.

Cooper, S. A Look at the Effect of Racism on Clinical Work. *Social Casework*, 1973, *54*, 76–84.

Cornely, P. B. The Health Status of the Negro Today and in the Future. *American Journal of Public Health*, 1968, *58*, 647–654.

Corning, P. A. The Evolution of Medicare . . . from Idea to Law. U.S. Department of Health, Education, and Welfare, Social Security Administration, Research Report No. 29. Washington, D.C.: U.S. Government Printing Office, 1969.

Cox, J. L. Aspects of Transcultural Psychiatry. *British Journal of Psychiatry*, 1977, *130*, 211–221.

Cray, E. In Failing Health: The Medical Crisis and the A.M.A. Indianapolis: Bobbs-Merrill, 1970.

Crowley, A. E. & Nicholson, H. C. Negro Enrollment in Medical Schools. *Journal of the American Medical Association*, 1969, *210*, 96–100.

Cuban Refugee Problem. Report of the Hearings Before the Subcommittee to Investigate Problems Connected with Refugees and Escapees, Committee on the Judiciary, United States Senate, in three parts. Washington, D.C.: U.S. Government Printing Office, 1966.

Cuban Refugees. *Newsweek*, May 26, 1980, 24–28.

Cuba's Children in Exile: The Story of the Unaccompanied Cuban Refugee Children's Program. U.S. Department of Health, Education, and Welfare, Children's Bureau, 1967.

Culliton, Barbara J. Health Care Economics: The High Cost of Getting Well. *Science*, 1978, *200*, 883–885.

Dallek, G. Health Care for California's Poor/Separate and Unequal. National Health Law Program, July 13, 1979, pp. 3–4.

Danielson, R. Cuban Medicine. New Brunswick, New Jersey: Transaction Books, 1979.

The Darling Case. *Journal of the American Medical Association*, 1968, *206*, 1875.

Davis, M. M. & Haasis, B. A. The Visiting Nurse and the Immigrant. *Public Health Nurse*, 1920 , *12*, 823.

Davis, M. M. Immigrant Health and the Community. New York: Harper & Brothers, 1921. Reprinted Montclair, New Jersey: Patterson Smith Reprint Series, 1970.

Davitz, L. J., Sameshima, Y., & Davitz, J. Suffering as Viewed in Six Different Cultures. *American Journal of Nursing*, 1976, *76*, 1296–1297.

Deasy, L. C. Socio-Economic Status and Participation in the Poliomyelitis Vaccine Trial. *American Sociological Review*, 1956, *21*, 185–191.

DeGracia, R. T. Cultural Influences on Filipino Patients. *American Journal of Nursing*, 1979, *79*, 1412–1414.

Delgado, G., Brumback, C. L. & Deaver, M. B. Eating Problems Among Migrant Families. *Public Health Reports*, 1961, *76*, 349–355.

Delgado, M. Herbal Medicine in the Puerto Rican Community. *Health and Social Work*, 1979, *4*, 24–40.

Delgado, M. & Montalvo, S. Preventive Mental Health Services for Hispanic Preschool Children. *Child Today*, 1979, *8*, 6–8, 34.

Dellums, H.R. 2969, A Bill: To Establish a United States Health Service, 95th Congress, 2nd session. March 14, 1979.

de Tornyay, R. & Russell, M. L. Helping the High Risk Student Achieve. *Nursing Outlook*, 1978, *26*, 576–580.

Deutsch, M., Katz, I., & Jensen, A. R. (Eds.) Social Class, Race and Psychological Development. New York: Holt, 1968.

Dimock, E. & Riegel, B. Volunteering to Help Indians Help Themselves. *Children*, 1971, *18*, 23–27.

Division of Indian Health, Program Analysis and Special Studies Branch. Eskimos, Indians and Aleuts of Alaska. In U.S. Department of Health, Education, and Welfare Report, Indians on Federal Reservations. Washington, D.C.: U.S. Government Printing Office, 1963.

Dohrenwend, B. P. & Dohrenwend, B. S. Social Status and Psychological Disorder: A Causal Inquiry. New York: Wiley Interscience 1969.

Dohrenwend, B. S. & Dohrenwend, B. P. Stressful Life Events: Their Nature and Effects. New York: Wiley, 1974.

Dohrenwend, B. P. Sociocultural and Social-Psychological Factors in the Genesis of Mental Disorders. *Journal of Health and Social Behavior*, 1975, *16*, 365–392.

Donabedian, A. The Quality of Medical Care. *Science*, 1978, *200*, 856–864.

Dorson, N. Discrimination and Civil Rights. Boston: Little, Brown, 1969.

Douglas, J. The Social Meaning of Suicide. Princeton: Princeton University Press, 1967.

Dublin, L. I. Suicide: A Sociological and Statistical Study. New York: Ronald Press, 1963.

DuBois, W. E. B. The Souls of Black Folk. Crest reprint, Fawcett Publications, 1965.

Duff, R. S. & Hollingshead, A. B. Sickness and Society. New York: Harper, 1968.

Duffus, R. L. Lillian Wald: Neighbor and Crusader. New York: Macmillan, 1938.

Dumas, R. G. This I Believe . . . About Nursing and the Poor. *Nursing Outlook*, 1969, *17*, 47–49.

Dummett, C. O. The Growth and Development of the Negro in Dentistry. Chicago: Stanek Press for the National Dental Association, 1952.

Duncan, B., Smith, A. N., & Briese, F. W. A Comparison of Growth: Spanish-Surnamed with Non-Spanish-Surnamed Children. *American Journal of Public Health*, 1979, *69*, 903–907.

Dunham, H. W. Community and Schizophrenia: An Epidemiological Analysis. Detroit: Wayne State University Press, 1965.

Durkheim, E. Suicide: A Study in Sociology. Translated from the French by J. A. Spaulding and G. Simpson. Glencoe, Illinois: Free Press, 1951.

Dworkis, M. B. (Ed.). The Impact of Puerto Rican Migration on Governmental Services in New York City. New York: New York University Press, 1957.

Eaton, W. W. Residence, Social Class and Schizophrenia. *Journal of Health and Social Behavior*, 1974, *15*, 289–299.

Ehrenreich, B. & Ehrenreich, J. The American Health Empire: Power, Profits and Politics. A Health PAC Book. New York: Random House, 1970.

Eilers, R. D. National Health Insurance: What Kind and How Much. *New England Journal of Medicine*, 1971, *284*, 945–954.

Eisinger, P. The Community Action Program and the Development of Black Political Leadership. Research on Poverty, Discussion Paper No. 493–78. Madison, Wisconsin: Institute for Research on Poverty, 1979.

Elling, R. H. National Health Care: Issues and Problems in Socialized Medicine. Chicago: Aldine-Atherton, 1971.

Elling, R. H. Cross-National Study of Health Systems: Concepts, Methods, and Data Sources: A Guide to Information Sources. Detroit: Gale, 1980.

Ellwood, P. M. Health Maintenance Organizations: Concept and Strategy. *Hospitals*, 1971, *45*, 53–56.

Elman, R. M. The Poorhouse State: The American Way of Life on Public Assistance. New York: Delta Book, 1966.

Erkel, E. A. The Implications of Cultural Conflict for Health Care. *Health Values: Achieving High Level Wellness*, 1980, *4*, 51–57.

Fagen, R. R., Brody, R. A., & O'Leary, T. J. Cubans in Exile: Disaffection and the Revolution. Stanford: Stanford University Press, 1968.

Falk, I. S. Beyond Medicare. *American Journal of Public Health*, 1969, *59*, 608–619.

Falkner, F. Key Issues in Infant Mortality, Report of a Conference April 16–18, 1969, Washington, D.C. Washington, D.C.: U.S. Government Printing Office, 1969.

Faris, R. E. L. & Dunham, H. W. Mental Disorders in Urban Areas: An Ecological Study of Schizophrenia and other Pychoses. Chicago: University of Chicago Press, 1939.

Federal Regulation of Services to the Poor Under the Hill-Burton Act: Realities and Pitfalls. *Northwestern Law Review*, June 1, 1975.

Feldman, R., Deitz, D. M., & Brooks, E. The Financial Viability of Rural Primary Health Care Centers. *American Journal of Public Health*, 1978, *68*, 981–987.

Ferenczi, I. International Migrations, Volume 1, Statistics. New York: Arno Press, 1929. Republished, 1970.

Fey, H. E. & McNickel, D. Indians and Other Americans: Two Ways of Life. New York: Harper & Brothers, 1959.

Fischman, S. H. & Palley, H. A. Adolescent Unwed Motherhood: Implications for a National Family Policy. *Health and Social Work*, 1978, *3*, 30–46.

Floriani, C. M. Southeast Asian Refugees: Life in a Camp. *American Journal of Nursing*, *1980*, *80*, 2028–2030.

Fogelson, R. M. & Hill, R. B. Who Riots? A Study of Participation in the 1967 Riots. In Supplemental Studies for the National Advisory Commission on Civil Disorders. Otto Kerner, Chairman. Washington, D.C.: U.S. Government Printing Office, 1968.

Forbes, J. D. (Ed.). The Indian in America's Past. Englewood Cliffs, New Jersey: Prentice-Hall, 1964.

Ford, T. R. (Ed.). The Southern Appalachian Region: A Survey. Lexington: University of Kentucky Press, 1962.

Foster, G. M. Relationships Between Spanish and Spanish-American Folk Medicine. *Journal of American Folklore*, 1953, *66*, 201–217.

Frackelton, D. L. & Faville, K. Opportunities in Nursing for Disadvantaged Youth. *Nursing Outlook,* 1966, *14,* 26–28.

Franklin, J. H. From Slavery to Freedom (3rd ed). New York: Alfred A Knopf, 1967.

Frazier, E. F. Black Bourgeoisie. New York: Collier Books, 1962.

Frazier, E. F. The Negro Family in the United States. Chicago: University of Chicago, 1939.

Frazier, H. S. & Hiatt, H. H. Evaluation of Medical Practices. *Science,* 1978, *200,* 875–878.

Fredericks, M. A. & Mundy, P. Health Care Professionals: A Model for Teaching the Components of Society-Culture-Personality in the Delivery of Care. *Journal of the National Medical Association,* 1978, *70,* 585–589.

Frerichs, R. R., Webber, L. S., Srinivasan, S. R., & Berenson, G. S. Hemoglobin Levels in Children From a Biracial Southern Community. *American Journal of Public Health,* 1977, *67,* 841–845.

Freidson, E. Client Control and Medical Practice. *American Journal of Sociology,* 1960, *65,* 374–382.

Freidson, E. Patient's View of Medical Practice. New York: Russell Sage Foundation, 1961.

Freidson, E. Profession of Medicine, A Study of the Sociology of Applied Knowledge. New York: Dodd, Mead, 1970.

Freidson, E. & Lorber, J. (Eds.). Medical Men and Their Work: A Sociological Reader. Chicago: Aldine-Atherton, 1971.

Freidson, E. Professional Dominance: The Social Structure of Medical Care. New York: Atherton Press, 1970.

Frost, F. & Shy, K. K. Racial Differences Between Linked Birth and Infant Death Records in Washington State. *American Journal of Public Health,* *1980, 70,* 974–976.

Furman, S. S., Sweat, L. G., & Crocetti, G. M. Social Class Factors in the Flow of Children to Outpatient Psychiatric Facilities. *American Journal of Public Health,* 1965, *55,* 385–392.

Galarza, E. Merchants of Labor: The Mexican Bracero Story. Santa Barbara: McNally & Loftin, 1964.

Galarza, E., Gallegos, H., & Samora, J. Mexican-Americans in the Southwest. Santa Barbara: McNally & Loftin, in cooperation with the Anti-Defamation League of B'nai B'rith, 1969.

Garcia, J. A. & Juarez, R. Z. Utilization of Dental Services by Chicanos and Anglos. Journal of Health and Social Behavior, 1978, *19,* 428–436.

Garfinkel, I. & Haverman, R., with assistance of D. Betson. Earning Capacity, Poverty and Inequality. Madison, Wisconsin: Institute for Research on Poverty 1978. Also Academic Press, 1978.

Geiger, H. J. The Endlessly Revolving Door. *American Journal of Nursing,* 1969, 2435–2445.

Gerber, A. A Swedish Prescription: Socialized Medicine Works, but It's No Cure-All. *Los Angeles Times,* December 11, 1977.

Gibbs, J. P. & Martin, W. T. Status Integration and Suicide. Eugene, Oregon: University of Oregon, 1964.

Gibson, C. D. The Neighborhood Health Center: The Primary Unit of Health Care. *American Journal of Public Health, 1968, 58,* 1188–1191.

Ginzberg, E., with Ostow, M. *Men, Money and Medicine. New York: Columbia University Press, 1969.*

Glaser, W. A. Paying the Doctor: Systems of Remuneration and Their Effects. Baltimore: Johns Hopkins Press, 1970.

Glazer, N. Y. & Moynihan, D. P. Beyond the Melting Pot: The Negroes, Puerto Ricans, Jews, Italians, and Irish of New York City (2nd Ed.). Cambridge, Massachusetts: M.I.T. Press, 1970.

Gliebe, W. A. & Malley, L. R. Use of the Health Care Delivery System by Urban Mexican-Americans in Ohio. *Public Health Report,* 1979, *94,* 226–230.

Goetzl, U. Mental Illness and Cultural Beliefs in a Southern Italian Immigrant Family. A Case Report. *Canadian Psychiatry Association Journal,* 1973, *18,* 219–222.

Goffman, E. Asylums: Essays on the Social Situations of Mental Patients and Other Inmates. New York: Anchor Books, 1961.

Goldscheider, C. & Uhlenberg, P. R. Minority Group Status and Fertility. *American Journal of Sociology,* 1969, *74,* 361–372.

Goldschmid, M. L. (Ed.). Black Americans and White Racism, Theory and Research. New York: Holt, 1970.

Goldstein, M. S. Longevity and Health Status of the Negro American. *Journal of Negro Education,* 1963, *32,* 337–348

Gonzalez, H. H. Health Care Needs of the Mexican-American. In Ethnicity and Health Care. pp. 21–28. New York: National League for Nursing, 1976, p. 21–28.

Goode, E. (Ed.). Marijuana. New York: Atherton Press, 1969.

Goode, E. The Marijuana Smokers. New York: Basic Books, 1970.

Goode, W. J. Illegitimacy in the Caribbean Social Structure. *American Sociological Review,* 1960, *25,* 21–30.

Goodman, M. E. Race Awareness in Young Children. Cambridge, Massachusetts: Addison-Wesley Press, 1952.

Gordon, C. C., Matousek, I. M., & Lang, T. A. Southeast Asian Refugees: Life in America. *American Journal of Nursing,* 1980, *80,* 2031–2036.

Gordon, M. Assimilation in American Life: The Role of Race, Religion, and National Origin. New York: Oxford University Press, 1964.

Gori, G. B. & Richter, B. J. Macroeconomics of Disease Prevention in the United States: Prevention of Major Causes of Mortality Would Alter Life Table Assumptions and Economic Projections. *Science,* 1978, *200,* 1124–1130.

Bullough, V. & Bullough, B. What Color Are Your Germs? Chicago: The Committee to End Discrimination in Chicago Medical Institutions, 1955.

Bullough, V. & Bullough, B. The Untouchables. Chicago: Committee Against Discrimination and the Southern Conference on Education, 1955.

Bullough, V. & Bullough, B. Care of the Sick: Emergence of Modern Nursing (3rd ed.). New York: Prodist, 1978.

Bunker, J. P., Hinkley, D., & McDermott, W. V. Surgical Innovation and Its Evaluation. *Science*, 1978, *200*, 937–941.

Bureau of Maternal and Child Health, California State Department of Public Health. Health for the Harvesters: A Ten Year Report by the Farm Workers Health Service. State of California, 1970.

Burgess, E. W. Urban Areas. In T. V. Smith & L. White (Eds.), Chicago: An Experiment in Social Science Research. Chicago: University of Chicago Press, 1929, pp. 113–138.

Burrell, L. & Rayder, N. F. Black and White Students Attitudes Toward White Counselors. *Journal of Negro Education*, 1971, *40*, 48–52.

Cabot, R. C. Social Service and the Art of Healing. New York: Dodd, Mead, 1931.

Cahalan, D., Cisin, I., & Crossley, H. M. American Drinking Practices: A National Survey of Behavior and Attitudes Related to Alcoholic Beverages. Washington, D.C.: Social Research Group, George Washington University, Report No. 3, 1967.

California Legislative Assembly Committee on Health and Welfare. Malnutrition: One Key to the Poverty Cycle. January 1970.

Campbell, A. A. Fertility and Family Planning Among Non-White Married Couples in the United States. *Eugenics Quarterly*, 1961, *12*, 124–131.

Cannon, M. S. & Locke, B. Z. Being Black is Detrimental to One's Mental Health: Myth or Reality? *Phylon*, 1977, *38*, 408–428.

Cappannori, S. C. et al. Voodoo in the General Hospital, A Case of Hexing and Regional Enteritis. *Journal of the American Medical Association*, 1975, *232*, 939–940.

Carkuff, R. R. & Pierce, R. Differential Effects of Therapists' Race and Social Class Upon Patient Depth of Self Exploration in the Initial Interview. *Journal of Consulting Psychology*, 1967, *31*, 632–634.

Carnegie Commission on Higher Education. Higher Education and the Nation's Health: Policies for Dental and Medical Education. New York: McGraw-Hill, 1970.

Carnegie, M. E. Are Negro Schools of Nursing Needed Today? *Nursing Outlook*, 1964, *12*, 52–56. Reprinted in Bullough, B. & Bullough, V. (Eds.), New Directions for Nurses, New York: Springer, 1971, pp. 292–303.

Carp, F. M. & Kataoka, E. Health Care Problems of the Elderly of San Francisco's Chinatown. *Gerontologist*, 1976, *16*, 30–38.

Hammond, E. I. Studies in Fetal and Infant Mortality. II-Differentials in Mortality by Sex and Race. *American Journal of Public Health*, 1965, *55*, 1152–1163.

Hampden-Turner, C. From Poverty to Dignity. Garden City, New York: Anchor Press/Doubleday, 1975.

Hand, W. D. Passing Through: Folk Medical Magic and Symbolism. *Proceedings of the American Philosophical Society*, 1968, *112*, 379–401.

Handler, J. F. Protecting the Social Service Client: Legal and Structural Controls on Official Discretion. New York: Academic Press, 1979.

Handler, O. The Uprooted. Boston: Atlantic Little, Brown, 1952.

Harburg, E., Gleibormann, L., Roeper, P., Schork, M. A., & Schull, W. Skin Color, Ethnicity and Blood Pressure. *American Journal of Public Health*, 1978, *68*, 1177–1183.

Harrington, M. The Other America: Poverty in the United States. Baltimore: Penguin Books, 1962.

Harris, L. How the Poor View Their Health. In Sources: A Blue Cross Report of Health Problems of the Poor. Chicago: Blue Cross Association, 1968, pp. 21–36.

Harris, F. R. & Harris, Mrs. F. R. Indian Health. In Sources: A Blue Cross Report of Health Problems of the Poor. Chicago: Blue Cross Association, 1968, pp. 38–43.

Harvey, L. H. Educational Problems of Minority Group Nurses. *Nursing Outlook*, 1970, *18*, 43–50.

Haveman, R. H. A Decade of Federal Antipoverty Programs: Achievements, Failures, and Lessons. New York: Academic Press, 1977.

Haynes, A. M. Distribution of Black Physicians in the United States. *Journal of the American Medical Association*, 1969, *210*, 93–95.

Health Advisory Committee to the Appalachian Regional Commission. Report. March 1966.

Health Care: What the Poor People Didn't Get from Kentucky Project. *Science*, 1971, *172*, 458–460.

Health Policy: The Legislative Agenda. An editorial research report. Washington, D. C.: Congressional Quarterly, Inc., 1980.

Health Programs: Slum Children Suffer Because of Low Fundings. *Science*, 1971, *172*, 921–924.

Health Service for American Indians. Prepared by the Office of the Surgeon General, U.S. Department of Health, Education, and Welfare, Public Health Service Publication No. 531. Washington, D.C.: U.S. Government Printing Office, 1957.

Health Status of Indochinese Refugees. *Journal of National Medical Association*, 1980, *72*, 59–65.

Hearings Before the Subcommittee on Health of the Elderly of the Special Committee on Aging, Costs and Delivery of Health Services to Older

Americans. United States Senate, Ninetieth Congress, First Session, Part I. Washington, D.C.: U.S. Government Printing Office, 1967.

Hearings Before the Subcommittee on Employment, Manpower and Poverty of the Committee on Labor and Public Welfare. United States Senate, Ninetieth Congress, July 11 and 12, 1967. Washington, D.C.: U.S. Government Printing Office.

Hearings Before the Subcommittee on Medicare-Medicaid, Committee on Finance. United States Senate, Ninety-first Congress, Part 2, April 14, 15, May 26, 27, June 2, 3, 15, 16, 1970. Washington, D.C.: U.S. Government Printing Office, 1970.

Hearings Before the Select Committee on Nutrition and Human Needs of the United States Senate. Ninetieth Congress, Second Session, Ninety-first Congress, Part 5B, Florida, Appendix. Washington, D.C.: U.S. Government Printing Office, 1969, p. 1835.

Heilbroner, R. L. Benign Neglect in the United States. *TransAction*, 1970, *7*, 15–22.

Hendin, H. Black Suicide. New York: Basic Books, 1969.

Henggeler, S. W. & Tavormina, J. B. The Children of Mexican-American Migrant Workers: A Population at Risk. *Journal of Abnormal Child Psychology, 1978, 6*, 97–106.

Herskovits, M. J. The Myth of the Negro Past. Boston: Beacon Press, 1941.

Herskovits, M. J. The New World Negro. Edited by F. S. Herskovits. Bloomington: Indiana University Press, 1966.

Hertz, H. Notes on Clay and Starch Eating Among Negroes in a Southern Community. *Social Forces*, 1957, *25*, 343–344.

Hertzberg, H. W. The Search for an American Indian Identity. Modern Pan—Indian Movements. Syracuse: Syracuse University Press, 1971.

Herzog, E. About the Poor. Some Facts and Some Fictions. U.S. Department of Health, Education, and Welfare, Children's Bureau, Publication No. 451. Washington, D.C.: U.S. Government Printing Office, 1967.

Heston, L. L. The Genetics of Schizophrenia and Schizoid Disease. *Science*, 1970, *167*, 249–256.

Hill, L. M. Sacramento Area Director, Bureau of Indian Affairs, as reported in the Progress Report to the Legislature by the Senate Interim Committee on Indian Affairs. Sacramento: California State Senate, 1955, pp. 241–242, 407–408.

Hirshfield, D. S. The Campaign for Compulsory Health Insurance in the United States from 1932 to 1943. Cambridge, Massachusetts: Harvard University Press, 1970.

Hochstim, J. R., Athanasopoulos, D. A., & Larkins, J. H. Poverty Area Under the Microscope. *American Journal of Public Health*, 1968, *58*, 1815–1827.

Hollingshead, A. B. & Redlich, F. C. Social Stratification and Psychiatric Disorders. *American Sociological Review*, 1953, *18*, 163–169.

Hollingshead, A. B. & Redlich, F. C. Social Class and Mental Illness. New York: Wiley, 1958.

Holm, D. Understanding Hypertension. In B. Bullough (Ed.), The Management of Common Human Miseries: A Text for Primary Health Care Practitioners. New York: Springer, 1979, pp. 249–269.

Holtan, N. R. Health Care Problems Among the Southeast Asian Refugees—The Boat People. *Minnesota Medicine*, 1979, *62*, 633–634.

Hongladarom, G. C. & Russell, M. An Ethnic Difference—Lactose Intolerance. *Nursing Outlook*, 1976, *24*, 764–765.

Hoppe, S. K. Alienation, Familism and the Utilization of Health Services by Mexican Americans. *Journal of Health and Social Behavior*, 1975, *16*, 304–314.

Hosten, A. O. Hypertension in Black and Other Populations: Environmental Factors and Approaches to Management. *Journal of the National Medical Association*, 1980, *72*, 111–117.

Howard, B. & Logue, J. American Class Society in Numbers. Kent, Ohio: Kent Popular Press, 1979.

Howard, J. & Holman, B. L. The Effects of Race and Occupation on Hypertension Mortality. *Milbank Memorial Fund Quarterly*, 1970, *48*, 263–296.

Huang, K. & Pilisak, M. At the Threshold of the Golden Gate: Special Problems of a Neglected Minority. *American Journal of Orthopsychiatry*, 1977, *47*, 701–713.

Hübotter, F. Chinesisch-Tibetische Pharmakologie. Ulm, Germany: K. F. Haug, 1957.

Hunger, U.S.A.: A Report by the Citizens' Board of Inquiry into Hunger and Malnutrition in the United States. Boston: Beacon Press, 1968.

Hyde, R. W. Socio-economic Aspects of Dental Caries. *New England Journal of Medicine*, 1944, *230*, 506–510.

The Impact of Title VI on Health Facilities. *The George Washington Law Review*, 1968, *36*, 980–993.

Indian Health Service. Suicide Among the American Indians. U.S. Public Health Service Publication No. 1903. Washington, D.C.: U.S. Government Printing Office, 1967.

Indian Health Service. To the First Americans: The Third Annual Report on the Indian Health Program of the U.S. Public Health Service. Washington, D.C.: U.S. Government Printing Office, 1969, p. 13.

Indian Health Service. Trends and Services, 1969 Edition. U.S. Department of Health, Education, and Welfare. Washington, D.C.: U.S. Government Printing Office, 1969. p. 8.

Ingelfinger, F. J. Medicine: Meritorious or Meretricious. *Science*, 1978, *200*, 942–946.

Ingham, J. M. On Mexican Folk Medicine. *American Anthropologist*, 1970, *72*, 76–87.

Irelan, L. M. Low Income Life Styles. U.S. Department of Health, Education, and Welfare. Washington, D.C.: U.S. Government Printing Office, 1966.

Jackson, H. M. H. A Century of Dishonor. New edition, edited by Andrew F. Rolle. Reprinted New York: Harper, 1965.

Jaco, E. G. (Ed.). Patients, Physicians and Illness. Glencoe, Illinois: Free Press, 1958.

Jaco, E. G. Mental Health of the Spanish-American in Texas. In M. Opler (Ed.), Culture and Mental Health: Cross Cultural Studies. New York: Macmillan, 1959, pp. 467–485.

Jagdish, V. Community Medicine in the British National Health Service. *American Journal of Public Health*, 1978, *68*, 54–57.

James, G. Poverty and Public Health—New Outlooks: 1. Poverty as an Obstacle to Health Progress in Our Cities. *American Journal of Public Health*, 1965, *55*, 1757–1771.

Jensen, A. R. How Much Can We Boost I.Q. and Scholastic Achievement? *Harvard Educational Review*, 1969, *39*, 1–123.

Jensen, A. R. Bias in Mental Testing. New York: Free Press, 1980.

Jewell, D. P. A Case of a 'Psychotic Navaho Indian Male'. In J. K. Skipper & R. C. Leonard (Eds.), Social Interaction and Patient Care. Philadelphia: Lippincott, 1965.

Johnson, C. A. Nursing and Mexican American Folk Medicine. *Nursing Forum*, 1964, *3*, 100–112.

Johnson, C. A. Mexican-American Women in the Labor Force and Lowered Fertility. *American Journal of Public Health*, 1976, *66*, 1186–1188.

Johnson, D. G., Smith, V. C. & Tarnoff, S. T. Recruitment and Progress of Minority Medical School Entrants 1970–1972. *Journal of Medical Education*, 1975, *50*, 713–755.

Johnston, H. L. A Smoother Road for Migrants. *American Journal of Nursing*, 1966, *66*, 1752–1756.

Jones, J. H. Bad Blood: The Tuskegee Syphilis Experiment. New York: The Free Press, 1981.

Jones, M. A. American Immigration. Chicago: University of Chicago Press, 1960.

Josephy, A. M., Jr. The Indian Heritage of America. New York: Alfred A. Knopf, 1969.

Kandel, D., Single, E., & Kessler, R. C. The Epidemiology of Drug Use Among New York State High School Students: Distribution, Trends and Changes in Rates of Use. *American Journal of Public Health*, 1976, *66*, 43–53.

Kane, R. L. & Kane, R. A. Care of the Aged: Old Problems in Need of New Solutions. *Science*, 1978, *200*, 913–919.

Kane, R. L. Kasteler, J., & Grey, R. M. (Eds.). The Health Gap; Medical Services and the Poor. New York: Springer, 1976.

Karp, R., Fairorth, J., Kanofsky, P. et al. Effects of Rise in Food Costs on Hemoglobin Concentrations of Early School-Age Children, 1972–75. *Public Health Report*, 1978, *93*, 456–459.

Karp, R. J., Williams, C., & Grant, J. Increased Utilization of Salty Food with Age Among Preteenage Black Girls. *Journal of the National Medical Association*, 1980, *72*, 197–200.

Keaveny, T. J. & Hayden, R. L. Manpower Planning for Nurse Personnel. *American Journal of Public Health*, 1978, *68*, 656–662.

Keefe, S. E., Folk Medicine Among Urban Mexican Americans: Cultural Persistence, Change, and Displacement. *Hispanic Journal of Behavioral Sciences* 1981, *3*, 41–58.

Keil, J. E., Tyroler, H. A., Sandefer, S. H., & Boyle, E., Jr. Hypertension: Effects of Social Class and Racial Admixture. *American Journal of Public Health*, 1977, *67*, 634–639.

Keith, L., Rosenberg, C., Brown, E., & Webster, A. Amylophagia During Pregnancy: A Second Look. *Chicago Medical School Quarterly*, 1969, *28*, 109.

Kellogg, W. K. Foundation. Viewpoint: The Cost and Productivity of Health Care in the United States. A Summary Report on Current Programming in Health Care Cost/Productivity. Battle Creek, Michigan: W. K. Kellogg Foundation, September 1978.

Kelly, C. H. Fighting Poverty in Urban Areas. Fighting Poverty in Rural Areas. In B. Bullough & V. Bullough (Eds.), New Directions for Nurses. New York: Springer, 1971, pp. 248–259, 259–266.

Kelly, C. Health Care in the Mississippi Delta. *American Journal of Nursing*, 1969, *69*, 759–763.

Kennedy, J. H. Letter: Health Care in Jamaica. *Journal of Medical Education*, 1974, *49*, 211–212.

Kerner, O., Chairman. Report of the National Advisory Commission on Civil Disorders. Washington, D.C.: U.S. Government Printing Office, 1968.

Kershaw, D. & Fair, J. *The New Jersey Income-Maintenance Experiment: Vol. I Operations, Surveys and Administration* New York: Academic Press, 1981.

Kibrick, A. A Report on the Sealantic Projects Concerned with Recruiting the Disadvantaged into Schools of Nursing. New York: Sealantic Fund, n.d.

Kiev, A. Curanderismo: Mexican American Folk Psychiatry. New York: Free Press, 1968.

King, M. L. Stride Toward Freedom. New York: Harper, 1958.

Kitagawa, E. M. & Hauser, P. M. Differential Mortality in the United States, A Study in Socioeconomic Epidemiology. Cambridge, Massachusetts: Harvard University Press, 1973.

Kitzinger, S. Challenges in Antenatal Education. 1. Immigrant Women in Childbirth—an Anthropologist's View. *Nursing Mirror*, 1977, *144*, 19–22.

Kleinman, J. C. & Kopstein A. Who is Being Screened for Cervical Cancer. *American Journal of Public Health*, 1981, 73–76.

Kleinman, P. H. & Lukoff, I. F. Ethnic Factors Related to Drug Use. *Journal of Health and Social Behavior*, 1978, *19*, 190–199.

Kluckhohn, F. Variations in Value Orientations. Evanston, Illinois: Row, Peterson, 1961.

Knoch, H., Pasamanick, R., Harper, P. A., & Rider, R. The Effect of Prematurity on Health and Growth. *American Journal of Public Health*, 1959, *49*, 1164–1173.

Koos, E. L. The Health of Regionville. New York: Columbia University Press, 1954.

Kosa, J., Antonovsky, A., & Zola, I. K. (Eds.). Poverty and Health: A Sociological Analysis. Cambridge, Massachusetts: Commonwealth Fund Book, Harvard University Press, 1969.

Kotz, N. Let Them Eat Promises: The Politics of Hunger in America. New York: Anchor Books, 1971.

Kramer, M. Psychiatric Services and the Changing Institutional Scene 1950–1955. U.S. Department of Health, Education, and Welfare, National Institute of Mental Health Series B, No. 12. Washington, D.C.: U.S. Government Printing Office, 1977.

Kraus, B. S., with the collaboration of Jones, B. M. Indian Health in Arizona. Tucson: University of Arizona Press, 1954.

Kriesberg, L. Mothers in Poverty: A Study of Fatherless Families. Chicago: Aldine, 1970.

Kurth, A. Children and Youth of Domestic Agricultural Migrant Families. A survey paper reprinted from Children and Youth in the 1960's, with permission of the 1960 White House Conference on Children and Youth. Washington, D.C.: U.S. Department of Health, Education, and Welfare, 1965.

LaPouse, R., Monk, M. A., & Terris, M. The Drift Hypothesis and Socio-Economic Differentials in Schizophrenia. *American Journal of Public Health*, 1956, *46*, 978–986.

Lasagna, L. The Development and Regulation of New Medications. *Science*, 1978, *200*, 871–873.

Lave, J. R., & Leinhardt, S. An Evaluation of a Hospital Stay Regulatory Mechanism. *American Journal of Public Health*, 1976, *66*, 959–967.

Law, S. A. Blue Cross: What Went Wrong? New Haven: Yale University Press, 1974.

Leavitt, W. & Numbers, R. L. (Eds.). Sickness and Health in America. Madison: University of Wisconsin Press, 1978.

Lee, B. A. Residential Mobility on Skid Row: Disaffiliation, Powerlessness, and Decision Making. *Demography*, 1978, *15*, 285–300.

Lee, R. The Gypsies in Canada—An Ethnological Study. *Journal of Gypsy Lore Society*, 1967, *66*, 38–51; 1968, *67*, 12–28.

Leininger, M. M. Nursing and Anthropology: Two Worlds to Blend. New York: Wiley, 1970.

Leininger, M. Transcultural Nursing 1979. St. Paul, Minnesota: Masson Publishing, 1980.

Leong, L. Acupuncture. New York: Signet, 1974.

Lepper, M. H., Lashof, J. C., Lerner, M., German, J., & Adeleman, S. L. Approaches to Meeting Health Needs of Large Poverty Populations. *American Journal of Public Health*, 1967, *57*, 1153–1157.

Lewis, O. La Vida: A Puerto Rican Family in the Culture of Poverty. New York: Random House, 1965.

Lewis, O. The Children of Sanchez. New York: Vintage Books, 1961.

Lewis, O. The Culture of Poverty. *Scientific American*, October 1966, 19–25.

Li, Frederick P. et al. Health Care for the Chinese Community in Boston. *American Journal of Public Health*, April 1972, 536–539.

Lincoln, C. E. The Black Muslims in America. Boston: Beacon Press, 1961.

Lincoln, C. E. The Negro Pilgrimage in America. New York: Bantam Books, 1967.

Linden, G. The Influence of Social Class in the Survival of Cancer Patients. *American Journal of Public Health*, 1969, *59*, 267–274.

Lindes, C. Intestinal Parasites in Laotian Refugees. *Journal of Family Practice*, 1979, *9*, 819–822.

Lindesmith, A. R. Addiction and Opiates. Chicago: Aldine, 1968.

Lindesmith, A. R. Basic Problems in the Social Psychology of Addiction and Theory. In J. A. O'Donnell & J. C. Ball (Eds.), Narcotic Addiction. New York: Harper, 1966, pp. 91–109.

Lindsay, J. R. & Johnston, H. L. Health Programs for Migrant Workers. Excerpts from the proceedings of the Eighteenth National Conference on Rural Health, 1965, Miami Beach, Florida. Reprinted by the U.S. Department of Health, Education, and Welfare, 1966.

Liston, R. A. The American Poor: A Report on Poverty in the United States. New York: Dell, 1970.

Locke, B. Z., & Duvall, H. J. Alcoholism Among First Admissions to Ohio Public Mental Hospitals. *Quarterly Journal of Studies*, 1964, *25*, 521–534.

Lopez, A. The Puerto Ricans: Their History, Culture, and Society. Cambridge, Massachusetts: Schenkman, 1980.

Loughlin, B. W. Pregnancy in the Navajo Culture. *Nursing Outlook*, 1965, *13*, 55–58.

Lynds, B. G., Seyler, S. K., & Morgan, B. M. Relationship Between Elevated Blood Pressure and Obesity in Black Children. *American Journal of Public Health*, 1980, *70*, 171–173.

MacDonald, M. Food, Stamps, and Income Maintenance. New York: Academic Press, 1977.

Maddox, G. L. Drinking Among Negroes: Inferences from the Drinking Patterns of Selected Negro Male Collegians. *Journal of Health and Social Behavior*, 1967, *8*, 114–120.

Malhiot, G. & Ninan, M. A Seminar for Minority Students. *Nursing Outlook*, 1979, *27*, 473–475.

Malzberg, B. Mental Disease Among American Negroes: A Statistical Analysis. In O. Klineberg, Characteristics of the American Negro, New York: Harper, 1944.

Mann, F. Acupuncture: The Ancient Chinese Art of Healing. New York: Vintage Books, 1972.

Maris, R. W. Social Forces in Urban Suicide. Homewood, Illinois: Dorsey Press, 1969.

Marmor, T. The Politics of Medicare. Chicago: Aldine, 1970, 1973.

Martin, B. J. W. Ethnicity and Health Care: Afro-Americans. In Ethnicity and Health Care. New York: National League for Nursing, 1976, p. 53.

Martinez, C. & Martin, H. W. Folk Diseases Among Urban Mexican-Americans. *Journal of the American Medical Association*, 1966, *196*, 147–150.

Marx, G. T. Protest and Prejudice: A Study of Belief in the Black Community. New York: Harper, 1967.

McBroom, W. H. Illness, Behavior and Socioeconomic Status. *Journal of Health and Social Behavior*, 1970, *11*, 319–326.

McCarthy, B. J., Terry, J. et al. The Underregistration of Neonatal Deaths: Georgia 1974–77. *American Journal of Public Health*, 1980, *70*, 977–982.

McCarthy, M. A., Witte, E. J., & Gens, R. D. Indochinese Refugees Pose New Health Problems. *Pennsylvania Medicine*, 1980, *83*, 21.

McCoy, J. L. & Brown, D. L. Health Status Among Low-Income Elderly Persons: Rural-Urban Differences. *Social Security Bulletin*, 1979, *41*, 14–26.

McElroy, A. & Townsend, P. K. Medical Anthropology. North Scituate, Massachusetts: Duxbury Press, 1979.

McKenzie, J. L. & Chrisman, N. J. Healing Herbs, Gods, and Magic: Folk Beliefs Among Filipino-Americans. *Nursing Outlook*, 1977, *25*, 326–329.

McLemore, S. D. Ethnic Attitudes Towards Hospitalization: An Illustrative Comparison of Anglos and Mexican Americans. *Southwestern Social Science Quarterly*, March 1963, 341–346.

McWilliams, C. North From Mexico. The Spanish-Speaking People of the United States. Reprinted, New York: Greenwood Press, 1968.

Mechanic, D. Considerations in the Design of Mental Health Benefits Under National Health Insurance. *American Journal of Public Health*, 1978, *68*, 482–487.

Mechanic, D. Correlates of Frustration Among British General Practitioners, *Journal of Health and Social Behavior*, 1970, *11*, 87–104.

Mechanic, D. The English National Health Service: Some Comparisons with the United States. *Journal of Health and Social Behavior*, 1971, *12*, 18–29.

Mechanic, D. Mental Health and Social Policy. Englewood Cliffs, New Jersey: Prentice-Hall, 1969.

Menchik, P. Intergenerational Transmission of Inequality: An Empirical Study of Wealth Mobility. Institute for Research on Poverty, Discussion Paper No. 407, 1977.

Merton, R. K. Social Structure and Anomie. In Social Theory and Social Structure. Glencoe, Illinois: Free Press, 1957, pp. 131–160.

Milio, N. 9226 Kercheval: The Storefront That Did Not Burn. Ann Arbor: University of Michigan Press, 1970.

Milio, N. Values, Social Class and Community Health Services. *Nursing Research*, 1967, *16*, 26–31.

Milt, H. (Ed.). Health Care Problems of the Inner City: Report of the 1969 National Health Forum. New York: 1969.

Minuchin, Salvador et al. Families in the Slums. New York: Basic Books, 1967.

Montoya, R., Hayes-Bautista, D., Gonzales, L., & Smeloff, E. Minority Dental School Graduates: Do They Serve Minority Communities? *American Journal of Public Health*, 1978, *68*, 1017–1021.

Moon, M. L. *The Measurement of Economic Welfare: Its Application to the Aged Poor*, New York: Academic Press, 1977.

Moor, J. & Cuellar, A. Mexican Americans. Englewood Cliffs, New Jersey: Prentice-Hall, 1970.

Moore, E. C. Woman and Health: United States 1980. Public Health Reports. A Supplement to the September-October 1980 issue.

Morais, H. M. The History of the Negro in Medicine. New York: Publishers Company, 1968.

Morrill, R. L. The Negro Ghettos: Problems and Alternatives. *The Geographical Review*, 1965, *55*.

Morris, N. M., Hatch, M. H., & Chipman, S. S. Alienation as a Deterrent to Well-Child Supervision. *American Journal of Public Health*, 1966, *56*, 1874–1882.

Moustafa, A. T. & Weiss, G. Health Status and Practices of Mexican Americans. Mexican-American Study Project, Advance Report II. Los Angeles: University of California, 1968.

Moynihan, D. P. Maximum Feasible Misunderstanding: Community Action in the War on Poverty. New York: Free Press, 1969.

Munoz, R. Nursing in the North 1867–1967. The Alaska Nurses' Association, 1967.

Murphy, J. M. Psychiatric Labeling in a Cross-Cultural Perspective. *Science*, 1976, *191*, 1019–1028.

Murphy, P. R. Tuberculosis Control in San Francisco's Chinatown. *American Journal of Nursing*, 1970, *70*, 1044–1046.

Myers, J. K. & Bean, L. L., in collaboration with Pepper, M. P. A Decade Later: A Follow-Up of Social Class and Mental Illness. New York: Wiley, 1968.

Myers, J. K., Bean, L. L., & Pepper, M. P. Social Class and Psychiatric Disorders: A Ten Year Follow Up. *Journal of Health and Human Behavior*, 1965, *6*, 74–78.

Myers, J. K. & Roberts, B. N. Family and Class Dynamics in Mental Illness. New York: Wiley, 1959.

Myrdal, G., with the assistance of Sterner, R. & Rose, A. An American Dilemma: The Negro Problem and Modern Democracy. New York: Harper & Brothers, 1944.

Nakagawa, H. Family Health Care Patterns and Anomie. An unpublished Ph.D. dissertation. University of California at Los Angeles, 1968.

Nall, F. C., II & Speilberg, J. Social and Cultural Factors in the Responses of Mexican-Americans to Medical Treatment. *Journal of Health and Social Behavior*, 1967, *8*, 299–308.

Nash, R. M. Compliance of Hospitals and Health Agencies with Title VI of the Civil Rights Act. *American Journal of Public Health*, 1968, *58*, 246–251.

Nash, R. M. Integration in Health Facilities. *American Journal of Nursing*, 1966, *66*, 2480–2482.

National Center for Health Statistics. Differentials in Health Characteristics by Color, United States, July 1965–June 1967. U.S. Department of Health, Education, and Welfare, Public Health Service Publication No. 1000, Series 10, No. 56. Washington, D.C.: U.S. Government Printing Office, 1969.

National Center for Health Statistics. Medical Care, Health Status and Family Income. Vital and Health Statistics. U.S. Department of Health, Education, and Welfare, Public Health Service Publication No. 1000, Series 10, No. 9. Washington, D.C.: U.S. Government Printing Office, 1964.

National Center for Health Statistics. Selected Dental Findings in Adults by Age, Race and Sex, United States, 1960–1962. U.S. Department of Health, Education, and Welfare, Public Health Service Publication No. 1000, Series 11, No. 7. Washington, D.C.: U.S. Government Printing Office, 1965.

National Center for Health Statistics. Three Views of Hypertension and Heart Disease. U.S. Department of Health, Education, and Welfare, Public Health Service Publication No. 1000, Series 2, No. 22. Washington, D.C.: U.S. Government Printing Office, 1967.

National Institute of Mental Health and the Indian Health Service. Suicide Among the American Indians. Public Health Service Publication No. 1903. Washington, D.C.: U.S. Government Printing Office, 1967.

National League for Nursing. Ethnicity and Health Care. New York: National League for Nursing, 1976.

Naumer, J. N. American Indians: A Bibliography of Sources. *American Libraries*, 1970, *1* 861–864.

Nava, J. Mexican Americans: Past, Present, Future. New York: American Book, 1969.

Neale, A. The Health Care System vs Women and the Poor. *Hospital Progress*, 1979, *60*, 46–50.

Needham, J., assisted by Ling, W. Science and Civilization in China, Vol. 2. Cambridge, England: University Press, 1956, passim.

Nemeth, D. J. Nomad Gypsies in Los Angeles: Patterns of Livelihood. Unpublished master's thesis. Northridge: San Fernando Valley State College, 1970.

Neumann, H. H. Pica—Symptom or Vestigial Instinct?" *Pediatrics*, 1970, *46*, 441–444.

Norman, J. C. Medicine in the Ghetto. New York: Appleton, 1969.

Oakes, T. W. & Syme, S. L. Social Factors in Newly Discovered Elevated Blood Pressure. *Journal of Health and Social Behavior*, 1973, *14*, 198–204.

O'Donnell, J. A. & Ball, J. C. (Eds.). Narcotic Addiction. New York: Harper, 1966.

Okada. L. M. & Sparer, G. Dental Visits by Income and Race in Ten Urban and Two Rural Areas. *American Journal of Public Health*, 1976, *66*, 878–885.

Okada, L. M. & Wan, T. H. Impact of Community Health Centers and Medicaid on the Use of Health Services, *Public Health Reports* 1980, 95, 520–534.

Opler, M. K. Culture and Mental Health. New York: Macmillan, 1959.

O'Rourke, D. E., Quinn, J. G. et al. Geophagia During Pregnancy. *Obstetrics and Gynecology*, 1967, *29*, 581.

Orshansky, M. The Poverty Roster. In Sources. Chicago: The Blue Cross Association, 1968, pp. 4–19.

Orshansky, M. Who Was Poor in 1966? Research and Statistics Note, No. 23. Washington, D.C.: U.S. Department of Health, Education, and Welfare, 1967, Table 6.

Ortiz, J. S. The Prevalence of Intestinal Parasites in Puerto Rican Farm Workers in Western Massachusetts. *American Journal of Public Health*, 1980, *70*, 1103–1105.

Otterbein, K. F. Caribbean Family Organization: A Comparative Analysis. *American Anthropologist*, 1965, *67*, 66–79.

Padilla, A. M. (Ed.). Acculturation: Theory, Models and Some New Findings. Boulder, Colorado: Westview Press, 1980.

Paredes, A. & Stekert, E. J. The Urban Experience and Folk Tradition. Austin: American Folklore Society by University of Texas Press, 1971.

Parry, W. H. Discussion on Problems of an Immigrant Population: Health and Welfare of Immigrants. *The Practitioner*, 1970, *204*, 312–314.

Pasamanick, B. A Survey of Mental Disease in an Urban Population. In M. Grossack (Ed.), Mental Health and Segregation. New York: Springer, 1963, pp. 150–157.

Patterson, P. Miami Revisited One Year Later. *The Crisis*, 1981, *88*, 168–174.

Pavenstedt, E. A Comparison of the Child-Rearing Environment of Upper-Lower and Very Low-Lower Class Families. *American Journal of Orthopsychiatry*, 1965, *35*, 89–98.

Pelton, W. J., Dunbar, J. B. et al. The Epidemiology of Oral Health. Cambridge, Massachusetts: Harvard University Press, 1969.

The People Left Behind: The Rural Poor, A Report by the President's Commission on Rural Poverty. In L. A. Ferman, J. L. Kornblugh, & A. Haber (Eds.), Poverty in America. Ann Arbor: University of Michigan Press, revised ed., 1968, pp. 152–153.

Petitti, D. B. & Cates, W., Jr. Restricting Medicaid Funds for Abortions: Projections of Excess Mortality for Women of Childbearing Age. *American Journal of Public Health*, 1977, *67*, 860–862.

Pettigrew, T. F. A Profile of the Negro American. Princeton, New Jersey: D. Van Nostrand, 1964.

Pilisak, M. & Pilisak, P. (Eds.). Poor Americans: How the Poor White Live. Chicago: Aldine, 1971.

Piven, F. F. & Cloward, R. A. The Relief of Welfare. *Transaction*, 1971, *8*, 31–39, 52–53.

Primeaux, M. Caring for the American Indian. In J. R. Folta & E. S. Deck (Eds.), Sociological Framework for Patient Care (2nd ed.). New York: Wiley, 1979, pp. 31–38. Reprinted from *American Journal of Nursing*, 1977, *77*, 91–94.

Proshansky, H. & Newton, P. The Nature and Meaning of Negro Self-Identity. In M. Deutsch, I. Katz, & A. Jensen (Eds.), Social Class, Race and Psychological Development. New York: Holt, Rinehart & Winston, 1968, pp. 178–218.

Puckett, N. N. Folk Beliefs of the Southern Negro. Reprinted New York: Dover, 1969.

Quesada, G. M., Spears, M. W. & Ramos, P. Interracial Depressive Epidemiology in the Southwest. *Journal of Health and Social Behavior*, 1978, *19*, 77–85.

Quinn, J. B. The Affluent Elders. *Newsweek*, August 4, 1980, 53.

Rainwater, L. And the Poor Get Children. Chicago: Quadrangle Books, 1960.

Rainwater, L. Behind Ghetto Walls. Chicago: Aldine, 1970.

Rainwater, L. & Yancey, W. L. The Moynihan Report and the Politics of Controversy. Cambridge, Massachusetts: M.I.T. Press, 1967.

Ramirez, D. G. A Review of the Literature on the Underutilization of Mental Health Services by Mexican Americans: Implications for Future Research and Service Delivery. 1980. Intercultural Development Research Association, 5835 Callaghan, Suite 350, San Antonio, Texas 78228.

Randolph, V. Ozark Magic and Folklore. Reprinted New York: Dover Publications, 1964.

Ream, A. K. Advances in Medical Instrumentation. *Science*, 1978, *200*, 959–964.

Redding, J. S. They Came In Chains: Americans From Africa. Philadelphia: Lippincott, 1950, revised 1973.

Rehabilitating the Narcotic Addict. U.S. Department of Health, Education, and Welfare. Report of Institute on New Developments in the Rehabilitation of the Narcotic Addict, Fort Worth, Texas, February 16–18, 1966. Washington, D.C.: U.S. Government Printing Office, 1966.

Reinhold, R. America Has Plenty of Doctors But Many Americans Do Not. *New York Times*, September 14, 1980.

Reitzes, D. C. Negroes and Medicine. Cambridge, Massachusetts: Commonwealth Fund Study, Harvard University Press, 1958.

Reverby, S. & Rosner D. Health Care in America: Essays in Social History. Philadelphia: Temple University Press, 1979.

Rhoades, E. R. et al. Mental Health Problems of American Indians Seen in Outpatient Facilities of the Indian Health Service, 1975. *Public Health Reports*, 1980, *95*, 329–335.

Richard, M. P. The Negro Physician: Babbitt or Revolutionary. *Journal of Health and Social Behavior*, 1969, *10*, 265–274.

Riessman, F. Strategies Against Poverty. New York: Random House, 1969.

Riis, J. A. How the Other Half Lives. 1890. Reprinted New York: Sagamore Press, 1957.

Roach, J. L., Lewis, L. S., & Beauchamp, M. A. The Effects of Race and Socio-Economic Status on Family Planning. *Journal of Health and Social Behavior*, 1963, *4*, 40–45.

Robert, J. & Engel, E. Family Background, Early Development, and Intelligence of Children 6–11 Years. National Health Survey, Series 11, No. 142. Department of Health, Education, and Welfare, National Center for Health Statistics, August 1974.

Roberts, R. E. The Health of Mexican Americans: Evidence from the Human Population Laboratory Studies. *American Journal of Public Health*, 1980, *70*, 375–384.

Roberts, R. E. & Lee, E. S. Medical Care Use By Mexican-Americans: Evidence From the Human Population Laboratory Studies. *Medical Care*, 1980, *18*, 267–281.

Roberts, R. E. Prevalence of Psychological Distress Among Mexican Americans. *Journal of Health and Social Behavior*, 1980, *21*, 134–145.

Robertson, H. R. Removing Barriers to Health Care. *Nursing Outlook*, 1969, *17*, 43–46.

Robins, L. N. Social Correlates of Psychiatric Disorders. *Journal of Health and Social Behavior*, 1969, *10*, 95–104.

Robins, L. N. & Murphy, G. E. Drug Use in a Normal Population of Young Negro Men. *American Journal of Public Health*, 1967, *57*, 1580–1596.

Robins, P. K., Spiegelman, R. G., Weiner, S., and Bell, J. G. A Guaranteed Annual Income: Evidence from a Social Experiment. New York: Academic Press, 1981.

Roemer, M. I. Highlights of Soviet Health Services. *Milbank Memorial Fund Quarterly*, 1962, *15*, 381–385.

Roemer, M. I. Health Resources and Services in the Watts Area of Los Angeles. *California's Health*, February-March 1966, 123–143.

Roemer, M. I. The Organization of Medical Care Under Social Security. Geneva: International Labour Office, 1969.

Roemer, M. I. Health Care—Financing and Delivery Around the World. *American Journal of Nursing*, 1971, *71*, 1158–1163.

Roemer, M. I. Hospital Utilization and the Health Care System. *American Journal of Public Health*, 1976, *66*, 953–955.

Roemer, M. I. Rural Health Care. St. Louis: C. V. Mosby, 1976.

Roemer, M. I. & Axelrod, J. A National Health Service and Social Security. *American Journal of Public Health*, 1977, *67*, 462–465.

Roemer, R., Kramer, C., & Frink, J. E. Planning Urban Health Services from Jungle to System. New York: Springer, 1975.

Rosen, G. A History of Public Health. New York: M. D. Publications, 1958.

Rosen, G. The First Neighborhood Health Center Movement—Its Rise and Fall. *American Journal of Public Health*, 1971, *61*, 1620–1635.

Rosen, G. Preventive Medicine in the United States 1900–1975 Trends and Interpretations. New York: Science History Publications, 1975.

Rosenberg, C. E. Social Class and Medical Care in 19th-Century America: The Rise and Fall of the Dispensary. *Journal of the History of Medicine*, 1974, *29*, 32–54. Reprinted in J. W. Leavitt & R. L. Numbers (Eds.), Sickness and Health in America. Madison: University of Wisconsin, 1978, pp. 157–171.

Rosenblum, E. H. Conversation With a Navaho Nurse. *American Journal of Nursing*, 1980, *80*, 1459–1461.

Rosenthal, D., Goldberg, I. et al. Migration, Heredity, and Schizophrenia. *Psychiatry*, 1974, *37*, 321–339.

Rosenthal, R. & Jacobson, L. Pygmalion in the Classroom: Teacher Expectation and Pupils' Intellectual Development. New York; Holt, 1969.

Rosenthal, R. & Jacobson, L. Self Fulfilling Prophesies in the Classroom: Teacher's Expectations as Unintended Determinants of Pupils' Intellectual Competence. In M. Deutsch, I. Katz, & A. Jensen (Eds.), Social Class, Race and Psychological Development. New York: Holt, 1968, pp. 219–253.

Rowden, D. W., Michel, J. B., Dillehay, R. C., & Martin, H. W. Judgments About Candidates for Psychotherapy: The Influence of Social Class and Insight-Verbal Ability. *Journal of Health and Social Behavior*, 1970, *11*, 51–58.

Rubel, A. J. Concepts of Disease in Mexican-American Culture. *American Anthropologist*, October 1960, 795–814.

Rubel, A. J. Across the Tracks: Mexican-Americans in a Texas City. Austin: University of Texas Press, 1966.

Ruffin, J. E., in conjunction with members of the Affirmative Action Task Force of the American Nurses' Association. Affirmative Action Programming For the Nursing Profession Through The American Nurses' Association, Publication No. M-23 5M 11/75. Kansas City, Missouri: American Nurses' Association, 1975.

Sabagh, G. Fertility Planning Status of Chicano Couples in Los Angeles. *American Journal of Public Health*, 1980, *70*, 56–61.

Samet, J. M., Key, C. R., Kutvirt, D. M., & Wiggins, C. L. Respiratory Disease Mortality in New Mexico's American Indians and Hispanics. *American Journal of Public Health*, 1980, *70*, 492–497.

Samora, J., Bustamante, G., & Cardenas, G. Los Mojados: The Wetback Story. Notre Dame, Indiana: University of Notre Dame Press, 1966.

Samora, J. (Ed.). La Raza: Forgotten Americans. Notre Dame, Indiana: University of Notre Dame Press, 1966.

Sandifer, M. G., Jr. Social Psychiatry a Hundred Years Ago. *American Journal of Psychiatry*, 1962, *188*, 749–750.

Saunders, L. Cultural Differences and Medical Care: The Case of the Spanish-Speaking People of the Southwest. New York: Russell Sage Foundation, 1954.

Savitt, T. L. Medicine and Slavery. Urbana: University of Illinois, 1978.

Saward, E. & Sorensen, A. The Current Emphasis on Preventive Medicine. *Science*, 1978, *200*, 889–894.

Schaffner, W., Federspiel, C. F. et al. Maternal Mortality in Michigan: An Epidemiological Analysis, 1950–1971. *American Journal of Public Health*, 1977, *67*, 821–829.

Scheinfeldt, J. Opening Doors Wider in Nursing. *American Journal of Nursing*, 1967, *67*, 1461–1464.

Schmidt, W., Smart, R. G., & Moss, M. K. Social Class and the Treatment of Alcoholism: An Investigation of Social Class as a Determinant of Diagnoses, Prognosis and Therapy. Brookside Monograph for the Addiction Research Foundation, No. 7. Toronto: University of Toronto Press, 1968.

Schneider, R. L. Health Play and Politics of Health Priorities and Planning for Health Care in the United States Virgin Islands. *Journal of the National Medical Association*, 1981, *73*, 319–321.

Schulman, S. & Smith, A. M. The Concept of 'Health' Among Spanish Speaking Villagers of New Mexico and Colorado. *Journal of Health and Human Behavior*, 1963, *4*, 226–234.

Schulz, V. E. & Schwab, E. H. Arteriolar Hypertension in the American Negro. *American Heart Journal*, 1936, *11*, 66–74.

Schutte, J. E. Growth Standards for Blacks: Current Status. *Journal of the National Medical Association*, 1980, *72*, 973–978.

Schwarzweller, H. K., Brown, J. S., & Mangalem, J. J. Mountain Families in Transition. University Park: Pennsylvania State University Press, 1971.

Scrimshaw, N. S. & Gordon, J. E. Malnutrition, Learning and Behavior. Cambridge, Massachusetts: M.I.T. Press, 1971.

Seham, M. Discrimination Against Negroes in Hospitals. *New England Journal of Medicine*, 1964, *271*, 940–943.

Senior, C. Our Citizens from the Caribbean. New York: McGraw-Hill, 1965.

Senior, C. The Puerto Ricans. Chicago: Quadrangle Books, 1965.

Shapiro, S., Schlesinger, E. R., & Nesbitt, R. E. L., Jr. Infant, Perinatal, Maternal and Childhood Mortality in the United States. Cambridge: Harvard University Press, 1968.

Shelton, J. Very Young Adolescent Women in Georgia: Has Abortion or Contraception Lowered Their Fertility. *American Journal of Public Health*, 1977, *67*, 617–620.

Shih-Chen, L. Chinese Medicinal Herbs. Translated by F. P. Smith & G. A. Stuart. San Francisco: Georgetown Press, 1973.

Silver, G. A. Nixon's 'Gift' to the Poor; Balance Sheet on National Health. *The Nation*, March 12, 1973.

Simmons, O. G. Implications of Social Class for Public Health. In J. R. Folta & E. S. Deck (Eds.), New York: Wiley, 1966.

Simon, R. J., Fleiss, J. L. et al. Depression and Schizophrenia in Hospitalized Mental Patients. *Archives of General Psychiatry*, 1973, *28*, 509–512.

Smith, G. Nursing Beyond the Crossroads. *Nursing Outlook*, 1980, *28*, 540–545.

Sobey, F. The Nonprofessional Revolution in Mental Health. New York: Columbia University Press, 1970.

Somers, H. M. & Somers, A. R. Doctors, Patients and Health Insurance: The Organization and Financing of Medical Care. Washington, D.C.: Brookings Institution, 1961.

Sources: A Blue Cross Report on Health Problems of the Poor. Chicago: Blue Cross Association, 1968.

Spector, R. Cultural Diversity in Health and Illness. New York: Appleton, 1979.

Srole, L. Measurement and Classification in Socio-Psychiatric Epidemiology: Midtown Manhattan Study (1954) and Midtown Manhattan Restudy (1974). *Journal of Health and Social Behavior*, 1975, *16*, 347–363.

Srole, L., Langer, T. S. et al. Mental Health in the Metropolis: The Midtown Manhattan Study, Vol. 1. New York: McGraw-Hill, 1962.

Stamler, J. & Stamler, R. Psychological Factors and Hypertension Disease in Low-Income Middle Aged Negro Men in Chicago. *Circulation*, 1962, *26*, 790, Part 2.

Stamler, J., Stamler, R., & Curry, C. L. Symposium: Hypertension in the Inner City. Minneapolis, Minnesota: Proforum, 1974.

Stanley, J. C. Predicting College Success of the Educationally Disadvantaged. *Science*, 1971, *171*, 640–646.

Star, J. Cook County Hospital: The Terrible Place. *Look*, May 18, 1971, 24–33.

Steinbeck, J. The Grapes of Wrath. Many editions.

Stevens, J. & Meyers, R. Family's Persistence Pays Off: 45 Years of Confinement Finally Over. *Los Angeles Times*, November 23, 1978, Part XII 15.

Stewart, J. & Cratton, L. L. Delivery of Health Care Services to the Poor: Findings from a Review of the Current Periodical Literature with a Key to 47 Reports of Innovative Projects. San Antonio: University of Texas, 1975.

Stickle, G. The Health of Mothers and Babies: How Do We Stack Up? *The Family Coordinator*, 1977, *26*, 205–210.

Storlie, F. Nursing and the Social Conscience. New York: Appleton, 1970.

Strickland, S. P. Can Slum Children Learn? *American Education*, 1971, *7*, 3–7.

Suchman, E. A. Sociology and the Field of Public Health. New York: Russell Sage Foundation, 1963.

Suicide Among the American Indians: Two Workshops, Aberdeen, South Dakota, September 1967, Lewistown, Montana, November 1967. U.S. Department of Health, Education, and Welfare, Public Health Service Publication No. 1903. Washington, D.C.: U.S. Government Printing Office, 1969.

Suttles, G. D. The Social Order of the Slum: Ethnicity and Territory in the Inner City. Chicago: University of Chicago Press, 1968.

Taeuber, K. E. & Taeuber, A. F. Negroes in Cities. Chicago: Aldine, 1965.

Tancredi, L. R. & Barondess, J. A. The Problem of Defensive Medicine. *Science*, 1978, *200*, 879–882.

Tao-Kim-Nai, A. M. Orientals are Stoic, In J. Skipper & R. C. Leonard (Eds.), Social Interaction and Patient Care. Philadelphia: Lippincott, 1965.

Terris, M. The Epidemiological Revolution, National Health Insurance and the Role of Health Departments. In J. R. Folta & E. S. Deck (Eds.), A Sociological Framework for Patient Care (2nd ed.) New York: Wiley, 1979, pp. 89–111. Reprinted from the *American Journal of Public Health*, 1976, *66*, 1155–1164.

Terris, M. & Gold, E. M. An Epidemiological Study of Prematurity. *American Journal of Obstetrics and Gynecology*, 1969, *103*, 371–379.

Terris, M., Cornely, P. B., Daniels, H. C., & Kerr, L. E. The Case for a National Health Service. *American Journal of Public Health*, 1977, *67*, 1183–1185.

The Impact of Title VI on Health Facilities. *The George Washington Law Review*, 1968, *36*, 980–993.

Their Daily Bread: A Study of the National School Lunch Program. New York: Committee on School Lunch Participation, 1968.

Thernstrom, S., Orlov, A., & Handlin, O. (Eds.) Harvard Encyclopedia of American Ethnic Groups, Cambridge MA: Harvard University Press, 1981.

Thomas, T., Wan, H., & Gray, L. C. Differential Access to Preventive Services for Young Children in Low-Income Areas. *Journal of Health and Social Behavior*, 1978, *19*, 312–324.

Those Amazing Cuban Emigres. *Fortune*, 1966, *74*, 144–149.

Tomasson, R. F. The Mortality of Swedish and U.S. White Males: A Comparison of Experience, 1969–1971. *American Journal of Public Health*, 1976, *66*, 968–978.

Townsend, J. G. Indian Health—Past, Present, and Future. In O. LaFarge (Ed.), The Changing Indian. Norman: University of Oklahoma Press, 1942, pp. 28–41.

Trattner, W. I. From Poor Law to Welfare State: A History of Social Welfare in America. New York: Free Press, 1974.

Trevino, F. M., Bruhn, J. G., & Bunce, H. D. Utilization of Community Mental Health Services in a Texas-Mexico Border City. *Social Science Medicine*, 1979, *13A*, 331–334.

Tunley, R. The American Health Scandal. New York: Harper, 1966.

Turner, J. R. Social Mobility and Schizophrenia. *Journal of Health and Social Behavior, 1968, 9,* 194–203.

Tuttle, W. M., Jr. Race Riot. New York: Atheneum, 1970.

Udry, J. R., Bauman, K. E., Morris, N. M., & Chase, C. L. Social Class, Social Mobility, and Prematurity: A Test of the Childhood Environment Hypothesis for Negro Women. *Journal of Health and Social Behavior*, 1970, *11*, 190–195.

United Nations, Statistical Office. Statistical Yearbook, 1968. New York: United Nations Publishing Service, 1969, pp. 99–100.

U.S. Bureau of the Census. Current Population Reports, Series P-23, No. 28, Revision in Poverty Statistics, 1959–1968. Washington, D.C.: U.S. Government Printing Office, 1969.

U.S. Bureau of the Census. Current Population Reports, Series F-60, No. 76, 24 Million Americans—Poverty in the United States, 1969. Washington, D.C.: U.S. Government Printing Office, 1970.

U.S. Bureau of the Census. Statistical Abstract of the United States, 1970. Washington, D.C.: U.S. Government Printing Office, 1970.

U.S. Bureau of the Census. Statistical Abstracts of the United States, 1979. Washington, D.C.: U.S. Government Printing Office, 1979.

U.S. Center for Health Statistics. Dental Visits: Volume and Interval Since Last Visit, Public Health Services, Series 10, No. 76. Rockville, Maryland: Center for Health Statistics, 1972.

U.S. Commission on Civil Rights. Civil Rights '63. Washington, D.C.: U.S. Government Printing Office, 1963.

U.S. Commission on Civil Rights. Title VI . . . One Year After: A Survey of Desegregation of Health and Welfare Services in the South. Washington, D.C.: U.S. Government Printing Office, 1966.

U.S. Department of Commerce/Bureau of the Census Current Population Reports, The Social and Economic Status of Negroes in the U.S. 1970. Series P–23, No. 38, B.L.S. Report No. 394. Washington, D.C.: U.S. Government Printing Office.

U.S. Department of Health, Education, and Welfare, Indian Health Service. Health Careers for American Indians and Alaska Natives. Source Book, Educational Opportunities, and Financial Assistance. Washington, D.C.: U.S. Government Printing Office, 1970, 0–407–680.

U.S. Department of Health, Education, and Welfare, Health Services and Mental Health Administration. Health Service Use: National Trends and Variations—1953–1971, Publication No. HSM 73-3004. Rockville, Maryland: Health Services and Mental Health Administration, October 1972.

U.S. Department of Health, Education, and Welfare. Health Services for American Indians, Public Health Service Publication No. 531. Washington, D.C.: U.S. Government Printing Office, 1957.

U.S. Department of Health, Education, and Welfare. Health United States 1980, DHEW Publication No. (PHS) 81-1232. Public Health Service, Health Resources Administration. Rockville, Maryland: National Center for Health Statistics, 1980.

U.S. Department of Health Education and Welfare. Healthy People: The Surgeon Generals Report on Health Promotion and Disease Prevention. DHEW (PHS) Publication No 79-55071 Washington D.C. U.S. Government Printing Office, 1979.

U.S. Department of Health, Education, and Welfare. Human Investment Programs: Delivery of Health Services for the Poor, Public Health Service, December 1967, 12. Washington, D.C.: U.S. Government Printing Office, 1967.

U.S. Department of Health, Education, and Welfare, Indian Health Service. Indian Health Services: Trends and Services, 1969 Edition. Washington, D.C.: U.S. Government Printing Office, 1969.

U.S. Department of Health Education and Welfare, The Nation's use of Health Resources 1979. DHEW Publication No (PHS) 80-1240 Washington D.C.: U.S. Government Printing Office, 1980.

U.S. Department of Health, Education, and Welfare, Vital and Health Statistics. Selected Dental Findings in Adults by Age, Race and Sex, United States, 1960–1962, Public Health Publication, No. 1000, Series 11, No. 7. Washington, D.C.: U.S. Government Printing Office, 1969.

U.S. Department of Health, Education, and Welfare. Nursing Careers Among the American Indians. Public Health Service. Washington, D.C.: U.S. Government Printing Office, 1970.

U.S. Department of Health, Education, and Welfare. Medical Care, Health Status and Family Income, Vital and Health Statistics, Public Health Publication No. 1000, Series, 10, No. 9, p. 6. Washington, D.C.: U.S. Government Printing Office, 1964.

U.S. Department of Health, Education, and Welfare. The Impact of Medicare: An Annotated Bibliography of Selected Sources. Washington, D.C.: U.S. Government Printing Office, 1969.

U.S. Department of Health, Education, and Welfare. Variations in Birth Weight: Legitimate Live Births, United States, 1963, Vital and Health Statistics, Public Health Service Publication No. 1000, Series 22, No. 8. Washington, D.C.: U.S. Government Printing Office, 1964.

U.S. Department of Health, Education, and Welfare. Volume of Physician Visits, United States, July 1966–June 1967, Vital and Health Statistics, Series 10, No. 49, p. 21. Washington, D.C.: National Center for Health Statistics, 1969.

U.S. Department of Health, Education, and Welfare. Vital Statistics of the United States, Vol. II, Mortality. Washington, D.C.: U.S. Government Printing Office, 1968.

U.S. Department of Health, Education, and Welfare. Differentials in Health Characteristics by Color, Vital and Health Statistics, July 1965–June 1967, Public Health Publication No. 1000, Series 10, No. 56, p. 5. Washington, D.C.: U.S. Government Printing Office, 1969.

U.S. Department of Health, Education, and Welfare. Health United States 1979, Publication No. PHS 80–1232. Hyattsville, Maryland: National Center for Health Statistics.

U.S. Department of Health and Human Services, National Center for Health Statistics, Monthly Vital Statistics Report 30, 2, Births, Marriages, Divorces, and Deaths for February 1981. Washington D.C. U.S. Government Printing Office, 1981.

U.S. Department of Health and Human Services, Socioeconomic Differentials and Trends in Timing of Births, DHHS Publication No (PHS) 81–82. Hyattsville Maryland, 1981.

U.S. Department of Labor. The Negro Family: The Case for National Action. Washington, D.C.: U.S. Government Printing Office 1965.

U.S. Division of Indian Health. Indians on Federal Reservation in the United States, Phoenix Area: Arizona, California, Nevada, Utah. U.S. Department of Health, Education, and Welfare, Public Health Service Publication No. 615, Part 6. Washington, D.C.: U.S. Government Printing Office, January 1961.

U.S. Division of Indian Health, Program Analysis and Special Studies Branch. Eskimos, Indians, and Aleuts of Alaska—A Digest. U.S. Department of Health, Education, and Welfare. Washington, D.C.: U.S. Government Printing Office, 1963.

United States Government Expands Migrant Health Programs. *American Journal of Nursing*, 1968, *68*, 1405–1406.

U.S. Social Security Administration. Social Security Programs Throughout the World. Washington, D.C.: U.S. Government Printing Office, 1967.

Valentine, C. A. Culture and Poverty; Critique and Counter Proposals. Chicago: University of Chicago Press, 1968.

Vance, R. B. The Region: A New Survey. In T. R. Ford (Ed.), The Southern Appalachian Region: A Survey. Lexington: University of Kentucky Press, 1962, pp. 4–5.

Vaughn, J. C. & Johnson, W. L. Educational Preparation for Nursing—1978. Nursing Outlook, 1979, 27, 608–614.

Vesey, B. & Fitzgerald, F. Gypsy Medicine. Journal of the Gypsy Lore Society, 1944, 23, 21–33.

Vladeck, B. C. Interest Group Representation and the HSA's: Health Planning and Political Theory. American Journal of Public Health, 1977, 67, 23–29.

Wakefield, D. Island in the City: Puerto Ricans in New York. New York: Corinth Books, 1960.

Wald, L. The House on Henry Street. New York: Henry Holt, 1915.

Waldman, S. & Peel, E. National Health Insurance: A Comparison of Five Proposals. Research and Statistics Note, U.S. Department of Health, Education, and Welfare, Social Security Administration Office of Research and Statistics, July 23, 1970, Note No. 12, 1970.

Waldman, E. B., Lege, S. B., Oseid, B., & Carter, J. P. Health and Nutritional Status of Vietnamese Refugees. Southern Medical Journal, 1979, 72, 1300–1303.

Walker, B. The Hindu World: An Encyclopedia Survey of Hinduism, 2 vols. New York: Praeger, 1968.

Walker, G. M., Jr. The Utilization of Health Care: The Laredo Migrant Experience. American Journal of Public Health, 1979, 69, 667–672.

Wallnofer, H. & von Rottauscher, A. Chinese Folk Medicine. Translated by Marion Palmedo. New York: Crown Publishers, 1965.

Walsh, J. Stanford School of Medicine (1) Problems over More than Money. Science, February 12, 1971, 551–553.

Walsh, J. Federal Health Spending Passes the $50-Billion Mark. Science, 1978, 200, 886–887.

Walsh, J. Britain's National Health Service: It Works and They Like It, But—Science, 1978, 201, 239–241.

Walsh, J. Britain's National Health Service: The Doctors' Dilemmas. Science, 1978, 201, 325–329.

Warheit, G. J., Holzer, C. E., III, & Schwab, J. An Analysis of Social Class and Racial Differences in Depressive Symptomatology. Journal of Health and Social Behavior, 1973, 14, 291–299

Warheit, G. J., Holzer, C. E., III, & Arey, S. A. Race and Mental Illness: An Epidemiological Update. Journal of Health and Social Behavior, 1975, 16, 243–256.

Warne, F. J. The Tide of Immigration. New York: D. Appleton, 1916.

Warshauer, M. E. & Monk, M. Problems in Suicide Statistics for Whites and Blacks. *American Journal of Public Health*, 1978, *68*, 383–388.

Watkins, E. L. Low-Income Negro Mothers—Their Decision to Seek Prenatal Care. *American Journal of Public Health*, 1968, *58*, 655–667.

Watts: Everything Has Changed—and Nothing. *Newsweek*, August 24, 1970, 58–60.

Watts, H. & Rees, A. (Eds.). Expenditures, Health, and Social Behavior; and the Quality of the Evidence, Vol. 3. New York, San Francisco, and London: Academic Press, 1977.

Watts, W. Social Class, Ethnic Background and Patient Care. *Nursing Forum*, 1967, *6*.

Waxman, C. J. The Stigma of Poverty: A Critique of Poverty Theories, New York: Pergamon Press, 1977.

Waybur, A. Analysis of Diverse Modes of Organization for Medical Care of the Poor. Doctoral dissertation, University of California, Los Angeles, School of Public Health, Spring 1974.

Weiner, G., Rider, R. V. et al. Correlates of Low Birth Weight: Psychological Status at Six to Seven Years of Age. *Pediatrics*, 1965, *35*, 434–444.

Weiner, G., Rider, R. V. et al. Correlates of Low Birth Weight: Psychological Status at Eight to Ten Years of Age. *Pediatric Research*, 1968, *2*, 110–118.

Weise, F. E. Health Statistics: A Guide to Information Sources. Detroit: Gale, 1980.

Welch, S., Comer, J., & Steinman, M. Some Social and Attitudinal Correlates of Health Care Among Mexican Americans. *Journal of Health and Social Behavior*, 1973, *14*, 205–213.

Weller, J. E. Yesterday's People: Life in Contemporary Appalachia. Lexington: University of Kentucky Press, 1965.

Wendkos, M. H., Soudack, M., & Fischer, G. A Novel Rehabilitation Program for the Non-Institutional Disadvantaged Elderly Residing in an Urban Community. *Journal of the American Geriatric Society*, 1972, *20*, 116–120.

West, K. M. Diabetes in American Indians and Other Native Populations of the New World. *Diabetes*, 1974, *21*, 841–855.

Westoff, C. F., Potter, R. C., Jr., & Sagi, P. C. The Third Child. Princeton: Princeton University Press, 1963.

Westoff, C. F., Potter, R. C., Jr., Sagi, P. C., & Mishler, E. Family Growth in Metropolitan America. Princeton: Princeton University Press, 1961.

Whelpton, P. K. & Kiser, C. V. Social and Psychological Factors Affecting Fertility, Vol. V. New York: Milbank Memorial Fund, 1958.

White House Conference on Food, Nutrition and Health, Final Report. Jean Mayer, Chairman. Washington, D.C.: U.S. Government Printing Office, 1970.

Whiteman, M. & Deutsch, M. Social Disadvantage as Related to Intellective and Language Development. In M. Deutsch, I. Katz, & A. R. Jensen (Eds.), Social Class, Race and Psychological Development. New York: Holt, 1968, pp. 86–114.

Williams, K. N. & Lockett, B. A. Migration of Foreign Physicians to the United States: The Perspective of Health Manpower Planning. *International Journal Health Service*, 1974, *4*, 213–243.

Willie, C. V. A New Look at Black Famillies, Bayside New York: General Hall, 1980.

Willie, C. V. The Social Class of Patients that Public Health Nurses Prefer to Serve. *American Journal of Public Health*, 1960, *50*, 1126–1136.

Wilson, H. S. & Heinert, J. Los Viejitos: The Old Ones. *Journal of Gerontology Nursing*, 1977, *3*, 19–25.

Winikoff, B. Nutrition, Population, and Health: Some Implications for Policy. *Science*, 1978, *200*, 895–902.

Winter, A. E. Why Young Black Women Don't Enter Nursing. *Nursing Forum*, 1971, *4.*

Wirth, L. The Ghetto. Chicago: University of Chicago Press, 1928.

Wirth, L. The Problem of Minority Groups. In R. Linton, (Ed.), The Science of Man in the World Crisis. New York: Columbia University Press, 1945, pp. 347–372.

Woodson, C. G. The Negro Professional Man and the Community. Johnson Reprint Co., 1934.

Yamamoto, J. & Steinberg, A. Ethnic, Racial and Social Class Factors in Mental Health, *Journal of the National Medical Association*, 1981, *73*, 231–240.

Yates, J. A. Breakthrough in Minnesota. *American Journal of Nursing*, 1970, *70*, 563–565.

The Yellow Emperor's Classic of Internal Medicine. Edited and translated by I. Veith. Berkeley: University of California Press, 1972.

Yerby, A. S. Improving Care for the Disadvantaged. *American Journal of Nursing*, 1968, *68*, 1044.

Yost, E. The U.S. Health Industry—The Costs of Acceptable Medical Care. New York: Praeger, 1969.

Young, W. M. To Be Equal. New York: McGraw-Hill, 1964.

Zborowski, M. Cultural Components in Responses to Pain. *Journal of Social Issues*, August 1954, 21–25.

Zborowski, M. People in Pain. San Francisco: Jossey-Bass, Inc., 1969.

Index

Accidents, fatal
  among blacks, 172
  among Mexican American, 77–78
  among Native Americans, 103–104,
    107
Acculturation, definition of, 105
Acupuncture, 121
Adams, Jane, 32
Agnew, Spiro T., 22
Agricultural revolution, 138–139
Alaskan natives, 102
Alcoholism
  among blacks, 172
  among immigrant minority groups,
    28
  among Native Americans, 106–107,
    172
Aleuts, 102
Alienation, 57, 58, 135, 169
Alinsky, Saul, 135, 136
American Association for Labor Legis-
    lation, 211–212
American College of Surgeons,
    214
American Hospital Association, 195,
    206, 214, 216

American Medical Association, 11, 181,
    195, 205–206, 211, 212, 213, 214,
    215
Anemia, 54, 147, 148, 149
Anger, and mental health, 170–171
Anomie, 57, 104, 106, 171
Appalachia, poverty in, 140–143
Appalachian migrants, 21, 35, 141, 142
Arab immigrants, 118, 123–124
Armenian Church, 129
Armenian immigrants, 36, 118
Asian Americans, 36
  and immigration policy, 24, 25
  suicide among, 172
Assimilation
  definition of, 105
  of European ethnic minorities, 17
  of immigrants, 16
  of Jews, 23
  and Native Americans, 96–100
  rate of, 19
Assimilationist minority, 17
Astrology, 143
Ataque, 88
Autopsies, 129
Avicenna, 123

267

Back to Africa movement, 44
Bad air, 86–87
Bakke case, 186
Batista, Fulgenico, 75
Bertholf, Connie, 128
Better Jobs and Income Programs, 152
Bilis, 87
Birth rate, in Puerto Rico, 73
Black Americans
  accidents among, 172
  alcoholism among, 172
  and anger, 170–171
  discrimination against, 4–5, 41–43,
    46, 48, 51–52, 56, 58
  education of, 43, 45, 47, 48, 182, 183
  employment of, 45, 47–49
  folk medicine of, 39, 40–41, 52–
    54
  health of, 12, 46, 53, 54–55, 171, 172
  and health care, 4–8, 49–52, 189–
    196
  health professionals, 43, 182–183,
    191, 193
  integration of, 43, 44, 45, 46
  and intelligence, 166
  life expectancy of, 46, 47
  and mental illness, 164, 165
  northern migration of, 21, 35, 42, 45
  and personality damage, 168–169
  pica among, 53
  political power of, 42, 45, 136
  poverty among, 46–47, 55–60
  segregation of, 42–43, 48, 51, 58,
    181–182, 183
  and suicide, 172
Black Muslims, 124
Black power movement, 45, 168
Blindness, 100, 101
Blood transfusions, 129
Blue Cross, 214, 216
Blue Shield, 215
Bohemian immigrants, 22
Bolita, 85
Braceros, 69–70
Brauche, 130
Brewster, Mary, 31
Buckley, John, 185
Buddhists, 129
Bureau of Indian Affairs, 92, 93, 98,
    100, 101
Butler, Patricia, 195

Cabot, Richard, 30
Cambodian refugess, 26, 36
Capitation, 209
Carkuff, R. R., 165
Carter, Jimmy, 152, 154
Cash benefit system, 208–209
Castro, Fidel, 75
Catholics, 21–22, 128, 129
Century of Dishonor, A, 96
Child health care, 13, 31
Childbirth, 8, 9, 129
Chinese Americans, 18, 24, 25, 36, 59
Chinese Exclusion Act, 24, 25
Chinese medicine, 120
Chiropractors, 131
Cholera, 29
Christian Scientists, 130–131
Christians, 128, 129
Chronic illness, 50–51
Circumcision, 129
Cirrhosis, 104, 172
Cities, immigrant minority groups in,
    27, 28–29
Citizens Crusade Against Poverty, 147
Civil Rights Act, 46, 192–193
Civil rights movement, 45, 46
Clark, Joseph S., 146
Clark, Kenneth, 168
Clark, Mamie, 168
Clark, Margaret, 84, 87
Clay eating, 53, 149
Clean Eagle, West Virginia, 141–142
Cobbs, Price, 170
Coleman, James, 169
Collier, John, 99, 108
Committee on Economic Security, 213
Community Action Programs, 135–136
Conjurers, 39, 40–41, 52
Consensual unions, 82
Constitution, U. S., 15, 16, 42
Contagious diseases, 1, 12, 28, 29, 95,
    96, 145. *See also specific disease*
Contract labor, 37, 68, 70
Cubans, 74–77
  folk medicine, 84
  immigration of, 25, 26, 74–76, 117,
    118
Culture, traditional. *See* Traditional
    culture
Culture contact, types of, 105–106
Culture of poverty, 56–58, 59, 134, 135

Cunningham, Baily, 40
Cupping, 143
Curandero(a), 82–83, 84, 85, 89

Darling case, 7
Dawes General Allotment Act, 97
De Funis, Marco, 186
Death and dying, 129
Demonstration health centers, 205
Dental caries, racial differences, in, 59
Dental education, 181, 182–183, 188
Dentistry, 59, 101, 179, 181
Diabetes, 78
Diarrhea, infant, 85–86, 108
Diet
  of blacks, 171
  of immigrant groups, 120
  and religion, 123, 124, 128
Diffusion, 105
Diphtheria, 29
Discrimination. *See also under specific
    ethnic group*
  and anger, 170–171
  in dental education, 182–183, 188
  in health care, 4–8, 51–52, 147, 189–
    196
  in housing, 5, 21
  in medical education, 181–182, 183–
    184, 185–188
  in nursing education, 182, 183, 188
    and personality damage, 166–170
  in pharmacist education, 183
Dispensaries, 29–30
Dohrenwend, Barbara, 158, 165
Dohrenwend, Bruce, 158, 165
Drug addiction, 172–173
Drug therapy, 30
Dublin, Louis, 171
DuBois, W. E. B., 43, 45
Dunbar, Leslie, 147
Dunham, H. Warner, 157, 158
Durkheim, Emile, 104, 171
du Sable, Jean Baptiste Point, 36
Dutch immigrants, 19
Dysentery, 81

East Los Angeles Health Task Force,
    78, 79
Eastern European refugees, 26, 118

Education, 167–168. *See also specific
    type*
  of blacks, 43, 45, 47, 48
  of Cubans, 75, 76
  of European immigrants, 21
  of Mexican Americans, 71
  of Native Americans, 71
  of Puerto Ricans, 74
  of rural poor, 139 ˙
  segregated, 169
Einstein College of Medicine, 182
Eisenhower, Dwight D., 9, 22
Elderly
  and food stamps, 151
  health care of, 13, 195–196. *See also
    Medicare*
  poverty of, 137–138
Emigration, 18–19
Empacho, 85
Employment
  of blacks, 45, 47–49
  of Cubans, 75, 76
  of immigrant minority groups, 27–
    28, 48
  of Native Americans, 106
  and poverty, 204
  of Puerto Ricans, 74
  of rural poor, 139
  of Russian Jews, 119
Episcopalians, 129
Eskimos, 102
Ethnic enclaves, 19, 20, 21, 23, 70, 71,
    142
Ethnicity, and mental illness, 164–166
Europe
  ethnic minorities in, 17–18
  immigration to, 34
Evil eye, 86, 123–124, 126–127

Fair Employment Practice Acts, 45
Fallen fotanel, 85–86
Family
  African, weakening of, 38
  disorganized, 162–164, 172
  extended, 81–82, 162
  and mental illness, 162–164
  nuclear, 162
  rural, 139
Family planning, 57–58, 129
Faris, Robert E. L., 157, 158

Farm workers, 69–70, 139–140, 141
  migrant, 143–145, 148, 150
Farming, Native American, 100
Fasting, 124, 128
Fee-for-service system, 207–208
Filariasis, 81
Filipino-American medicine, 124–125
Filipino immigrants, 36
Fishbein, Morris, 213
Florida, Cubans in, 74, 76
Folk diseases
  of Old Order Amish, 130
  of Spanish-speaking people, 84–89
Folk medicine
  Appalachian, 142–143
  black, 39, 40–41, 52–54
  Chinese, 120–122
  combined with modern medicine,
    109, 110, 111–112, 117
  Cuban, 84
  Filipino-American, 124–125
  Gypsy, 125–127
  Indian, 122–123
  Islamic, 123–124
  Mexican American, 82–83, 89
  Native American, 100, 108–112
  Old Order Amish, 130
  Puerto Rican, 83–84, 89
Food stamps, 31, 151–152
Forand bill, 215–216
Foreign medical graduates, 186–187
France, national health insurance in,
  209
Frazier, Franklin, 38
Freidson, Eliot, 52
French Canadian immigrants, 118
French Huguenot immigrants, 19
Freud, Sigmund, 160
"Fright," 87

Garvey, Marcus, 44, 45
Geiger, H. Jack, 150, 151
Generational differences, 116, 119
Geophagia, 53
German immigrants, 19–20, 22, 117
Germany, national health insurance
  in, 206–208
Ghetto, definition of, 22
Ginseng root, 121
Gompers, Samuel, 212

Gradualism, 43, 45
Grandy, Charles, 40
Grapes of Wrath, The, 139
Graves, Mildred, 41
Great Britain, national health insur-
  ance in, 207, 209
Gregg, Elinor D., 102–103, 108
Grier, William, 170
Group Health Association, 214–215
Gypsy medicine, 125–127, 128

Haitian refugees, 117
Hall, Sam, Jr., 117
Hand trembler, 109
Hayes, Rutherford B., 42
Haymarket Riot, 24
Head Start, 167
Health
  of blacks, 12, 46, 53, 54–55, 171, 172
  of Cubans, 76
  of Mexican Americans, 12, 77–80,
    82, 165
  of Native Americans, 12, 95, 96,
    100–104, 106–108
  and poverty, 145–154
  of Puerto Ricans, 80–82
  and religion, 122–123, 124, 126
  self-assessment of, 50
Health care
  of blacks, 4–8, 49–52, 189–196
  changing nature of, 8–13
  costs, 1, 10, 11, 145, 152–153, 218–
    219, 220
  discrimination in, 147, 189–196
  of elderly, 195–196
  of immigrant minority groups, 29–
    32
  and language barriers, 78–79, 120,
    188–189
  levels of utilization of, 55–56
  of Mexican Americans, 78–80
  of Native Americans, 100–104, 108,
    109–112
  preventive. *See* Preventive health
    care and religion, 127–131
  of rural poor, 142
  of slaves, 39–41
  specialization in, 2, 181, 199–201, 221
  technology, 201
  tertiary, 2

Health care team, 180, 181
Health insurance, 49, 211–217, 220–225
Health insurance industry, 206
Health Insurance Plan (HIP), 222, 223–224
Health maintenance organizations, 222–224
Health practitioners. *See also specific type*
  and cooperation with folk practitioners, 88–89
  folk. *See* Folk medicine
  foreign-trained, 118–119
  prejudice of, 30–31, 161
  socioeconomic status of, 161, 165, 178–179, 225–226
  unorthodox, 131
Health Services Agencies, 219–220
Heart disease, 78
Heilbroner, Robert, 203
Henry Street Settlement, 32
Herb doctors, 39
Herbs
  in Chinese medicine, 121
  in Native American medicine, 109–110
Herskovits, Melville, 39
Hill-Burton Act, 51, 191–192, 193, 194
Hindus, 122, 129
Holidays, and health care, 129
Hollingshead, August, 158
Home health aides, 204
Homicide, 104
Hookworm, 81
Hopkins, Harry, 213
Hospital insurance, 9, 212, 213, 214, 217
Hospitalization
  of Mexican Americans, 79–80, 82
  of Native Americans, 110
  of Puerto Ricans, 81, 82
Hospitals
  and Alaskan natives, 102
  changing nature of, 9, 29, 180–181, 217
  and discrimination, 51–52, 189–195
  mental, 160, 161, 164–165
  and Native Americans, 102, 103
  and nursing, 11, 29, 30
  profit-making, 10

Hospitals *(cont.)*
  religious, 127
  and segregation, 51, 52, 190–192, 193, 194
  and university affiliation, 11, 218
Hot-cold theory of illness, 84–85
Housing conditions
  of blacks, 406
  of European immigrants, 21, 22, 28–29
  and infectious disease, 145
  and mental illness, 157–158
  of Native Americans, 106
  of Puerto Ricans, 74, 80
Howard University Medical School, 182, 183
Hull House, 32
Hungarian immigrants, 22, 25, 26
Hyde, R. W., 59
Hypertension, 55, 171

Illegal aliens. *See* Undocumented aliens
Immigrant minority groups, 15–33, 117–132. *See also specific group*
  assimilation of, 16
  and discrimination, 16, 21, 23
  education of, 21
  employment of, 27–28, 48
  exploitation of, 20–21
  and health care, 29–32
  housing conditions of, 21, 22, 28–29
  in-group identification of, 16
  literacy test for, 24–25
  poverty of, 20, 21, 22
  and racism, 23–24
  reactions of health care practitioners to, 30–31
  sea voyage of, 26–27
Immigrants, preference, 25–26
Immigration policy, 23, 24–26, 34, 68, 69, 70, 75, 118
Immigration Restriction League, 24
Immunization, 12, 58–59
Indian Health Service, 102
Indian immigrants, 36
Indian medicine, 122–123
Indian Reorganization Act, 99
Indochinese refugees, 26. *See also specific ethnic group*

Industrialization, 34–35
Infant baptism, 129–130
Infant diarrhea, 85–86, 108
Infant mortality
  among blacks, 55
  among Mexican Americans, 77, 78
  among Native Americans, 103, 108
  and poverty, 2, 145
  racial differences in, 2
  U. S., compared with other nations,
    1, 2, 3
Infertility, 86
Influenza, 77
Institute for Research on Poverty, 134
Intellectual development, and mater-
  nal malnutrition, 150
Intelligence, and race, 166
Iranian immigrants, 36, 118
Irish immigrants, 20–21, 30, 117
Ishi, 104–105
Islamic medicine, 123–124, 128
Isoniazid, experimental use of, 107,
  108
Italian immigrants, 22

Jackson, Helen Hunt, 96
Jaco, E. Gartly, 88, 165
Jamaican immigrants, 118
Japanese, 25, 36
Jehovah's Witnesses, 129
Jensen, Arthur, 166
Jews
  discrimination against, in medical
    education, 182
  in Europe, 22
  immigration of, 22
  orthodox, 128, 129
  Russian, 23, 36, 119
"Jim Crow" legislation, 42
Jinn, 124
Johnson, Lyndon B., 134, 170, 204, 216

Kaiser-Permanente, 222–223
Kaplan, Harold I., 187
Kennedy, John F., 22, 216
Kerr-Mills Bill, 216
King, Martin Luther, Jr., 46
Kingsbury, John A., 214
Knights of the White Camelia, 42
Koch, Robert, 12

Koos, E. L., 59
Korean immigrants, 25, 36, 118
Kosa, John, 56
Kroeber, Theodore, 104
Ku Klux Klan, 42
Kwashiorkor, 148–149

Labor supply, 34–36, 37, 67, 68–70
Lactose intolerance, 54, 120
Lambert, Alexander, 211
Language barriers, 78, 120, 188–189
Laotian immigrants, 26, 118
Last rites, 129
Latin American immigrants, 26
Lay referral system, 52
Lead poisoning, 53
Leininger, Madeline, 116
Lewis, Oscar, 56, 134
Life expectancy
  of blacks, 46, 47
  of Native Americans, 103
Life support systems, 225
Literacy test, for immigrants, 24–25
Liver-growed, 143
Livergrown, 130
Los Angeles, Mexican Americans in, 66

Mal aire, 86–87
Mal ojo, 86
Malaria, 81
Malnutrition
  among Native Americans, 103, 108
  and poverty, 145–152
  among Puerto Ricans, 81
Malpractice, 6–8
Malthus, Thomas, 202
Malzberg, B., 164
Marasmus, 148, 149
March of Dimes, 12
Marine Hospital Health Service, 101
Maternal health, 31, 77
Maternal mortality, 59, 145
Mather, Increase, 95
Mays, Benjamin E., 147
Measles, 95
Medicaid, 10, 13, 49, 134, 153–154,
  195, 216, 217, 220–221
Medi-Cal, 152

Medical Care for the American People,
    212
Medical Committee for Human Rights,
    206
Medical education, 178–179, 180–181,
    206
    changing nature of, 8, 10, 11, 217–
        218
    discrimination in, 181–182, 183–
        184, 185–188
    recruitment of minorities in, 184–
        186
Medical experimentation, 107–108
Medical industrial complex, 9, 10, 218
Medicare, 10, 13, 49, 51, 134, 137, 152,
    154, 193, 215–217, 220
Medicine, changing nature of, 8–11, 180
Medicine man, Native American, 109,
    110, 111–112
Meharry Medical College, 182, 183
Mennonites, 19
Mental hospitals, 160, 161, 164–165
Mental illness, 157–177
    and anger, 170–171
    and ethnic identity, 28, 164–166
    and family, 162–164
    folk, 87–88
    and personality damage, 166–170
    and poverty, 157–161
Meriam, Lewis, 98, 99, 101
Mexican Americans, 18, 65–72
    and discrimination, 70, 71, 72
    folk diseases of, 84–88
    folk medicine of, 82–83, 89
    health of, 12, 77–80, 82, 165
    and health care, 78–80
    and mental illness, 165
    suicide among, 172
    and traditional culture, 66, 68, 71–
        72, 79
Mexico, Indians of, 93
Middle-Eastern immigrants, 36
Midwives, 8, 41, 83
Migrant farm workers, 143–145, 148,
    150
Migration
    of Appalachians, 21
    northern, 21, 35, 42, 45
    Puerto Rican, 21
    rural-urban, 34, 35, 139, 141, 142
    western, 35

Milbank, Albert G., 214
Milbank Fund, 214
Militant minority, 17
Military industrial complex, 9–10
Milk stations, 31
Minorities, *See also specific group*
    classification of, 17
    definition of, 15
    types of, 15–16
Mississippi, 146–147
Mobile Infirmary, 194
Mollera ciada, 85–86
Mormons, 24, 27, 128
Mortality, *See also* Infant mortality;
        Maternal mortality
    among blacks, 171
    among immigrant minority groups,
        27, 28–29
    among Mexican Americans, 77, 78
    among Native Americans, 95, 103
    among slaves, 37, 40
Mount Sinai College of Medicine, 182
Moynihan, Daniel P., 135, 136
Muhammad, Elijah, 124
Murphy, George, 146
Muslims, 128, 129
Myrdal, Gunnar, 51

National Association for the Advance-
        ment of Colored People (NAACP),
        44, 45
National health insurance, 2, 206–211
    in France, 209
    in Germany, 206–208
    in Great Britain, 207, 209
    struggle for, in U. S., 211–215, 224–
        225
    in Sweden, 209
    in USSR, 207, 210
National Health Law Program, 194–
    195
National Health Planning and Re-
    sources Development Act, 219
National Medical Association, 191
National Urban League, 44
Native American Church, 106
Native Americans, 92–115
    alcoholism among, 172
    classification of, 92–93
    conferral of citizenship on, 98

Native Americans *(cont.)*
  cultural differences among, 94, 98, 109
  education of, 96, 97–98, 106
  employment of, 106
  folk medicine of, 100, 108–112
  government policy toward, 95–100
  health of, 12, 95, 96, 100–104, 106–108
  and health care, 100–104, 108, 109–112
  as health workers, 103, 111
  housing conditions of, 108
  impact of European settlement on, 18, 94–95
  physical appearance of, 94
  protein deficiency among, 148
  reservations of, 95–96, 99–100, 106
  and social change, 103–107
  suicide among, 171, 172
  and traditional culture, 105–106
  unemployment among, 100, 106
Naturopaths, 131
Navaho hand trembler, 109
Neighborhood organizations, 32
New York Diet Kitchen, 31
New York Infirmary for Women and Children, 31
Niagara Movement, 44
Nino, Pedro Alonzo, 36
Nixon, Richard, 134, 151
Nonverbal communication, 189
Nurses
  foreign-trained, 118–119
  importance of, 9
  in settlement house movement, 31
  socioeconomic status of, 179, 180
Nursing
  changing nature of, 11, 30, 179, 180
  of slaves, 39–40, 41
Nursing education, 179
  changing nature of, 11
  discrimination in, 182, 183
  recruitment of minority students in, 185
  sex segregation in, 188
Nursing homes, 10, 193
Nutritional knowledge, 149

ODWIN, 185
Office of Economic Opportunity, 48, 147, 204, 205

Office of Equal Health Opportunity, 193, 194
Old Order Amish, 19, 130
Organic Act, 72
osteopathic schools, 182

Pain, reaction to, 125
Parasitic diseases, 81, 148
Parole authority, 26
Parsi, 129
Partera, 83
Pasamanick, Benjamin, 164
Pasteur, Louis, 12, 29
Pavenstedt, E., 163
Pennsylvania, ethnic enclaves in, 19
Periodontal disease, 59
Perkins, Frances, 213
Personality damage, and mental illness, 166–170
Peyote ceremony, 106
Pharmacists, socioeconomic status of, 179
Pharmacy, changing nature of, 181
Phillips, Elsie, 31
Phillips, Wilbur, 31
Physical development, and malnutrition, 149, 150
Physician-patient relationship, 8
Physician visits, racial differences in number of, 50
Physicians. *See also* Health professionals
  businesses owned by, 10
  class background of, 8, 30
  foreign-trained, 118–119
  income of, 8, 11
  prejudice of, 30–31
Physicians for Social Responsibility, 206
Pica, 53
Pierce, R., 165
Pluralistic minority, 17
Pneumonia, 77, 108
Poliomyelitis, 12
Polish immigrants, 22, 118
Political power, 135, 136
Population growth, in Puerto Rico, 73
Poverty, 133–145, 203–205
  of blacks, 46–47, 55–60
  of European immigrants, 20, 21, 22

Poverty *(cont.)*
  and health, 142, 154
  and health care, 194–195
  and infant mortality, 2
  and malnutrition, 145–152
  and mental illness, 157–161
  of Native Americans, 103, 106, 107
  rural, 138–145
  and suicide, 170
Poverty index, 46–47, 145–146
Preference immigrants, 118
Pregnancy
  medical care in, 13
  pica in, 53
  toxemia in, 53
Prejudice
  and immigrant minority groups, 30–31
  of health practitioners, 161
  and mental health, 168–169
Prematurity, 150
Prepaid medical care, 214–215, 222–224
Preventive care, 50, 55–56, 57–59, 126, 169, 223, 224, 226–227
Primary care practitioners, 221–222
Profit-making companies, 10
Protein deficiencies, 148
"Pseudoscience" and racism, 23–24
Psychiatric treatment, 160–161
Psychological factors, and poverty, 56–58
Psychotherapy, 160, 161
Public health movement, 11–13
Public health nurses, 30, 101
Public Health Service, 101, 102, 108, 192, 193
Public health services, 1–2
Puerto Ricans, 72–74
  employment of, 35, 74
  folk diseases of, 88
  folk medicine of, 83–84, 89
  health of, 80–82
  housing condition of, 74, 80
  migration of, 21, 73
Puerto Rico, 72–73, 80

Race riots, 46, 170–171
Racism, 23–24
Radicalism, fear of, 24
Rat bites, 4–5, 80

Reagan, Ronald, 152, 154
Redlich, Fredrick, 158
Refugees, 25. *See also specific group*
Religion. *See also specific religion*
  as coping mechanism, 128
  and health care, 127–131
  and medicine, 122–123, 124, 126
  Native American, 106
  and prejudice, 21–22
Relman, Arnold S., 9, 10
Reservation system, 95–96, 99–100, 106
Respiratory diseases, 78. *See also specific disease*
Rheumatic fever, 77
Roemer, Milton, 199–200, 201
Roosevelt, Franklin D., 12, 99, 213
Roosevelt, Theodore, 211
Root doctors, 39
Rubinow, I. M., 211
Rural poor, 138–145
Russian immigrants, 22, 26, 118
Russian Jews, 23, 36, 119

Salary system, 210
Samoan immigrants, 36, 118
Savitt, Todd L., 40
Scarlet fever, 29
Schistosomiasis mansoni, 81
Schizophrenia, 157–158, 160, 165
Scotch Irish, 19
Secessionist minority, 17
Seeman, Melvin, 135
Segregation, 42–43, 45, 58
  in education, 48, 169
  in health care, 51, 52, 189–194
  in medical education, 181, 182
  in nursing education, 188
Señora, 83
Settlement house movement, 31–32
Seventh Day Adventists, 128
Sickle cell anemia, 54
Sickle cell trait, 54
Simkins vs. *Moses H. Cone Memorial Hospital*, 192
Simon, R. J., 164
Skin color, and observation of illness-related changes, 54–55
Slavery, 36–38, 164
  and health care, 39–41

Slavery *(cont.)*
  impact of, 38–41, 56
  reactions to abolishment of, 41–43
Smallpox, 95
Snow, Jensey, 41
Snyder Act, 98
Social change, and Native Americans,
  103–107
Social problems, of immigrants, 23–24
Social Security, 137, 214
Social Security Act, 1–2
  1972 amendment to, 10
Social work, 32
Social work assistants, 204
Society for Krishna Consciousness,
  122–123
Sovador, 84
Spanish-speaking minority groups. *See
  also* Cubans; Mexican Americans;
  Puerto Ricans; Spanish-speaking
  people, indigenous
  and mental illness, 165
Spanish-speaking people, indigenous,
  35
Specialization, in medicine, 2, 18,
  199–201, 221
Spiritualists, 83–84, 131
Spotted Tail, 96
Srole, Leo, 57, 159
Starch eating, 53
Steinbeck, John, 139
Strauss, Nathan, 31
Suicide
  and anomie, 171–172
  among Native Americans, 104, 171,
  172
  and poverty, 171
Susto, 87
Sweden, national health insurance in,
  209
Swedish immigrants, 19, 22
Syphilis, 95

Teachers, expectation of, 167–168
Tertiary care, 2
Thailand immigrants, 36
Tilden, Samuel J., 42
Time orientation, 57, 110
Trachoma, 100–101
Traditional culture
  black, 38, 39, 54

Traditional culture *(cont.)*
  and emigration, 19
  Mexican American, 66, 68, 71–72, 79
  Native American, 105–106
Transcultural health care, elements of,
  116–117
Transcultural nursing, 116
Trinidadian immigrants, 118
Tuberculosis
  among Alaskan natives, 102
  among blacks, 12, 55
  among immigrant minority groups,
  28
  among Mexican Americans, 12, 82
  among Native Americans, 12, 95,
  102, 107, 108
  among Puerto Ricans, 80–81, 82
Tuskegee Institute, 43

Ukranian immigrants, 118
Undocumented aliens, 70, 71
Unemployment, 48, 49, 100
Universal Negro Improvement Associa-
  tion, 44
Urbanization, 199, 201
USSR, national health care in, 207,
  210
Utilization review, 195

Vascular diseases, 78
Vietnamese immigrants, 25, 26, 118
Voodoo practitioners, 52–53

Wagner-Murray-Dingell bill, 215
Wald, Lillian, 31, 32
War on Poverty, 134–136, 137, 204
Warmer, 120
Washington, Booker T., 43, 45
Washington Conference on the Eco-
  nomic Factors Affecting the Or-
  ganization of Medicine, 212
Well-baby care, 12
Wheeler Howard Act, 99
White poverty, 47, 133, 138–
  145
Wilbur, Roy Lyman, 212
Wilson, Woodrow, 24

Wirth, Louis, 17
Witch doctors, Yoruba, 88
Women
    black, health care by, 54
    and discrimination, 187–188
    Mexican American, health care by,
        83
    minority status of, 15
    Puerto Rican, health care by, 83–84

Women *(cont.)*
    slave, health care by, 40, 41
Workmen's compensation, 211

Yellow fever, 29
Yerby, Alonzo, 202
Yin/yang, 120–121
Yoruba witch doctors, 88